Critical Thinking to Achieve Positive Health Outcomes

Nursing Case Studies and Analyses

Critical Thinking to Achieve Positive Health Outcomes

Nursing Case Studies and Analyses

Margaret Lunney, RN, PhD
and Contributors

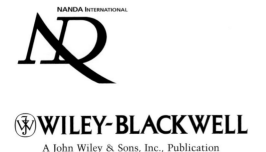

A John Wiley & Sons, Inc., Publication

Edition first published 2009
© 2009 NANDA International

Blackwell Publishing was acquired by John Wiley & Sons in February 2007.
Blackwell's publishing program has been merged with Wiley's global
Scientific, Technical, and Medical business to form Wiley-Blackwell.

Editorial Office
2121 State Avenue, Ames, Iowa 50014-8300, USA

For details of our global editorial offices, for customer services, and
for information about how to apply for permission to reuse the
copyright material in this book, please see our website at
www.wiley.com/wiley-blackwell.

Library of Congress Cataloging-in-Publication Data

Critical thinking to achieve positive health outcomes : nursing case studies
and analyses / edited by Margaret Lunney. – 2nd ed.
        p. ; cm.
    Rev. ed. of: Critical thinking & nursing diagnosis / edited by Margaret
Lunney. 2001.
    Includes bibliographical references and index.
    ISBN 978-0-8138-1601-2 (pbk. : alk. paper)
    1. Nursing diagnosis–Case studies.   2. Critical thinking.   I. Lunney,
Margaret.   II. NANDA International.   III. Critical thinking & nursing
diagnosis.
    [DNLM: 1. Nursing Diagnosis–Case Reports.   2. Outcome Assessment
(Health Care)–Case Reports.   3. Thinking–Case Reports.
WY 100.4 C9345 2009]
    RT48.6.C75 2009
    616.07'5–dc22

                                                        2009005670

A catalog record for this book is available from the U.S. Library of Congress.

Set in 10 on 12 pt Palatino by SNP Best-set Typesetter Ltd., Hong Kong
Printed in Singapore by Markono Print Media Pte Ltd

1   2009

Contents

*Additional resources are published on the book's website
(www.wiley.com/go/lunney).*

Contributors

Miriam de Abreu Almeida
RN, PhD
Professor
Universidade Federal
Rio Grande do Sul

Bernadette Amicucci
RN, MS, CNE
Instructor
Cochran School of Nursing
Yonkers, New York

Ilva Marico Mizumoto Aragaki
RN, MNS
Chief of the Maternity Unit
University Hospital of the University of São Paulo,
Brazil

Alba Lucia Bottura Leite de Barros
RN, NS, PhD
Professor and Dean
Paulista School of Nursing
São Paulo, Brazil

Steven L. Baumann
RN, PhD, GNP-BC, PMHNP-BC
Professor and GNP/ANP Program Coordinator
Hunter-Bellevue School of Nursing, CUNY
New York, NY

Judy M. Carlson
RN, EdD
Nurse Researcher
Tripler Army Medical Center
Honolulu, HI

Roberta Cavendish
RN, PhD, CPE
Adjunct Professor
College of Staten Island, CUNY
Staten Island, NY

Gail Champagne
RN, BSN
Staff Nurse
Home and Hospice Care of Rhode Island
Pawtucket, RI

June Como
RN, MSA, MS, CCRN, CCNS
Faculty
College of Staten Island, CUNY
Staten Island, NY

Diná de Almeida Lopes Monteiro da Cruz
RN, PhD
Professor
School of Nursing
University of São Paulo
São Paulo, Brazil

Jeanne Cummings
RN, MS, PMHNP-BC, PMHCNS-BC
Adult Nurse Practitioner
Psychiatric Clinic
New York, NY

Cynthia Degazon
RN, PhD
Professor Emerita
Hunter-Bellevue School of Nursing
New York, NY

Annemarie Dowling-Castronovo
RN, MA, GNP
Assistant Professor
Evelyn L. Spiro School of Nursing
Wagner College
Staten Island, NY

Menay Drake
RN, MS, IBCLC
Adjunct Faculty
College of Staten Island, CUNY
Staten Island, NY

Joyce Dungan
RN, MSN, EdD
Professor Emerita; Consultant
University of Evansville
Evansville, IN

MaryAnn Edelman
RN, MS CNS
Associate Professor
Kingsborough Community College, CUNY
Brooklyn, NY

Carme Espinosa-Fresnedo
RN, MS
Professor
Blanquerna School of Nursing
Ramon Lluill University
Barcelona, Spain

Dawn Fairlie
RN, MS, APRN-BC
Instructor
College of Staten Island, CUNY
Staten Island, NY

Arlene Farren
RN, PhD
Assistant Professor
College of Staten Island, CUNY
Staten Island, NY

Maria Aurora Fernandez–Roibas
RN, BS
Palliative Care Nurse
Complexo Hospitalario de Ourense
Ourense, Spain

Sandra Frick-Helms
RN, PhD
Registered Play Therapist Supervisor
University of South Carolina School of Medicine
Columbia, SC

Paul G. Germano
RN, BS
Staff Nurse
Veterans Administration
New York Harbor Health Care
Brooklyn, NY

Eileen Gigliotti
RN, PhD
Professor
College of Staten Island, CUNY
Staten Island, NY

Marie Giordano
RN, MS
Instructor
College of Staten Island, CUNY
Staten Island, NY

Alda Valéria Neves Soares Gomes
RN, MNS
Director, Maternal-Child Division
University Hospital of the University of São Paulo
São Paulo, Brazil

Debra Guss
RN, BS
Staff Nurse
St. Vincent's Home Care
Staten Island, NY

Tomoko Hasegawa Katz
RN, MPH, PhD
Professor
Univesity of Fukui
School of Nursing
Fukui, Japan

Atsuko Higuchi
RN
Chief Nurse
Fukui Kosei Hospital
Fukui, Japan

Betty A. Jensen
RN, PhD
Assistant Professor of Clinical Nursing
The University of Texas at Austin

Rick Jepson
RN
Nurse Supervisor
Inpatient Dialysis
Utah Valley Regional Medical Center
Provo, UT

Gloria Just
RN, PhD, ANP-BC
Adjunct Professor
Radford University
Radford, VA

Andrea Karolys
MSN, MPH, CNS
District Nurse
Health Services
San Juan Capistrano, CA

Arlene Kasten
RN, MSN, GNP, BC
Nurse Practitioner
Zablocki Veteran Affairs Medical Center
Milwaukee, WI

Edmont Katz
MA
Assistant Professor of Linguistics
University of Fukui
School of Nursing
Fukui City, Japan

Emma Kontzamanis
RN, MA
Assistant Professor
New York City College of Technology, CUNY
New York, NY

Maryanne Krenz
RN, MS
Associate Professor
Brookdale Community College
Lincroft, NJ

Coleen Kumar
RN, MS,
Assistant Professor
Kingsborough Community College, CUNY
Brooklyn, NY

MaryAnne Levine
RN, PhD, SCM
Professor
Humboldt State University
Arcata, CA

Juliana de Lima Lopes
RN, MS
Nurse
Heart Institute
São Paulo, Brazil

Amália de Fátima Lucena
RN, PhD
Professor
Universidade Federal do Rio Grande do Sul School of Nursing
Brazil

Barbara Kraynyak Luise
RN, EdD
Associate Professor
College of Staten Island, CUNY
Staten Island, NY

Anne T. Lunney
MS, MD
Anesthesiologist
National Children's Hospital
Washington, DC

Leo Lunney
RN
Director of Cardiopulmonary Services
Hackettstown Regional Medical Center
Hackettstown, NJ

Margaret Lunney
RN, PhD
Professor and Graduate Programs Coordinator
College of Staten Island
City University of New York
Staten Island, NY

Nora Maloney
RN, MS
Substitute Lecturer
College of Staten Island, CUNY
Staten Island, NY

Fabiana Gonçalves de Oliveira Azevedo Matos
RN, MNS
Faculty
University of São Paulo, School of Nursing
São Paulo, Brazil

Ann Mayo
RN, DNSc, CNS
Professor
Philip Y. Hahn School of Nursing
University of San Diego
San Diego, CA

Mary McCaffery-Tesoro
MS, RN, C, OCN
Lecturer
Lehman College Department of Nursing
New York, NY

Mary Ellen McMorrow
RN, EdD, APN
Professor
College of Staten Island, CUNY
Staten Island, NY

Susan Mee
RN, MS
Assistant Professor
College of Staten Island, CUNY
Staten Island, NY

Ellen Mitchell
RN, MA
Advanced Practice Nurse Case Manager
St. Vincent's Catholic Medical Center
New York, NY

Maria Müller Staub
RN, PhD
Nurse Scientist
Nursing PBS
Swtizerland

Roseann Nahmod
RN, MS, NE-BC
Substitute Lecturer
College of Staten Island, CUNY
Staten Island, NY

Chie Ogasawara
RN, Med, PhD
Professor
Department of Nursing
Hiroshima International University
Hiroshima, Japan

Catherine Paradiso
RN, MS, APRN, BC
Chief Clinical Officer
Staten Island Physician's Practice
Staten Island, NY

Alsacia Pasci
RN, MS, CEN, CCRN, FNP
Lecturer
Lehman College
City University of New York
New York, NY

Janice Pattison
RN, MS, ANP-C
Distinguished Lecturer
College of Staten Island
City University of New York
Staten Island, NY

Bobbie Jean Perdue
RN, PhD
Professor
South Carolina State University
Orangeburg, SC

Mary Pilossoph
RN, MA, APRN-BC
Oncology Nurse Practitioner
Women's Oncology and Wellness Practice
New York, NY

Margaret Reilly
RN, MS, APRN-BC
Associate Professor of Nursing
Queensborough Community College
City University of New York
New York, NY

Sondra Rivera
RN, MSN-Ed
Assistant Professor
New York City College of Technology, CUNY
New York, NY

Deborah Hein Seganfredo
RN, BS
Master's Student
Universidade Federal do Rio Grande do Sul School of Nursing
Brazil

Gilcéria Tochika Shimoda
RN, MNS
Staff Nurse
University Hospital of the University of São Paulo
São Paulo, Brazil

Danna Sims
RN, MS
Instructor
College of Staten Island, CUNY
Staten Island, NY

Margaret M. Terjesen
RN, MS, FNP-BC
Adjunct Faculty
College of Staten Island, CUNY
Staten Island, NY

Michiyo Yagi
RN
Assistant Head Nurse
Fukui Kosei Hospital
Fukui City, Japan

Riyako Yoshikawa
RN
Head Nurse
Fukui Kosei Hospital
Fukui, Japan

Saori Yoshioka
RN, MSN
Assistant Professor and Doctoral Candidate
Hiroshima International University
Department of Nursing
Hiroshima, Japan

Preface

This is a second edition of the book *Critical Thinking and Nursing Diagnosis: Case Studies and Analyses*, published by NANDA (2001). This edition differs from the first in that the nursing process, from assessment to evaluation, is represented, not just the diagnostic process. The three nursing languages of NANDA International (NANDA-I, 2009), Nursing Outcomes Classification (NOC, Moorhead, Johnson, Mass, and Swanson, 2008), and Nursing Interventions Classification (NIC, Bulechek, Butcher, and Dochterman, 2008) are used with each and every case study. Another difference is that the submitters' analyses are presented immediately after the case studies, rather than in a different chapter. This is to enable nurses to learn application of these three languages. Each case study has been edited to achieve consistency in use of the languages.

This book was written for nurses and nursing students to develop or enhance their thinking processes related to the achievement of positive health outcomes. The nursing care elements of nursing diagnosis, nursing interventions, and health outcomes serve as the basis for discussion of the work of nurses to help people to achieve positive health outcomes.

The focus of this book is the application of critical thinking to make accurate diagnoses of human responses and select the most appropriate outcomes and interventions to achieve positive patient care results. Accuracy of nurses' diagnoses is considered critical to the success of nursing care. Without accurate diagnoses, nurses would select inappropriate interventions. Once the intention of accuracy and strategies for achieving accuracy are included in the process of diagnosing, nurses are transformed to diagnosticians, which includes the responsibility of selecting outcomes and interventions. When nurses understand thinking, and are able to consider their thinking to achieve accuracy, they gain insight on how to incorporate the behaviors of a diagnostician into daily practice.

The four chapters in Part I focus on how and why knowledge of critical thinking and the concept of accuracy in selecting diagnoses and deciding on outcomes and interventions can help nurses to achieve high quality nursing care. Chapter 1 describes Sternberg's theory of intelligence in order to understand intelligence in nursing. Critical thinking is an aspect of nursing intelligence. A definition of critical thinking developed through nursing research is discussed in Chapter 1 and serves as a guide for nurses' thinking.

Even though the thinking of nurses is addressed throughout this book, it is important to remember that consumers also think about their responses to health problems and life processes. People know what they experience and why interventions may be needed. This book is based on the premise that the nursing process is interactive and collaborative with consumers of health care. The term consumer is used to illustrate the mutually collaborative nature of the diagnostic process in nursing. Consumers are "the experts" in respect to their own experiences. Nurses are resources to help consumers name their experiences as the basis for nursing interventions and projected outcomes.

Chapter 2 explains diagnostic reasoning and the concept of accuracy of nurses' diagnoses. The meaning of accuracy and factors that affect accuracy provide a foundation for understanding use of critical thinking in diagnostic processes. Chapter 3 presents 10 principles for use of NANDA-I diagnoses and explains how to use the NOC and NIC classifications. Chapter 4 provides examples of application of the content of Chapter 3.

Part II, chapters 5 through 8, consists of 56 case studies and analyses, some of which were in the first edition of this book. All of these cases were written by practicing nurses who based these cases on actual consumers of nursing care. All identifying data were changed to protect consumers' privacy. For some case studies, the NANDA-I, NOC, and NIC classifications were not actually used at the time of nursing care, but they are used here to illustrate their usefulness in guiding and documenting nursing care.

These case studies provide opportunities for nurses and nursing students to use critical thinking in their use of standardized nursing languages to help people achieve positive health outcomes. Readers can compare their own thinking with that of the nurses who wrote the case studies. The submitters' analyses explain the thinking that occurred in the clinical cases. The case studies and analyses provide fertile resources for learning about the complexities of diagnosing human responses and selecting outcomes and interventions.

The history and traditions of nursing have not included the nurse as diagnostician. In general, much work still needs to be done before nurses routinely acknowledge, describe, and implement the responsibilities of diagnosticians, which include identifying feasible outcomes and implementing nursing interventions. To be a diagnostician means to attend to the accuracy of diagnoses and to examine the thinking processes involved with making diagnoses. This book can be used as a reference for development of these thinking skills.

Margaret Lunney, RN, PhD

References

Bulechek, G.M., Butcher, H.K., and Dochterman, J.M. (2008). *Nursing Interventions Classification (NIC)* (5th ed.). St. Louis, MO: Mosby.

Lunney, M. (2001). *Critical thinking and nursing diagnosis: Case studies and analyses*. Philadelphia: NANDA.

Moorhead, S., Johnson, M., Maas, M.L., and Swanson, E. (2008). *Nursing Outcomes Classification (NOC)* (4th ed.). St Louis, MO: Mosby.

NANDA International. (2009). *Nursing diagnosis: Definitions and classification, 2009–2011*. Ames, IA: Wiley-Blackwell.

Acknowledgments

The emotional and tacit support of my husband, John H. Lewis, was most important to enable me to write and edit this book. I thank him profusely for making it possible for me to easily pursue my professional interests.

I particularly thank the authors of the case studies for their dedication to nursing and health care. The task of writing a case study and analysis is a difficult one but they met this challenge in order to share their experiences with other nurses and to benefit the consumers of nursing care. The reviewers listed below made it possible for this book to reflect the latest knowledge in use of standardized nursing languages and in specialty areas of nursing. Because my background is community health, they advised me on cases that were not within my specialty knowledge.

These ideas were developed through ongoing discussions with my good friends and professional colleagues at the College of Staten Island and beyond, e.g., Judy Carlson in Hawaii. My association with NANDA International and its members has inspired me since 1982. Students at baccalaureate, masters, and doctoral levels who challenged some of the prevailing ideas about use of standardized nursing languages helped to refine the explanation of how to use NANDA-I, NOC, and NIC.

Thank you to the Wiley-Blackwell editors who were so helpful and kind at every stage of writing and book development, especially Susan Farmer, Carrie Sutton, and Tracy Petersen.

Margaret Lunney, RN, PhD

Reviewers

Kay Avant
Diná de Almeida Lopes Monteiro da Cruz
Carme Espinosa-Fresnedo
Arlene Farren
T. Heather Herdman
MaryAnne Levine
Leo M. Lunney
Mary Ellen McMorrow
Janice Pattison
Leann Scroggins
Danna Sims
Maria Müller Staub

How to Use this Book

The standardized nursing languages of NANDA International (I), NOC, and NIC (NNN) are used throughout the book because they represent research-based knowledge in nursing. These or other standardized nursing languages are needed for documentation in electronic health records. Learning how to use NNN also helps nurses to use other standardized nursing languages when needed.

The case study examples in Part II give nurses opportunities to develop and "practice" critical thinking with real individual and family clinical situations. The findings of previous research studies on development of critical thinking show that repeated experiences or practice is needed for those who want to integrate their current thinking skills with specific types of knowledge such as NANDA-I, NOC, and NIC. (for more information, see the NANDA-I and Center for Nursing Classifications websites, which appear in the Webliography.)

To effectively use this book, read the first four chapters as a source of knowledge on how to think and act like a diagnostician. The NNN books (NANDA-I, 2009; Moorhead, Johnson, Mass, and Swanson, 2008; Bulechek, Butcher, and Dochterman, 2008) can be used as reference materials, but in the beginning, the main focus should be to identify the main concepts or ideas that underlie use of these languages, not necessarily the exact NANDAI, NOC, and NIC terms.

A goal of the book is for readers to practice using the various types of thinking that are defined in Chapter 1, e.g., analyzing, logical reasoning, and developing the related thinking habits. I assume that everyone comes into nursing with the basic thinking skills that are needed to function well as a nurse, but research shows that adults in any professional field, including nurses, vary widely in thinking abilities. Research findings show that repeated practice is necessary to build thinking competencies for application in specific types of problem solving. These case studies, when used for this purpose, will help readers to develop the thinking processes needed to diagnose and treat cases such as those in this book. Unfortunately, the book cannot help readers to develop the communication skills needed to work in partnership with consumers. The authors of the case studies, however, provide role models of the partnership process.

For each case study:

1. List as many nursing diagnoses as you would consider relevant to the case study.
2. Decide which of the diagnoses you identified should be ruled out based on principles of diagnosis in nursing.
3. Of the remaining diagnoses, which diagnosis(es) is (are) likely to yield a positive change in health status through the use of nursing interventions? Would the consumer be likely to agree with the selected diagnosis and associated nursing interventions?
4. Consider the most likely outcomes and interventions for the diagnoses you selected. Think about whether the consumer and other nurses would agree that, in the context of the situation, these choices would be the most appropriate outcomes and interventions.
5. After validating your thinking by reading the submitter's discussion of how NANDAI, NIC, and NOC were used, consider:
    a) What are the indications in the case study of the author's use of specific cognitive skills and habits of mind?
    b) Which cognitive skills and habits of mind did you use to accurately diagnose the case?
    c) What types of standards were applied by the nurse(s)? What additional standards could be applied?

Website: Online Learning Resources

The companion website, www.wiley.com/go/lunney, can be used to further your knowledge about related topics.

Background materials that were published in many different sources from 1990 to 2008 are on the website. The website content includes relevant journal articles, presentation slides, and other learning resources, and is organized as follows:

Importance of Using Standardized Nursing Languages in the Electronic Health Record
Understanding Accuracy of Nurses' Diagnoses
Facilitating the Development of Intelligence and Critical Thinking Skills
Helping Students and Nurses to Develop as Diagnosticians
Developing Case Studies for Teaching, Testing, and as Research Tools
Examples of Research Studies

The email address is provided for readers who wish to make comments regarding the contents of the book. Please email us if you have something important to say about these topics.

Critical Thinking to Achieve Positive Health Outcomes

Nursing Case Studies and Analyses

Strategies for Critical Thinking to Achieve Positive Health Outcomes

Use of Critical Thinking to Achieve Positive Health Outcomes

Margaret Lunney, RN, PhD

Chapter Objectives

By completion of this chapter, readers will be able to:

1. Describe the importance of quality-based nursing care;
2. Explain the relation of intelligence and critical thinking to quality-based care;
3. Describe the need for case studies to facilitate development of critical thinking for quality-based care.

The most important indicator of the quality of health care, including nursing care, is the health outcomes of consumers (Committee on Quality of Health Care in America, Institute of Medicine [IOM], 2001, 2004). The identification of consumer health outcomes is a priority so that the effectiveness of provider interventions can be described, explained, and predicted. Three assumptions related to the focus on health outcomes are: (1) the effectiveness of interventions varies among health care professionals, (2) knowledge development of the effectiveness of interventions is the responsibility of health care providers, and (3) when effectiveness is compromised, people may be "better off" without providers.

Health care providers can only provide quality-based care when they have sufficient intelligence and critical thinking competencies to use existing knowledge to provide health care services. Knowledge is necessary but not sufficient to provide the appropriate health care services; ability to think about and effectively use knowledge is also essential. The purposes of this chapter are to (a) review the importance of quality-based nursing care, as demonstrated in the processes and outcomes of care; (b) explain the relation of intelligence and thinking to the achievement of quality-based care; and (c) describe the need for case studies to develop critical thinking competencies.

Importance of Quality-Based Care

The quality of health care services has become a major focus of health care providers, professional organizations, accrediting agencies, and other stakeholders such as governmental agencies, foundations, and insurance companies (e.g., Al-Assaf and Sheikh, 2004; Committee on Reviewing Evidence to Identify Highly Effective Clinical Services, IOM, 2008; Donabedian, 2002; Mechanic, 2008; Montalvo and Dunton, 2007). On its web page, the Robert Wood Johnson Foundation (2008) summarized the issue of quality care in the United States with the following statement: "Americans receive only about half of the recommended care they should receive. Adopting quality improvement strategies, reducing racial and ethnic disparities in care, and changing how care is delivered at the local level can improve the care all Americans receive."

A major reason for the current emphasis on quality is that research findings have shown that quality varies widely among localities, health care agencies, and providers (Committee on Quality of Health Care in America, IOM, 2001, 2004). When the quality of care varies widely, many consumers are not receiving quality-based services. For example, the results of a recent U.S. study of the quality of care provided in 73 hospital systems that represented 1,510 hospitals showed substantial variability in system quality for pneumonia, surgical infection prevention, acute myocardial infarction, and congestive heart failure (Hines and Joshi, 2008). Medication errors is an example of the problems that exist with quality. In the U.S., "medication errors harm at least 1.5 million people every year" (Institute of Medicine, 2008). The current emphasis on quality-based services is intended to establish accountability for the quality of health care services provided to the public and to make significant improvements in quality.

Nurses have a significant role in providing quality care (Aiken, 2005). According to Henderson's definition of nursing (1964), nurses help consumers as needed with the health behaviors that they would ordinarily do for themselves, e.g., eating, breathing, moving, obtaining nutrition, and taking medications. Nurses help people with their responses to health problems and life processes (NANDA International (I), 2009). Nurses are legally and professionally responsible for any interventions that they use to support consumer health, even when those interventions have been prescribed by physicians (Aiken, 2005). Because nurses make up the largest number of health care workers, any efforts of nurses to improve quality-based care will probably have broad positive effects on health care in general.

Evidence-Based Practice

It is widely accepted that the quality of care is best achieved by using the best available research evidence for health care decisions (Committee on Reviewing Evidence to Identify Highly Effective Clinical Services, IOM, 2008; Melnyk and Fineout-Overholt, 2005). In many types of health care, variance in quality exists because there is insufficient evidence to establish consensus on the best way to approach the problem, risk state, or need for health promotion. In other types of health care, sufficient research evidence is available, but providers do not use the available evidence.

Nurse leaders collaborate with leaders from other disciplines to promote evidenced-based practice for improved quality of care. Strategies for nurses to learn how to critique research studies for possible use are taught in bachelor's and master's degree programs and in health care agencies (American Association of Colleges of Nursing, 2006; Ireland, 2008; Leasure, Stirlen, and Thompson, 2008). Methods to develop evidence-based practice projects and protocols are included in master's degree programs and implemented in clinical agencies.

Impact of Electronic Health Records on Quality-Based Care

Electronic health records (EHR) are being implemented everywhere in the world (Committee on Quality of Health Care in America, IOM, 2004; Olsson, Lymberts, and Whitehouse, 2004) and will eventually be mandated for all health care events. The advantage is that when health care events are electronically recorded the individual health records can be aggregated with other health records to measure the outcomes of care provided in specific localities and by specific agencies and providers. Health care data can be compared from one place to another to determine the quality of care provided (Committee on Quality of Health Care in America, IOM, 2004).

For decades, nurse leaders have been expecting and preparing for the EHR. For example, NANDA-I was started in 1973 at the first meeting to classify nursing phenomena for computerized documentation (Gordon, 1982). This meeting was initiated by Drs. Kristine Gebbie and MaryAnne Levine to identify the phenomena that should represent the focus of nursing care. Since that time, many nurse leaders have been involved in health technology and informatics. For example, nursing specialty groups have a strong presence within the international and national informatics associations (see Appendix A, Webliography). These are the professional leaders who are planning for and working toward worldwide implementation of EHRs. Judith Warren, a past president of NANDA-I, is one of 18 members of the most important U.S. government group for planning an EHR system, the National Committee on Vital and Health Statistics.

Need for Standardized Nursing Languages (SNLs)

Standardized nursing languages are organized systems of labels, definitions, and descriptions of the three nursing care elements of diagnosis (assessment is subsumed within diagnosis), outcomes, and interventions—key aspects of the nursing process (Wilkinson, 2007). These three elements are considered essential for establishing a nursing minimum data set (NMDS) (Delaney and Moorhead, 1995). Some SNLs are combinations of all three elements, e.g., the Omaha System (Martin and Norris, 1996). NANDA-I, NOC, and NIC, the SNLs used in this book, are three separate systems that are used together to represent diagnosis of human responses (NANDA-I), the results or outcomes of nursing care (NOC), and nursing interventions (NIC) (Bulechek, Butcher, and Dochterman, 2008; Moorhead, Johnson, Maas, and Swanson, 2008; NANDA-I, 2009). These three systems are used for this book because they are the most comprehensive of all nursing language systems and have strong research support.

SNLs are needed to achieve quality-based nursing care for three reasons: (1) they represent three nursing care elements considered essential for the NMDS, (2) they represent evidence-based nursing, and (3) they serve as the file names for documentation in computerized systems. The elements of an NMDS were described by nurse leaders as the minimum data that should be available and communicated to determine the quality of nursing care.

SNLs such as NANDA-I, NOC, and NIC represent evidence-based nursing. Each of these languages was developed using nursing research. The individual labels and descriptions of the NANDA-I classification are based on research studies (NANDA-I, 2009). The NOC and NIC labels and descriptions were developed and organized by research teams, partially funded with millions of dollars from the National Institute of Nursing Research. To develop these systems, the research teams organized previous nursing knowledge, both research and practical, that had evolved over decades.

SNLs provide the file names with which to record consumer data in EHRs. Organized systems of file names are needed to organize and retrieve data from electronic systems. The three systems of NANDA-I, NOC, and NIC were developed with the EHR in mind; each label, for example, is coded for the EHR. Consistent use of these labels enables health care agencies to describe the services they provide and determine the quality of care. A medical-surgical unit, for example, can describe the number of patients in a day, week, month, or year for which the diagnosis of *disturbed body image** was made and treated. Inferences about the quality of care are made by comparing interventions to evidence-based standards and measuring the outcomes of nursing interventions.

Because SNLs are so useful to evidence-based clinical practice and implementation of EHRs, nurses need to learn how to use critical thinking for selecting diagnoses, outcomes, and interventions. The following section explains intelligence and critical thinking for application in clinical practice.

Intelligence and Critical Thinking to Achieve Quality Care

For nurses to help people achieve positive health outcomes, they need intelligence to think about, interpret, and act on clinical situations. Sternberg's theory of intelligence (1988, 1997) provides a framework for understanding this concept. From this perspective, intelligence is described as the ability to function well in the external world of work, home, play, and so forth, not by performance on an intelligence test. Critical thinking is a dimension of nursing intelligence that is necessary for using the nursing care elements of diagnosis and selecting appropriate outcomes and interventions. Nurse clinicians and students have the potential to continuously improve the quality of nursing care if they know about thinking processes and critical thinking.

Sternberg's Theory of Intelligence: The Triarchic Mind

Sternberg's Theory of the Triarchic Mind (1988) focuses on intelligence as it pertains to "everyday" matters in the lives of people. Sternberg identified five major problems associated with previous theories of intelligence. First, there was too much emphasis on the use of intelligence in unusual and bizarre situations rather than in ordinary problem solving. Second, positions pertaining to intelligence were politicized (e.g., the argument about which was more important, genetics or environment) before there was sufficient evidence about how people think. Third, technology was driving the science of intelligence—people were being tested for intelligence without knowing what intelligence was all about. Fourth, the belief that a single test score, the intelligence quotient (IQ), revealed people's intelligence was given too much credence in the

---

*Italics will be used throughout the book for the official NANDA-I, NOC, and NIC labels.

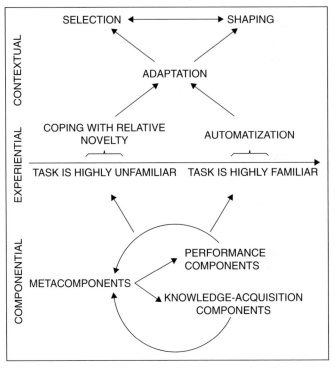

Figure 1.1. Relationships among the various aspects of the triarchic theory of human intelligence. Source: From *The triarchic mind: A new theory of human intelligence* (p. 68) by R.J. Sternberg, 1988, New York: Penguin Books. Reprinted with permission.

face of evidence that intelligence was much more complex than an IQ score could indicate. Fifth, the idea that intelligence is a "fixed entity" was promulgated and believed while research and experience demonstrated that intelligence can be improved through guided instruction and practice. Sternberg's theory counteracts previous views and provides a more optimistic view of intelligence.

According to Sternberg's theory, intelligence in everyday life is mental self-management consisting of "the purposive adaptation to, selection of, and shaping of ... environments relevant to one's life and abilities" (p. 65). The process of mental self management makes it possible to continuously develop intelligence for functioning well within our daily environments, for example, nursing care. Intelligence develops as an interaction or relation among three components: the internal world of the individual, the external world of the individual, and the person's experience of the resultant interchange between internal and external worlds (Figure 1.1). It is through these interrelationships that people can improve their own intellectual functioning, including critical thinking.

The Internal World of the Individual

The internal world of the individual is comprised of three components: metacomponents, knowledge-acquisition components, and performance components. The metacomponents activate the other two components, which in turn provide feedback to the metacomponents. Metacomponents are the executive processes used to plan, monitor, and evaluate problem solving. The knowledge-acquisition components are processes used to learn how to solve problems. Performance components are the lower order (intellectual) processes used to implement the commands of the metacomponents. The performance components refer to performance of the person's mind (e.g., making a decision after more complex thinking processes have led you to that decision), not visible performance of the whole person.

Metacomponents are used to think about the nurses' role in relation to the clinical situation. Nurses need to think about whether a consumer has a problem that should be treated, the severity of the problem, the priority of the problem, the prognosis of the problem, the interventions that are needed, how the problem should be communicated to others for a plan of care, the accuracy of the problem's identification, and the effectiveness of the interventions in responding to the problem.

Knowledge-acquisition components are used to select related knowledge. Examples of knowledge acquisition are use of books on nursing diagnoses, nursing-sensitive patient outcomes, and nursing interventions; checking an agency policy manual; seeking a family member to obtain more information; and collaborating with another nurse to understand the meaning of data.

In the performance components, when data are available for making an accurate diagnosis, the diagnosis is selected in partnership with the consumer, if possible. When a diagnosis is considered to be highly accurate, an outcome is selected, a baseline score is assigned, and interventions are chosen. These three components are continuously interactive in the internal world of the nurse diagnostician. Each aspect of the internal world of a nurse provides feedback to the other two aspects and has the potential to improve intelligence for the practical world of nursing.

The External World of the Individual

The external world of an individual consists of all of the individual's environments. The individual uses intelligence to exist in these environments. Intelligence serves three functions in the person's external world: (1) adapting to existing environments, (2) selecting new environments, and (3) shaping existing environments into new environments. For example, a woman who is being battered by a male partner can use her intelligence to adapt to the situation, leave the situation, or change the situation to fit her needs. The environments in which people live and work are the contexts within which intelligence exists. When intelligence is developing, the person considers the contexts of the external world and develops a fit within these contexts. People in various contexts use a wide variety of strategies to function in the external world. People who function well in relevant environments seem to capitalize on their strengths and compensate for limitations by using other resources and seeking consultations.

Nurses must use their intelligence to function well in a variety of environments or contexts. Sometimes there are serious time constraints for health assessments and thinking about diagnostic and intervention possibilities. Other times, the clinical situation is extremely complex with multiple interacting variables related to pathophysiology, emotional states, family processes, and so forth. With the complexity and diversity of environments that form the context of nursing, nurses can capitalize on their strengths to help them function well in a variety of environments (e.g., ability to conduct interviews and physical examinations, ability to collaborate effectively with families). They can also compensate for weaknesses by collaborating with other nurses on making diagnoses and validating diagnostic impressions with health care consumers.

The Experience of the Individual
The three components of the individual—metacomponents, knowledge-acquisition components, and performance components—are applied at various levels of experience (i.e., from new experiences to routine experiences) in the external world. There are differences in the use of metacomponents, knowledge-acquisition components, and performance components when a task in the external world is novel as opposed to routine. After a task is performed a number of times, it becomes routine or automatic. For example, brushing teeth is novel to an infant but becomes routinized as the mother helps the child to practice this skill. The ability to cope with novelty, including checking whether aspects of the situation are familiar enough to rely on previous knowledge and techniques, is considered an aspect of intelligence.

In nursing situations, for example, the first time that a specific diagnosis is used, it may require more emphasis on knowledge-acquisition components than metacomponents. The performance components of a nurse who is familiar with the human experience being diagnosed are more competent or efficient than those of a nurse who is unfamiliar with the experience. The three mental processes of intelligence are improved with repeated exposures to particular nursing diagnoses in a variety of contexts. This aspect of Sternberg's theory was supported by nursing research conducted on the development of competence (Benner, 1984). Benner showed that years of nursing experience was a critical factor in development from the novice stage to more advanced stages of competence.

Critical thinking involves specific types of thinking that occur in the internal world of the individual (i.e., in the three components). Knowledge of critical thinking, as it applies in nursing practice, and reflection on thinking processes (metacognition) enable nurses to improve these aspects of the internal world.

Critical Thinking

A definition of critical thinking in nursing that was produced by a study of expert nurse opinions serves as a basis for understanding the subject (Scheffer and Rubenfeld, 2000; Rubenfeld and Schaffer, 2006). Critical thinking in nursing is an essential component of professional accountability and quality nursing care. Critical thinkers in nursing exhibit these habits of the mind: confidence, contextual perspective, creativity, flexibility, inquisitiveness, intellectual integrity, intuition, open-mindedness, perseverance, and reflection. Critical thinkers in nursing practice the cognitive skills of analyzing, applying standards, discriminating, seeking information, logical reasoning, predicting, and transforming knowledge (Scheffer and Rubenfeld, 2000, p. 357).

This definition was developed through five rounds of a Delphi study with 51 nurse experts in critical thinking. The definition includes the characteristics of critical thinking from previous theoretical and research-based activities considered important for nursing.

It is assumed that nurses, like other adults, vary widely in thinking abilities; numerous studies have shown that adults demonstrate a wide variance in thinking abilities of all types (Gambrill, 2005; Sternberg, 1988, 1997; Willingham, 2007a, 2007b). Lunney (1992) substantiated that nurses vary widely in the divergent thinking abilities of fluency, flexibility, and elaboration. Fluency is the ability to think of many units of information. Flexibility is the ability to mentally change from one category of information to another. Elaboration is the ability to identify many implications from a unit of information. Some nurses scored very high, while others scored very low on fluency, flexibility, and elaboration. These thinking abilities, however, can be improved through instruction and practice (Gambrill, 2005; Sternberg, 1997; Willingham, 2007a). One of the purposes of selecting diagnoses, outcomes, and interventions for the case studies in this book is to further develop thinking skills for application to future clinical cases.

The seven cognitive skills of critical thinking—analyzing, applying standards, discriminating, seeking information, logical reasoning, predicting, and transforming knowledge—are applied during the nursing process (Scheffer and Rubenfeld, 2000; Table 1.1). The 10 habits of mind developed by critical thinkers in nursing are evident in each of the cognitive skills. Intuition as a habit of mind seems to be associated with increased experience and may be related to fewer of the cognitive skills than other habits of mind. The seven cognitive skills

Table 1.1. Critical thinking in nursing: definitions of terms.*

Dimensions of Critical Thinking	Definitions
Cognitive skills	
Analyzing	Separating or breaking a whole into parts to discover the nature, function, and relationships
Applying standards	Judging according to established personal, professional, or social rules or criteria
Discriminating	Recognizing differences and similarities among things or situations and distinguishing carefully as to category or rank
Information seeking	Searching for evidence, facts, or knowledge by identifying relevant sources and gathering objective, subjective, historical, and current data from those sources
Logical reasoning	Drawing inferences or conclusions that are supported in or justified by evidence
Predicting	Envisioning a plan and its consequences
Transforming knowledge	Changing or converting the condition, nature, form, or function of concepts among contexts
Habits of the mind	
Confidence	Assurance of one's reasoning abilities
Contextual perspective	Consideration of the whole situation, including relationships, background, and environment, relevant to some happening
Creativity	Intellectual inventiveness used to generate, discover, or restructure ideas; imagining alternatives
Flexibility	Capacity to adapt, accommodate, modify, or change thoughts, ideas, and behaviors
Inquisitiveness	An eagerness to know by seeking knowledge and understanding through observation and thoughtful questioning in order to explore possibilities and alternatives
Intellectual integrity	Seeking the truth through sincere, honest processes, even if the results are contrary to one's assumptions and beliefs
Intuition	Insightful sense of knowing without conscious use of reason
Open-mindedness	A viewpoint characterized by being receptive to divergent views and sensitive to one's biases
Perseverance	Pursuit of a course with determination to overcome obstacles
Reflection	Contemplation upon a subject, especially one's assumptions and thinking, for purposes of deeper understanding and self-evaluation

*Scheffer, B.K., and Rubenfeld, M.G. (2000). A consensus statement on critical thinking. *Journal of Nursing Education, 39*, 352–359.

and the 10 habits of mind are mental processes of the internal world of nurses.

Use of Cognitive Skills and Habits of Mind

The use of cognitive skills and habits of mind are discussed here in relation to deciding on a diagnosis because that is the foundation for selecting outcomes and interventions. The two aspects of critical thinking, cognitive skills and habits of mind, are interrelated (Scheffer and Rubenfeld, 2000); cognitive skills are the context in which the habits of mind are useful. Nurses can develop both aspects as they learn to diagnose and intervene for diagnoses to achieve positive health outcomes. To illustrate these relationships, the 10 habits of mind are explained in relation to each of the cognitive skills. The cognitive skills are presented in alphabetical order because most likely the order in which they are used differs for various aspects of the nursing process.

Cognitive Skill of Analyzing

When a person presents with cues (signs and symptoms) that indicate a nurse should assess that person's health status, the nurse (internal world, metacomponent) analyzes the presenting data and determines what additional data are needed and which diagnoses are probable. During the assessment process, the nurse synthesizes information and analyzes how well the cues fit with particular diagnoses.

Habits of Mind
A contextual perspective is needed to analyze cues in the context of the whole situation (e.g., if a woman is smiling, it may not mean that she is happy; rather, she may have been taught to smile to cover up bad feelings). The nurse needs confidence to trust the data analysis and seek further consensus through mutual collaboration with health care consumers and other providers. Creativity, flexibility, inquisitiveness, intuition, and open-mindedness are needed to consider a variety of possible meanings of data. Intellectual integrity is also required for analysis along with a commitment to spend professional time and energy on the analysis process. Perseverance and reflection are essential when the analysis is more difficult and time consuming than expected.

Cognitive Skill of Applying Standards

The nurse (internal world, metacomponent) applies standards related to the diagnostic process by: (a) using the principles of good communication during the health history, (b) working collaboratively with the consumer throughout the diagnostic process, (c) conducting physical examinations using valid and reliable techniques, and (d) using research and theory when making diagnoses. The nurse draws these standards from memory or identifies standards during information seeking.

Habits of Mind
Confidence is required when selecting the best standard for use in the diagnostic process. A contextual perspective is needed to discern the relevance of standards to the whole situation, e.g., the culture of the individual. Creativity, flexibility, inquisitiveness, intuition, and open-mindedness are needed when the usual standards may not apply. Intellectual integrity is essential when the applied standards are not well accepted by others. Perseverance and reflection are needed to identify standards for application in unusual or difficult situations.

Cognitive Skill of Discriminating
The nurse (internal world, metacomponent) notices or discriminates those cues or data in a clinical situation that are important to consider. These cues are discerned in relation to the possible meanings of cues (diagnoses) and the relevance of cues, e.g., low, moderate, high. This process narrows the selection of cues for consideration during analysis and other mental processes (internal world, performance component intellectual).

Habits of Mind
Because cues and diagnoses are only meaningful in the context of the whole situation, a contextual perspective is essential. Confidence in self is needed to isolate important cues. Creativity, flexibility, inquisitiveness, intuition, and open-mindedness are required to notice unusual or unexpected cues. Intellectual integrity is needed to follow up on cues, despite the time, energy, and effort involved. Perseverance and reflection are needed to discriminate cues that fit with other cues for making decisions about the diagnosis.

Cognitive Skill of Information Seeking
The nurse (internal world, knowledge-acquisition component) seeks information to assist with and support the interpretation of cues as they relate to diagnoses. Information sources may be the health care consumer, the family, the health care record, the literature on a particular health problem, the literature on human response concepts, and the literature related to developmental or cultural aspects of the consumer.

Habits of Mind
The mental habit of reflection is needed to guide the nurse's search for new information. Intellectual integrity is needed to seek the most appropriate source of information, even when the task is difficult or unrewarding. It is important that nurses use creativity, flexibility, and inquisitiveness as they consider sources of information that are unusual

for the situation. Perseverance is needed when the required knowledge is elusive, difficult to find, or difficult to interpret.

Cognitive Skill of Logical Reasoning

The nurse (internal world, metacomponent) uses logical reasoning to consider the meaning and relevance of cues in relation to diagnoses and to converge to the most accurate diagnoses. Logical reasoning is a process of evaluating, comparing, and judging existing data against expected data. In previous decades, logical reasoning, inductive and deductive, was considered to be the primary method of interpreting data (e.g., Bandman and Bandman, 1995). Additional thinking strategies such as intuition were acknowledged and accepted as seen in the definition of critical thinking (Scheffer and Rubenfeld, 2000). The cognitive skills of analysis, discrimination, and applying standards are intimately involved with logical reasoning in making diagnoses.

Habits of Mind

Confidence is needed to select the most appropriate diagnoses for a data set. A contextual perspective enables the nurse to interpret data in the context of the whole situation. Intellectual integrity is required to select the most accurate diagnosis when the decision is a difficult one. Intuition and open-mindedness are needed to recognize and accept that logical reasoning may not be the most appropriate way to make a diagnosis in a specific situation. Perseverance and reflection are needed when logical reasoning is more difficult than expected.

Cognitive Skill of Predicting

The nurse (internal world, metacomponents, and performance components) predicts possible diagnoses from clusters of cues, anticipates human responses for particular health states, and prioritizes diagnoses for interventions and outcomes. Thinking abilities, clinical experience in nursing, and knowledge are the basis for such predictions.

Habits of Mind

Confidence is needed to make predictions. A contextual perspective or consideration of the whole situation, not just the parts, improves the validity of predictions. When the most accurate predictions are different than the routine, the nurse needs to be open-minded enough to accept explanations that are unusual, inquisitive enough to explore alternative explanations, and flexible enough to change from one category of explanation to another. Creativity may be needed when explanations are unusual or novel. Intellectual integrity is needed to accept the predictions that are best indicated by the data. Intuition is needed to discern cues and predict that which may not be evident through logical reasoning. Perseverance and reflection are needed when predictions are more difficult to develop than usual.

Cognitive Skill of Transforming Knowledge

The nurse transforms knowledge by using the processes described above to apply the general knowledge of diagnostic concepts to clinical situations of varying contexts. Knowledge is transformed from one form to another when general knowledge of diagnostic concepts is used to help an individual, family, group, or community. For example, general knowledge of self-esteem must be transformed for use with people of various cultures. The meaning of self-esteem varies among cultures so the concept cannot be universally applied. The nurse transforms knowledge by integrating knowledge gained through clinical experiences (practical knowledge) with theoretical knowledge (research and theory). For example, the nurse with five years of clinical experiences working with post-operative patients with ineffective airway clearance applies theoretical knowledge of this concept differently than a nurse with one year of experience.

Habits of Mind

Without self-confidence, the nurse cannot transform knowledge to make a diagnosis, especially when the diagnosis is not one that is routine. An inquisitive nurse is more likely to recognize opportunities for transforming knowledge. Being able to incorporate the context of a clinical situation with highly relevant data enables nurses to be more accurate in diagnosis generation and transformation of knowledge. With flexibility, the nurse can mentally search multiple categories of knowledge as indicated. Creativity supports the transformation of knowledge through identification of unusual connections or relationships. Intuition is needed when the specific data for knowledge transformations cannot be identified. Perseverance and reflection are needed when knowledge transformations are more challenging than usual. Intellectual integrity may be needed to accept knowledge transformations despite conflicts with assumptions and beliefs and to be able to validate diagnoses with others.

Metacognition

Nurses' intelligence and critical thinking are improved through metacognition (Pesut and Herman, 1999). Metacognition involves thinking about thinking and is a tool for self-improvement. Development of this skill provides a basis for growth as a professional. The seven cognitive skills and 10 habits of mind provide the language, meanings, and framework for nurses to think about their own thinking. Each of the cognitive skills and habits of mind can be thought about and analyzed independently, discussed with other nurses or instructors, or written about in a journal for examination later.

An independent process of thinking about the diagnostic process was referred to as self-monitoring of diagnostic reasoning (Carnevali,

1984; Lunney, 1989). It can be likened to having a bird sitting on your shoulder and whispering in your ear: what are you thinking? how are you thinking? (Carnevali, 1984). Reflection, or reflective practice (Johns, 2006), includes self-monitoring of thinking processes. Self-monitoring can be described for self or others (e.g., an instructor) through a clinical journal (Degazon and Lunney, 1995). Teachers can require students to write clinical journals so they can reflect on the thinking processes that occurred during a clinical event. A course requirement to use metacognition in clinical journals can stimulate ongoing use of thinking about thinking.

Need for Case Studies to Develop Critical Thinking Skills for Quality-Based Care

Case studies are needed for nurses and nursing students to learn critical thinking for diagnosis, outcomes, and interventions because metacognition only achieves skill development when it is combined with repeated practice of the thinking processes with the specific skill, e.g., use of NANDA-I, NOC, and NIC (Lunney, 2008; Willingham, 2007a). Many studies have substantiated that critical thinking skills only advance when metacognition is combined with repeated experiences of applying the requisite skills (Willingham, 2007a, 2007b).

In the real world of nursing, there are not enough clinical experiences that can be offered to nurses and student nurses for them to become proficient in applying the cognitive skills and habits of mind to diagnose clinical cases and use NANDA-I, NOC, and NIC. Case studies offer low-risk opportunities to use critical thinking and metacognition to achieve evidence-based practice. The case studies and analyses in this book stimulate metacognition by providing challenges to the thinking processes of nurses and nursing students. Readers can diagnose the clinical cases and match their diagnoses and thinking processes with those of the case study authors.

References

Aiken, L. (2005). Improving quality through nursing. In D. Mechanic, *Policy challenges in modern health care* (pp. 177–188). Piscataway, NJ: Rutgers University Press.

Al-Assaf, A.F., and Sheikh, M. (2004). *Quality improvement in primary health care: A practical guide.* Geneva: WHO Regional Office for the Eastern Mediterranean.

American Association of Colleges of Nursing. (2006). *AACN Position Statement on Nursing Research.* Washington, DC: Author.

Bandman, E.L., and Bandman, B. (1995). *Critical thinking in nursing* (2nd ed.). Upper Saddle River, NJ: Prentice Hall.

Benner, P. (1984). *From novice to expert: Excellence and power in clinical nursing practice*. Menlo Park, CA: Addison-Wesley.

Bulechek, G.M., Butcher, H.K., and Dochterman, J.M. (2008). *Nursing interventions classification (NIC)* (5th ed.). St. Louis: Mosby.

Carnevali, D.L. (1984). Strategies for self-monitoring of diagnostic reasoning behaviors: Pathway to professional growth. In D.L. Carnevali, P. Mitchell, N. Woods, and C. Tanner, *Diagnostic reasoning in nursing* (pp. 225–228). Philadelphia: Lippincott.

Committee on Quality of Health Care in America, Institute of Medicine. (2001). *Crossing the quality chasm: A new health system for the 21st Century*. Washington, DC: National Academies Press.

Committee on Quality of Health Care in America, Institute of Medicine (2004). *Keeping patients safe*. Washington DC: National Academies Press.

Committee on Reviewing Evidence to Identify Highly Effective Clinical Services, Institute of Medicine. (2008). *Knowing what works in health care: A roadmap for the nation*. Washington, DC: National Academies Press.

Degazon, C., and Lunney, M. (1995). Clinical journal: A tool to foster critical thinking for competence in advanced practice. *Clinical Nurse Specialist: The Journal of Advanced Nursing Practice, 9*, 270–274.

Delaney, C., and Moorhead, S. (1995). The nursing minimum data set, standardized languages, and health care quality. *Journal of Nursing Care Quality, 10*, 16–30.

Donabedian, A. (2002). *An introduction to quality assurance in health care*. London, UK: Oxford University Press.

Gambrill, E. (2005). *Critical thinking in clinical practice: Improving the quality of judgment and decisions* (2nd ed.). Hoboken, NJ: John Wiley and Sons.

Gordon, M. (1982). Historical perspective: The National Conference Group for Classification of Nursing Diagnoses. In M.J. Kim and D.A. Moritz, *Classification of nursing diagnoses: Proceedings of the third and fourth national conferences* (pp. 2–8). New York: McGraw-Hill.

Henderson, V. (1964). The nature of nursing. *American Journal of Nursing, 64*(8), 62–68.

Hines, S., and Joshi, M.S. (2008). Variation in the quality of care within health systems. *Joint Commission Journal of Quality and Patient Safety, 34*, 326–322.

Institute of Medicine. (2008). *News: Medication errors injure 1.5 million people and cost billions of dollars annually*. Retrieved on 7/15/08 from http://www8. nationalacademies.org/onpinews/newsitem.aspx?RecordID=11623

Ireland, M. (2008). Assisting students to use evidence as part of reflection on practice. *Nursing Education Perspectives, 29*, 90–93.

Johns, C. (2006). *Engaging reflection in practice: A narrative approach*. London: Blackwell.

Leasure, A.R., Stirlen, J., and Thompson, C. (2008). Barriers and facilitators to the use of evidence-based best practices. *Dimensions of Critical Care Nursing, 27*(2), 74–82.

Lunney, M. (1989). Self monitoring of accuracy using an integrated model of the diagnostic process. *Journal of Advanced Medical-Surgical Nursing, 1*(3), 43–52.

Lunney, M. (1992). Divergent productive thinking factors and accuracy of nursing diagnoses. *Research in Nursing and Health, 15*, 303–311.

Lunney, M. (2008). Current knowledge related to intelligence and thinking and implications for development and use of case studies. *International Journal of Nursing Terminologies and Classifications, 19*(4), 358–362.

Martin, K., and Norris, J. (1996). The Omaha System: A model for describing practice. *Holistic Nursing Practice, 11,* 75–83.

Mechanic, D. (2008). *The truth about health care in America: Why reform is not working.* New Brunswick, NJ: Rutgers University Press.

Melnyk, B.M., and Fineout-Overholt, E. (2005). *Evidenced-based practice in nursing and healthcare: A guide to best practice.* Philadelphia: Lippincott Williams and Wilkins.

Montalvo, I., and Dunton, N. (Eds.). (2007). *Transforming nursing data into quality care: Profiles of quality improvement in U.S. healthcare facilities.* Washington: Nursesbooks.org

Moorhead, S., Johnson, M., Maas, M.L., and Swanson, E. (2008). *Nursing outcomes classification (NOC)* (4th ed.). St Louis: Mosby.

NANDA International. (2009). *Nursing diagnosis: Definitions and classification, 2009–2011.* Hoboken, NJ: Wiley-Blackwell.

Olsson, S., Lymberts, A., and Whitehouse, D. (2004). European Commission activities in ehealth. *International Journal of Circumpolar Health, 63,* 310–316.

Pesut, D.J., and Herman, J.A. (1999). *Clinical reasoning: The art and science of critical and creative thinking.* Albany, NY: Delmar.

Robert Wood Johnson Foundation. (2008). *Quality.* Retrieved on July 15, 2008 from http://www.rwjf.org/pr/topic.jsp?topicid=1053

Rubenfeld, M.G., and Scheffer, B.K. (2006). *Critical thinking TACTICS for nurses.* Boston: Jones and Bartlett.

Scheffer, B.K., and Rubenfeld, M.G. (2000). A consensus statement on critical thinking. *Journal of Nursing Education, 39,* 352–359.

Sternberg, R.J. (1988). *The triarchic mind: A new theory of human intelligence.* New York: Penguin Books.

Sternberg, R.J. (1997). *Successful intelligence: How practical and creative intelligence determine success in life.* New York: Plume Books.

Wilkinson, J.M. (2007). *Nursing process and critical thinking.* (4th ed.). Upper Saddle River, NJ: Prentice Hall.

Willingham, D.T. (2007a). Critical thinking: Why is it so hard to teach? *American Educator, 31*(2), 8–19.

Willingham, D.T. (2007b). *Cognition: The thinking animal* (3rd ed.). Upper Saddle River, NJ: Prentice Hall.

Diagnostic Reasoning and Accuracy of Diagnosing Human Responses

Margaret Lunney, RN, PhD

Chapter Objectives

By completion of this chapter, readers will be able to:

1. Explain diagnostic reasoning in nursing;
2. Discuss the goal of accuracy of nurses' diagnoses, including (a) historical perspective of knowledge development, and (b) reasons why accuracy is a concern;
3. Describe three reasons to develop diagnostic reasoning for accuracy of nurses' diagnoses;
4. Describe the relation of nursing diagnoses to consumer outcomes and nursing interventions; and
5. Discuss the professional accountability for accuracy.

Since the time of Nightingale, leaders in nursing recognized the need for intelligence in making decisions for nursing care (Kelly, 1966). Then, in 1967, the first description of the nursing process by Yura and Walsh addressed the intellectual aspects of nursing and highlighted intelligence as a significant dimension of the nursing process. Prior to the 1980s, discussions about the intellectual aspects of nursing focused predominately on development of knowledge for clinical practice, i.e., the content of thinking. Since the late 1980s, however, greater emphasis has been placed on both the processes and the content of thinking (Bandman and Bandman, 1995; Facione and Facione, 1996; Narayan, Corcoran-Perry, Drew, Hoyman, and Lewis, 2003; Rubenfeld and Scheffer, 2006; Tanner, 2006; Walsh and Seldomridge, 2006). The content of thinking for nursing care reflects the knowledge that has accrued in more than 100 years of nursing practice, theory development, and research. The processes of thinking are known through the research and theories of psychology, philosophy, and nursing. This chapter explains the thinking processes involved with diagnostic reasoning and the goal of accuracy of nurses' diagnoses.

Diagnostic Reasoning in Nursing

The diagnosis of human responses is a complex process involving the interpretation of human behavior related to health. Webster (1984), a philosopher of science, noted that the complexity of nursing's phenomena of concern is "unrivaled" (p. 14). This relates to the focus of nursing, which addresses the holistic nature of people and health. "The patient looks to the nurse for recognition as a person and not just as an example of a kind of disease or problem" (Webster, 1984, p. 15). In addition, nurses help people to achieve health in the context of how they live their lives.

Diagnostic reasoning in nursing involves an interaction of interpersonal, technical, and intellectual processes. Interpersonal processes include communicating with health care consumers and other providers for data collection, data analyses, and decision making. Technical processes include using specific tools and skills such as taking a person's health history (see Appendix B, Assessment tool: Functional Health Patterns) and conducting individual, family, and community assessments and physical examinations. Intellectual processes include developing intelligence and using critical thinking for data collection, data analyses, and decision making. Diagnostic reasoning has been described as a step-by-step process, an iterative process, a heuristic process, and an intuitive process (Carnevali and Thomas, 1993; Gordon, 1994; O'Neill, 1995; O'Neill and Dluhy, 1997; Rew, 1988). The discussion to follow outlines critical elements of diagnostic reasoning and reflects the complexity of decision making in nursing. The content from this point through the section on validating diagnoses was also published in Chapter 1 of NANDA-I (2009, pp. 10–12).

Recognizing the Existence of Cues

Nurses mentally recognize cues early in the diagnostic process and continue to integrate cue recognition throughout the process. Cues are units of data, for example, a person's rate of breathing, that a nurse collects during intentional or unintentional assessment. Intentional assessment involves deliberate collection of data as a foundation for nursing actions. Unintentional assessment involves noticing cues that are important without planning to do so. In clinical situations, nurses notice cues to diagnoses by thinking about what they see, hear, smell, touch, and taste. Information pertaining to the health care consumer is thought about in relation to the nurse's knowledge of the consumer's health state or life situation. Nurses attend to information based on established ideas of what should occur in various situations. A nurse may not notice a person's rate of breathing, for example, unless it looks unusual in the context of a health problem, e.g., the individual is one day post-operative abdominal surgery, or other aspects of the clinical situation, e.g., the individual has just completed a vigorous exercise. A nurse's recognition of a unit of data as a cue with special meaning depends on knowledge stored in memory. Knowledge bases in memory are used to compare current data with expected data.

Mentally Generating Possible Diagnoses

The meaning that nurses assign to cues noticed early in the diagnostic process can only be understood if there are possible and plausible explanations for the cues within the context of the situation. This is an *active* thinking process whereby the nurse explores knowledge in memory for possible explanations of data. Often, many possible diagnoses or explanations may be considered. Sometimes, there is only one plausible meaning for cues noticed early in the diagnostic process. For example, if a woman who is newly admitted to a hospital unit for a surgical procedure is rapidly asking the nurse many questions, and exhibits a fast rate of breathing, the cues are not specific enough to consider only one possible diagnosis. The nurse in this instance would consider a number of possible explanations for this set of cues such as fear, anxiety, ineffective breathing pattern, and others. A nurse diagnostician avoids deciding on a diagnosis prematurely, that is, before there are sufficient data to support a diagnostic judgment. A broad search of the mind is needed to identify possible diagnoses and other cues to explore.

Comparing Cues to Possible Diagnoses

Cues are analyzed in relation to possible diagnoses through a mental process of evaluation, which involves matching existing cues with the expected cues for the diagnoses being considered. Information about the expected cues to diagnoses is found in a variety of sources such as NANDA International (NANDA-I, 2009) and current literature on specific phenomena such as pain, coping, and fluid volume. During the evaluation of cues and related diagnoses, nurses may decide that there is not enough evidence to make a diagnostic decision or that there is enough evidence for one likely diagnosis. If a nurse decides that there are not enough data, then the next step involves a focused search for additional cues. If a nurse decides that there is enough supporting evidence, a diagnosis is made and then validated.

Conducting a Focused Data Collection

In order to confirm or rule out diagnoses that are under consideration, additional cues may be collected by focusing questions to obtain data for one or more diagnoses. For example, with people who are pre-operative, as mentioned above, nurses might ask them how they feel about the surgical procedure. The answer to a broad question such as this can yield data to support many possible diagnoses in the psycho-social realm. If patients mention fear of death or fear of the unknown in relation to the surgery, nurses can begin to confirm "fear" as the diagnosis and eliminate some of the other possibilities such as anxiety. When the nurse conducts a health history and physical examination, biological reasons for the fast rate of breathing can also be confirmed or ruled out. A focused data collection concludes when the nurse synthesizes available data and selects one of the diagnoses being considered, rules out all of the diagnoses being considered, or revises the diagnoses being considered to incorporate new diagnoses. If a diagnosis under consideration is supported through focused data collection, the next step is to validate the diagnosis. Other scenarios to consider include: all of the diagnoses are ruled out or not confirmed, new diagnoses are considered, or the nurse concludes that there is no diagnosis. If new diagnoses are considered, then a focused data collection continues until the revised set of diagnoses are confirmed or ruled out through supporting evidence (cues).

Validating Diagnoses

With the complexity of human behavior, nurses cannot truly "know" what other people are experiencing (Munhall, 1993). It is important, then, that nurses' thinking and technical processes be accompanied by collaborative interpersonal processes with consumers and other providers. In most instances nurses validate diagnoses with health care consumers. For example a nurse may say: "From the information you have just given me, it seems that you are experiencing fear associated with surgery. Is that correct?" Based upon the person's response, the nurse validates or refutes the diagnosis. When people are unable to collaborate with nurses because they are too sick, developmentally unable, or mentally incompetent, nurses can validate diagnoses with family members or other providers. For example a nurse may say: "From the information, you have given me about your son, it seems that he is having difficulty coping with the stress of the illness. Is that correct?" To validate with another provider, a nurse may say: "From my physical examination, I concluded that Mary's airway clearance is impaired. Do you agree?"

Validating diagnoses with others helps to ensure the accuracy of diagnoses as the bases for subsequent stages of the nursing process. To save the time, energy, and costs associated with interventions for diagnoses, diagnoses generally should be validated as highly accurate. Three exceptions are (a) when there is a crisis situation and the diagnosis should be immediately treated, (b) the person is not likely to be able to discern accuracy, as in physiological diagnosis such as decreased cardiac output, and (c) the person is not mentally able to discern accuracy.

The responses of people to health problems and life processes are routinely interpreted by health care providers. Nurses, physicians, dentists, social workers, and others interpret that patients experience fear, anxiety, pain, ineffective coping, or fluid volume deficit and provide interventions for these responses. Yet, in the past, the accuracy of these interpretations has not been considered or questioned. The discipline of nursing has taken responsibility for the diagnosis and treatment of human responses as indicated by Nurse Practice Acts (e.g., New York State) and the classification of nursing diagnoses developed by NANDA-I (2009).

Accuracy of Nurses' Diagnoses

Knowledge development in nursing for more than 30 years has shown that people's responses to health problems and life processes can easily be misinterpreted (Lunney, 2008). This is because interpreting human responses is a complex endeavor. A major influencing factor is that no human being can fully know or understand other human beings (Munhall, 1993). The risk of low accuracy is always present because nurses' interpretations of consumer responses are subjective impressions or diagnoses of other people's experiences. This section describes the historical perspective of knowledge development related to diagnostic reasoning and accuracy of nurses' diagnoses, and explains the reasons why accuracy is an issue of concern. These reasons are that (a) human responses are complex and diverse enough to be at risk for low degrees of accuracy, (b) selecting the most appropriate interventions depends on high degrees of accuracy, and (c) accountability for high accuracy is a professional behavior.

History of Knowledge Development Related to Diagnostic Reasoning and Accuracy of Nurses' Diagnoses

Since 1966, research findings have shown that there were broad variations in nurses' interpretations of responses such as pain, and thus broad variations of accuracy, even when the exact same data were available to each nurse (Kelly, 1966). In the 1960s through the 1980s, a major contributing factor to wide differences in data interpretations was a lack of consistency in definitions and defining characteristics of signs and symptoms. In 1973, 100 nurses from the United States and Canada attended the First National Conference on Classification of Nursing Diagnoses to identify and define the human responses that nurses diagnose (Gordon, 1982). The purpose was to begin knowledge development about these phenomena. These 100 nurses generated the first list of human responses to be labeled as nursing diagnoses. The original list formed by this group was the foundation for the current list of approved diagnoses in NANDA-I (2009). The goal of knowledge development has been realized to the extent that research findings serve as the basis for current diagnoses, definitions, defining characteristics, and related factors. The research evidence for diagnoses is one of the criteria used by the NANDA-I Diagnosis Development Committee when deciding whether to approve new diagnoses and revise previous diagnoses (NANDA-I, 2009).

Despite knowledge development of diagnostic concepts, however, accuracy is still a major issue to be addressed (Lunney, 2008). The threat of low accuracy is consistently present for every nursing diagnosis because nurses' impressions of the responses for which interventions are needed are intellectually developed or interpreted. The intellectual process of deciding on a diagnosis contributes to a range of accuracy from low to high.

The common sense idea of accuracy, that diagnoses are either accurate or inaccurate, was the basis of research studies until 1992. After an analysis of literature sources from the 1960s, 1970s and 1980s, Lunney (1990) concluded that accuracy of nurses' diagnoses of human responses is too complex and relative to be considered as a dichotomous (i.e., either/or) variable. It was found that this model of accuracy does not fit the complexity of interpreting human responses to health problems and life processes. Instead, diagnoses can be judged as:

- Highly accurate;
- Close to accurate;
- Representing the general idea but not precise enough;
- Reflecting some of the cues but not capturing highly relevant cues;
- Reflecting only one or a few cues;
- Not supported by the evidence;
- Should be refuted based on existing evidence.

A seven-point scale to measure accuracy as a continuous variable was developed and tested for judging accuracy and its validity was demonstrated (Lunney, 1990, 1992; Lunney, Karlik, Kiss, and Murphy, 1997, see Appendix C). Recently, this seven-point scale was reduced to fewer scale points for studies conducted in Brazil and Europe (Matos and Cruz, 2007; Hasegawa, Ogasawara, and Katz, 2007; Paquay,

Wouters, Debaille, and Geys, 2007). Matos and Cruz's scale to measure accuracy is in Appendix D. In the future, these researchers will collaborate to further develop a measurement scale that will be internationally useful for measuring accuracy.

Reasons Why the Degree of Accuracy is a Concern

Two major reasons for the previous lack of concern about accuracy are: (a) inadequate knowledge of the complexity of interpreting human responses, and (b) other priorities in health care. Before the concept of nursing diagnosis was broadly discussed and debated, nurses did not realize that interpretations of human responses such as pain, anxiety, and fluid volume deficit are complex because they are inferences.

Complexity of Human Responses

Inferences are the meanings that human beings attach to cues—units of information that are perceived through the five senses. For example, if you were to see a woman with hair roots that are white, you would perceive it through your senses; this is a cue. If you notice that the woman's hair roots are white, you might mentally consider "what does this mean?" Some meanings or inferences that you might consider are: "she is old," "she couldn't get to the store to buy hair dye," "she has gray hair so she has a great deal of experience and knowledge about life," or "she is sloppy." Many possible inferences are derived from such cues.

Thinking about the meaning of cues to make sense of them is a normal and usual process for human beings (Willingham, 2007a). Humans only retain seven units of data in short term memory, plus or minus two units (Newell and Simon, 1972). Therefore, units of data are converted to broader categories that encompass the meaning of the data in order to process large amounts of data. For example, while supervising a student on a home visit, the instructor noted that the patient's tone of voice and manner showed impatience with the student's questioning technique. The woman indicated that she wanted the student to finish the visit. Later the student referred to the woman as "hostile." The student was not able to recall the data that led to the inference that the woman was hostile. The woman's behavior was not hostile, however. When the student noted the woman's voice tone, abrupt manner, and short responses to the student's questions, the student interpreted these cues as "hostile" and stored the interpretation in her mind, not the cues. With the limited amount of storage in short term memory, this type of thinking process is expected.

Nurses, like other humans, interpret cues and use these interpretations as a basis for action. Interpretations are made whether or not they are labeled as nursing diagnoses. This means that nurses are at risk for low diagnostic accuracy whether or not they communicate their interpretations through diagnostic statements in a person's chart. Interventions are based on interpretations of data regardless of whether they are labeled as nursing diagnoses. Use of nursing diagnosis makes it possible to be more accurate by focusing attention on these interpretations.

In addition, when nurses do not know the meaning of human response concepts, they cannot be aware of the risk of low accuracy and are not likely to attend to the accuracy of interpreting, naming, and intervening for these phenomena. Studies have demonstrated, for example, that nurses do not understand the difference between fear and anxiety and these two concepts are used interchangeably as if they have the same meaning (Jones and Jakob, 1981, 1984; Yocum, 1984; Lunney et al., 1997). Yet these are different phenomena that require different interventions. The effects of this lack of knowledge on nursing care may be extensive, as indicated by the prevalence of *fear* and *anxiety* in a study of 159 newly admitted patients of three hospitals (Lunney et al., 1997). *Fear* and *anxiety* were the highest accuracy psychosocial diagnoses in 54.4% of 160 newly admitted persons in three hospitals.

Health Care Priorities
The second major reason that accuracy of nurses' diagnoses of human responses has been neglected is other health care priorities, for example, concern about medical diagnoses, selection and measurement of medical interventions, and cutting costs. The societal view that diagnoses of medical problems are more important to address than interpretations of human responses influences this pattern of priority setting. Also, nurses are more comfortable with medical knowledge because it has been developing for a longer period of time than nursing knowledge. Yet, nurses are not accountable for medical diagnosis and treatment, physicians are. The priority of cutting costs also makes it more difficult for nurses to have sufficient time to attend to accuracy.

Despite these difficulties, it is important at this point in time that nurses apply the knowledge that has been developing since the 1973 conference on nursing diagnosis by attending to the accuracy of human responses. Application of this body of knowledge will help health care consumers to achieve health-related goals. Health care consumers need nurses to work collaboratively with them for accurate interpretation of their responses to health problems and life processes.

Three Reasons to Develop Diagnostic Reasoning for Accuracy of Nurses' Diagnoses

The major reasons that nurses need to use diagnostic reasoning to accurately interpret human responses are that (a) human responses are complex and diverse enough to be at risk for low degrees of accuracy, (b) selecting the most appropriate interventions depends on high degrees of accuracy, and (c) accountability for high accuracy is a professional behavior. The complexity and diversity of human responses are described in numerous sources throughout the nursing literature, particularly sources on nursing diagnosis and cultural aspects of nursing. Selecting the most appropriate nursing interventions to achieve positive outcomes is the main reason that society needs and supports nurses, so it is the *raison d'être* of nursing's existence. In a health care market that emphasizes high efficiency, the discipline of nursing must demonstrate its accountability for all aspects of nursing care, including accurate interpretations of human responses.

Complexity and Diversity of Interpreting Human Responses

Three categories were identified as affecting the outcome or accuracy of interpreting human responses: the diagnostic task, the situational context, and the diagnostician. These categories were described by two major theorists on the diagnostic process in nursing, Doris Carnevali and Marjory Gordon. Books by these two theorists can be consulted for additional information on these topics (Carnevali and Thomas, 1993; Gordon 1994).

The Diagnostic Task
Diagnostic tasks consist of clinical situations (or simulations of clinical situations) that indicate a need for nursing or other health care services. Diagnostic tasks vary in many domains of the human condition: biological, psychological, social, cultural, spiritual, and others. Such variations contribute to the complexity and diversity of diagnostic tasks and the types of skills needed for interpretation. For example, a diagnostic task presented to an emergency department (ED) staff may be a woman who comes to the ED for treatment of a fractured arm. In the initial assessment, the woman says that she fell down the stairs in her home, so the ED nurse and other staff act on the problem as one that can be addressed by an orthopedic physician with no specific attention to the woman's responses to the fractured arm. But if the diagnostic task includes cues that the woman's response may be fear of battering by her husband, anxiety over who will provide care to her children, pain, concern about her mother who needs care giving, and/or mental confusion that may have precipitated the fall, the complexity of the diagnostic task is greatly increased. If other factors are added, such as the woman speaks a language that differs from the languages spoken by ED personnel, the complexity of interpreting human responses is further compounded.

The Situational Context

The context for clinical situations includes the health care setting, the people and other resources within the environment, and the policies and procedures that guide health care patterns. The specific mission and approach of health care settings as well as the acuity level of a situation can affect accuracy. For example, in acute care settings an obvious response that needs to be treated, such as fear of dying, may be ignored when there are other more pressing priorities.

The specialization of providers' knowledge in specific health care settings also affects accuracy. For example, a child on a surgical unit who experiences the abdominal pain of peritonitis after gastrointestinal surgery is more likely to be diagnosed accurately because providers on that unit are highly focused on preventing this complication of surgery. In contrast, a school nurse who assesses a child for the same type of pain may be less accurate because she or he usually attends to a much broader range of children's problems, not just gastrointestinal problems.

The availability of resources for diagnosing human responses affects the accuracy of interpreting human responses. Resources include (a) other providers who share accountability to help patients and (b) knowledge related to human responses. When other providers are not easily available (e.g., in-home care nursing), greater attention needs to be given to the accuracy of human response interpretations because the nurse may be the only provider to identify and treat specific responses. With institutional-based nursing, misdiagnosis or neglecting to diagnose a specific response may be corrected by other nurses, physicians, physical therapists, and so forth.

Knowledge related to human response concepts varies greatly among nurses. With the traditional emphasis in nursing schools and health care settings on the diagnosis and treatment of medical diagnoses, knowledge of human response concepts is often neglected. Nurses can attain this knowledge through in-service, continuing education programs, and self-directed learning such as using the case studies in this book. Studies of accuracy of nurses' diagnoses showed a relationship between nursing education on nursing diagnosis and accuracy of nurses' diagnoses (Lunney, 1992; Lunney et al., 1997).

Agency policies and procedures can have both positive and negative effects on accuracy. A policy that has positive effects is the expectation that nurses will name, or document, their diagnoses of human responses. The naming of a diagnostic concept draws attention to human experiences and contributes to cooperation and collaboration on, "What is the diagnosis?". Naming helps both the diagnostician and others to discern the phenomena of interest and provides an environment for them to work together toward a common understanding (Hayakawa and Hayakawa, 1990). Information on the interpretation of a human response acts as a "map" to understanding the patient. Just like maps of an area of land, diagnostic labels for human responses help nurses and others to think about and understand these human experiences. The naming of diagnoses of human responses also clarifies the focus of interventions. Words are needed to describe human responses because human beings think with words. Health care providers think about a phenomenon of concern through the use of words, which enhances their ability to sort out the data taken in through the senses and draw inferences. Nurses communicate with others through words and phrases, so use of nursing diagnoses improves the ability to communicate and cooperate with others.

Nurses' interpretations of clinical cases should be thought about, named, and validated with others because there is always a risk of low-accuracy interpretations. Validation means that the meanings of data are verified with others, which decreases the risk of inaccuracy. Just as the student who misdiagnosed the patient's behavior as "hostile," other nurses can make similar mistakes. To validate diagnoses, nurses can check the match of data with diagnoses in literature sources, determine the person's interpretation of the data, and collaborate with colleagues about the best diagnosis to guide nursing care. Validation of the accuracy of human responses supports the scientific nature of nursing practice, helps to ensure the quality of care, and is more likely to result in cost effectiveness. Consider, for example, a situation in which the nurse thinks that a person does not have sufficient knowledge to manage a health problem. If the nurse attempts to validate the diagnosis with the person and determines that he does in fact have sufficient knowledge, it saves the time, energy, and cost of teaching.

Two policies that can have negative effects are requirements to name nursing diagnoses in specified time periods and the use of assessment frameworks that do not include information on human responses. Agency requirements to name nursing diagnoses in a specified time period may interfere with and contradict the diagnostic process. For example, if hospital-based nurse administrators mandate staff nurses to state one or more nursing diagnoses on patient admission notes and ignore the fact that some patients may not have a problem, or that nurses may not have sufficient time to establish an accurate diagnosis, the diagnoses that are named by nurses may be inaccurate. Practicing nurses have shared many stories about writing nursing diagnoses on charts and care plans (e.g., anxiety and knowledge deficit) before patients are even admitted to the unit because of policies such as these. Such policies make no sense because they do not reflect the realities that a portion of patients may have no responses to report and, in some instances, it takes longer than an admission interview to identify the most accurate diagnosis.

With some assessment frameworks, nurses cannot derive accurate nursing diagnoses because the database is inadequate. A health history of biological systems, for example, provides information on the structural and functional status of body systems. Data on body systems is not holistic enough to identify human responses. To diagnose human responses, comprehensive information is needed on the health functioning of the whole person. Many schools of nursing and health care agencies have replaced the biological systems model of health assessment with that of the functional health patterns (FHP) (Gordon, 1994).

The Diagnostician

The specific knowledge and skills of diagnosticians can vary in three domains that affect accuracy of interpreting human responses: interpersonal, technical, and intellectual. The interpersonal domain includes the interpersonal aspects of interviewing, the ability to relate to people in general, and the ability to relate to people who are experiencing specific responses. The technical domain includes the ability to conduct an interview and physical examination under various conditions (e.g., comprehensive assessment, focused assessment). The intellectual domain includes the nurse's knowledge of human responses and thinking processes, use of the most appropriate thinking processes for making diagnoses, and development of perceptual abilities.

Diagnostician: Interpersonal Domain

Though the effects of various interpersonal abilities of nurses on accuracy of interpreting human responses have not been studied, the logic of this relationship is strongly supported. Human responses are subjective experiences that must be shared with providers by people who are seeking health care. These subjective experiences will not be shared unless the right questions or comments are made by providers to indicate an interest in the topic and unless the consumer-provider relationship is a positive one. Therapeutic communication is needed so nurses can collect valid and reliable data through interviews, that is, data that consistently match the actual experiences of consumers. People are not likely to share important information with nurses unless they trust nurses and want to share their thoughts and emotions with them.

A negative influence on the development of interpersonal skills for diagnosis of human responses has been the belief that the provider is the expert and decisions can be made about health care consumers without collaboration. It is likely, therefore, that the most accurate diagnoses of psychosocial responses will be made in collaboration with the person or family. In most cases, the diagnostic process should be a mutually collaborative process whereby nurses and health care consumers work together to identify the diagnosis. When a patient cannot collaborate with the nurse (e.g., the person has not reached a developmental stage of ability to conduct self care, is mentally incompetent, or is comatose), the nurse should put more emphasis on collaboration with other providers and family members.

Diagnostician: Technical Domain

The technical skills for accurate diagnosis are the ability to conduct a comprehensive health history, a problem-focused health history, an emergency health history, a complete physical examination, and partial physical examinations. These skills have become somewhat standardized as nurses study interviewing and physical examination skills in basic and advanced programs of education. Individually, however, nurses probably vary in personal development of these abilities. Data collection and analyses for accurate interpretation of human responses are influenced by individual abilities. The nurse who has developed strong skills in respiratory assessment will more accurately diagnose ineffective airway clearance, ineffective breathing pattern, and impaired gas exchange than nurses who have not developed these skills. The nurse who further develops interview skills for assessment of values and beliefs is more likely to accurately diagnose spiritual distress than a nurse who has not developed these skills.

Diagnostician: Intellectual Domain

The intellectual abilities of diagnosticians vary according to (a) the amounts and types of knowledge stored in memory, and (b) the specific thinking processes used by the diagnostician. Specific knowledge bases of human responses that can be stored in memory are definitions, defining characteristics, contributing factors, nursing interventions, and related outcomes. Because this type of knowledge is continuously developing through research, knowledge varies according to the clinician's basic education, continuing education, and personal accountability for keeping up with new knowledge. Revisiting the fear/anxiety example used above, research has shown that the experiences of fear and anxiety differ from one another and may be difficult to diagnose accurately (Whitley and Tousman, 1996). Knowledge of these two concepts is important because of the similarities of the two experiences, the frequency of these two experiences in health care settings, the difficulty of distinguishing the most accurate diagnosis, and the need to intervene appropriately. The interventions for fear should be focused on the object of the fear. The interventions for anxiety should focus on helping the person to deal appropriately with the experience of anxiety. Knowledge of human responses is continuously developing so nurses who keep up with knowledge development are more likely to be accurate than nurses who do not.

A diagnostician should use specific types of thinking processes for specific types of clinical cases. Yet studies have shown that abilities in various types of thinking processes vary for adults, including nurses (Lunney, 1992; Willingham, 2007a). The thinking processes used by a nurse may not match the type of thinking that is needed to solve the problem of the diagnosis. For example, a nurse with low ability to be mentally flexible, which is a habit of mind associated with critical thinking, may be required to diagnose a clinical case that requires a high ability to be mentally flexible. Knowledge of thinking processes contributes to optimum development of critical thinking as well as the use of critical thinking processes to diagnose human responses (Carnevali and Thomas, 1993; Gordon, 1994).

Relation of Nurses' Diagnoses to Interventions and Outcomes

Nurses' selections of interventions to address the health care needs of people are based on their impressions of what the diagnosis is. If a diagnosis is that a person has a specific problem, interventions are selected to resolve or mitigate the problem. These types of interventions are in the category of health restoration or disease and illness management. If a diagnosis is that a person is at risk for a specific problem, interventions are selected to address the risk state. These types of nursing interventions are in the category of health protection. If a diagnosis is that a person is relatively healthy but health promotion activities can be improved, the nurse uses health promotion interventions in the realms of nutrition, exercise, sleep, moderation in lifestyle, stress management, and social support. Inaccurate interpretations of the diagnosis can lead to inappropriate interventions and, subsequently, to undesired outcomes.

Professional Accountability for Accuracy

Because nursing is a profession and a science, nurses must be accountable to the public for the accuracy of their interpretations of clinical data. One of the criteria for being a professional is to be accountable for behavior (Chitty and Black, 2007). Accountability for nursing means answering to the public for the work of nursing (American Nurses Association, 2001). It means using critical thinking to achieve accurate interpretations of human responses so that interventions are the most appropriate and positive outcomes are achieved. Thinking abilities are improved through repeated use of appropriate thinking strategies (Sternberg, 1997; Willingham, 2007a, 2007b). By using the case studies in this book, nurses can practice critical thinking processes and check their own thinking processes against those of the case study authors and become more astute in thinking about the actual cases that they see in clinical practice.

References

American Nurses Association. (2001). *Code of ethics for nurses with interpretive statements*. Washington, DC: Author.

Bandman, E.L., and Bandman, B. (1995). *Critical thinking in nursing* (2nd ed.). Upper Saddle River, NJ: Prentice Hall.

Carnevali, D.L., and Thomas, M. D. (1993). *Diagnostic reasoning and treatment decision making*. Philadelphia: Lippincott.

Chitty, K.K., and Black, B.P. (2007). *Professional nursing: Concepts and challenges* (5th ed.). Philadelphia: Saunders.

Facione, N.C., and Facione, P.A. (1996). Externalizing the critical thinking in knowledge development and clinical judgment. *Nursing Outlook, 44*(3), 129–36.

Gordon, M. (1982). Historical perspective: The National Conference Group for Classification of Nursing Diagnoses. In M.J. Kim and D.A. Moritz, *Classification of nursing diagnoses: Proceedings of the third and fourth national conferences* (pp. 2–8). New York: McGraw-Hill.

Gordon, M. (1994). *Nursing diagnosis: Process and application* (3rd ed.). St. Louis: Mosby.

Hasegawa, T., Ogasawara, C., and Katz, E. C. (2007). Measuring diagnostic competency and the analysis of factors influencing competency using written case studies. *International Journal of Nursing Terminologies and Classifications, 18*(3), 93–102.

Hayakawa, S.I., and Hayakawa, A.R. (1990). *Language in thought and action* (5th ed.). San Diego: Harvest Original, Harcourt and Brace.

Jones, P., and Jakob, D.F. (1981) Nursing diagnosis: Differentiating fear and anxiety. *Nursing Papers: Perspectives in Nursing, 13*, 20–29.

Jones P., and Jakob, D.F. (1984). Anxiety revisited: from a practice perspective. In M.J. Kim, G. McFarland, and A.M. McLane (eds.). *Classification of nursing diagnoses: Proceedings of the fifth national conference* (pp. 285–290). St. Louis: Mosby.

Kelly, K. (1966). Clinical inference in nursing: A nurse's viewpoint. *Nursing Research, 15*, 23–26.

Lunney, M. (1990). Accuracy of nursing diagnoses: Concept development. *Nursing Diagnosis, 1*, 12–17.

Lunney, M. (1992). Divergent productive thinking factors and accuracy of nursing diagnoses. *Research in Nursing and Health, 15*, 303–311.

Lunney, M., Karlik, B., Kiss, M., and Murphy, P. (1997). Accuracy of nurses' diagnoses of psychosocial responses. *Nursing Diagnosis, 8*(4), 157–166.

Lunney, M. (2008). Critical need to address the accuracy of nurses' diagnoses. *OJIN: Online Journal of Issues in Nursing*. Available at http://www.nursingworld.org/MainMenuCategories/ANAMarketplace/ANAPeriodicals/OJIN/TableofContents/vol132008/No1Jan08/ArticlePreviousTopic/AccuracyofNursesDiagnoses.aspx

Matos, F.G.O.A., and Cruz, D.A.L.M. (April 2007). *Development of a tool for the evaluation of diagnostic accuracy*. Paper presented at the 6th European Conference of ACENDIO, Amsterdam, The Netherlands.

Munhall, P.L. (1993). "Unknowing": Toward another pattern of knowing in nursing. *Nursing Outlook, 41*, 125–128.

NANDA International. (2009). *Nursing diagnosis: Definitions and classification, 2009–2011*. Hoboken, NJ: Wiley-Blackwell.

Narayan, S.M., Corcoran-Perry, S., Drew, D., Hoyman, K., and Lewis, M. (2003). Decision analysis as a tool to support an analytical pattern-of-reasoning. *Nursing and Health Sciences, 5*, 229–243.

Newell, A., and Simon, H. (1972). *Human problem solving*. Englewood Cliffs, NJ: Prentice Hall.

O'Neill, E.S. (1995). Heuristics reasoning in diagnostic judgment. *Journal of Professional Nursing, 11*, 239–245.

O'Neill, E.S., and Dluhy, N.M. (1997). A longitudinal framework for fostering critical thinking and diagnostic reasoning. *Journal of Advanced Nursing, 26*, 825–832.

Paquay, L., Wouters, R., Debaille, R., and Geys, L. (April 2007). *Validity of nursing diagnoses in Flemish home care nursing*. Paper presented at ACENDIO conference, Amsterdam, The Netherlands.

Rew, L. (1988). Intuition in decision-making. *IMAGE: Journal of Nursing Scholarship, 20*, 150–154.

Rubenfeld, H.G., and Scheffer, B.K. (2006). *Critical thinking TACTICS for nurses*, Boston: Jones and Bartlett.

Sternberg, R.J. (1997). *Successful intelligence: How practical and creative intelligence determine success in life*. New York: Plume.

Tanner, C.A. (2006). Thinking like a nurse: A research-based model of clinical judgment in nursing. *Journal of Nursing Education, 45*, 204–211.

Walsh, C.M., and Seldomridge, L.A. (2006). Critical thinking: Back to square two. *Journal of Nursing Education, 45*, 212–219.

Webster, G. (1984). Nomenclature and classification system development. In M.J. Kim, G.K. McFarland, and A.M. McLane (eds.), *Classification of nursing diagnoses: Proceedings of the fifth national conference* (pp. 14–25). St. Louis: C.V. Mosby.

Whitley, G.G., and Tousman, S.A. (1996). A multivariate approach for the validation of anxiety and fear. *Nursing Diagnosis, 7*, 116–127.

Willingham, D.T. (2007a). *Cognition: The thinking animal*. (3rd ed.) New York: Prentice Hall.

Willingham, D.T. (2007b). Critical thinking: Why is it so hard to teach? *American Educator, 31*(2), 8–19.

Yocum, C. (1984). The differentiation of fear and anxiety. In M.J. Kim, G.K. McFarland, and A.M. McLane (eds.), *Classification of nursing diagnoses: Proceedings of the fifth national conference* (pp. 352–356). St. Louis: Mosby.

Yura, H., and Walsh, M. (1967). *The nursing process*. Washington, DC: Catholic University Press.

Guiding Principles for Use of Nursing Diagnoses and NANDA-I, NOC, and NIC

Margaret Lunney, RN, PhD

Chapter Objectives

By completion of this chapter, readers will be able to:

1. Describe 10 guiding principles for use of NANDA International nursing diagnoses that can be applied to select accurate and useful nursing diagnoses of both written simulations and real clinical cases;
2. Use the standardized nursing languages of NANDA International, NOC, and NIC to support the health of individuals and families and document nursing care.

In this chapter, a major focus is use of NANDA-I nursing diagnoses because identification of the best diagnoses to guide nursing care is the foundation of the nursing process. Correct use of the nursing languages of NANDA-I, NOC, and NIC is explained so these languages can be used with the case studies of this book and in clinical practice.

Use of NANDA-I Nursing Diagnoses

A nursing diagnosis is stated to provide additional information about individual, family, or community health experiences to provide health care services. This information guides nurses and other health care providers in addressing the health care needs of consumers. For example, in a study of battered women, Carlson-Catalano (1998) showed that when these women selected their own diagnoses of responses to battering, their health care needs far exceeded the diagnosis and treatment of their medical problems.

A nursing diagnosis is stated for the sole purpose of guiding nursing care. It is incorrect, then, to convert medical diagnoses to nursing diagnoses; the medical diagnosis is already available to guide nursing care. For example, if a person has renal calculi, the nurse should not necessarily use the nursing diagnosis of *impaired urinary elimination*. In this instance, the medical diagnosis of renal calculi provides guidance for nursing care and the nursing diagnosis may not add information, e.g., the case study by McCaffery-Tesoro (p. 273). Another example is when a person has had an amputation and nurses automatically use the nursing diagnosis of *impaired physical mobility*. In this instance, the diagnosis of *impaired physical mobility* should only be stated when nurses are helping the person to improve physical mobility. The goal of diagnosis in nursing is to name human responses and life processes for which interventions will be provided, not to name for the sake of naming or to change medical diagnoses to sound like nursing.

The following 10 guiding principles for use of NANDA-I nursing diagnoses were developed from a broad range of literature sources in nursing, primarily the theorists, Marjory Gordon (1994) and Doris Carnevali (Carnevali and Thomas, 1993). These guiding principles reflect knowledge development in nursing diagnosis over the last 37 years. Many thousands of nurses contributed to knowledge development of this topic.

The guiding principles for becoming a good diagnostician are discussed in this chapter and examples are provided in Chapter 4. After each guiding principle, some of the critical thinking concepts that apply from the framework discussed in Chapter 1 are stated in parentheses. The critical thinking terms in this framework provide one way to "think about thinking." Using these terms in relation to various nursing process activities helps nurses to improve critical thinking processes.

In the following descriptions of these guiding principles, the words "person" or "people" are used to represent the consumer of nursing care. Depending on the situation, the consumer can be an individual, family, group, or community. The cases in this book represent the care provided to individuals and families. Nursing care at the community level of analysis is specialized to the degree that it needs its own book of case studies.

Guiding Principles for Use of NANDA-I Nursing Diagnoses

See the box titled "Guidelines for Use of Nursing Diagnosis and NANDA-I."

Guidelines for Use of Nursing Diagnosis and NANDA-I

1. Use one or more nursing theories to guide your philosophical and theoretical approaches to nursing care.
2. In the context of the selected approach to nursing, conduct nursing assessments of the person to identify the problems, risk states, readiness for health promotion, and strengths that are appropriate to guide nursing care.
3. During assessments use the seven cognitive skills and 10 habits of mind of critical thinking along with the thinking processes of the person receiving nursing care.
4. Conduct focused assessments to identify the specific responses that the person may be experiencing, considering the situational context.
5. Obtain a sufficient amount of high and moderate relevance data to support or reject (rule in or rule out) the specific diagnoses being considered.
6. Compare the assessment data with the NANDA-I standardized nursing diagnoses, i.e., the labels, definitions, and defining characteristics.
7. Consider other possible diagnoses as you collect data.
8. Whenever possible, considering the situational context, validate diagnostic impressions with the individual or family.
9. If there is more than one diagnosis, identify the priority diagnosis or diagnoses.
10. Communicate, verbally and in writing, the selected priority diagnosis or diagnoses to others as a basis for planning outcomes and interventions.

---

1. Use one or more nursing theories to guide your philosophical and theoretical approaches to nursing care (*applying standards*). Nursing is a science and a profession that differs from all others. As a science, nursing is guided by many broad and middle-range conceptual models and theories. Examples of broad models and theories are those of Martha Rogers (1992), Sr. Callista Roy (Roy and Andrews, 2009), Betty Neuman (Neuman and Fawcett, 2002), and Dorothea Orem (2001). Examples of mid-range theories are those of Elizabeth A.M. Barrett (1990, 2000), Nola J. Pender (Pender, Murdaugh, and Parsons, 2006), and Madeleine Leininger (Leininger and McFarland, 2006). These theories explicate the unique aspects of nursing science and are used by nurses worldwide to guide their approaches to nursing care and communicate to others the unique dimensions of nursing practice. The complexity of nursing as a discipline is evident in the wide variety of possible theories for nurses' use.

These theories should be integrated with nursing diagnoses, outcomes, and interventions. It is beyond the scope of this book to explain in detail how specific broad conceptual models and middle-range theories of nursing are integrated with nursing diagnoses, but, in this book, some of the case studies illustrate the process. For example, Gigliotti is a well known expert on the Neuman Systems Model, so Gigliotti's case study can be used as an example of integrating Neuman's model with NANDA-I, NOC, and NIC (p. 247). Farren is an expert in using Martha Rogers' model, so the description in the Farren and Champagne case study helps readers integrate Rogers with NANDA-I, NOC, and NIC (p. 206).

The NANDA-I classification of nursing diagnosis represents the human responses to health problems and life processes that people experience (NANDA-I, 2009); nurses may have opportunities to help people with these experiences. Such responses are named to provide direction for nursing care and communicate to others the focus of nursing care. For optimum clinical practice in nursing, nursing diagnoses should be integrated with one or more general approaches as described in nursing's conceptual models and mid-range theories.

The basic philosophical approach of caring, (e.g., Watson, 2005), guides the integration of broad conceptual models and middle-range theories with nursing diagnoses. Nurses can use a wide variety of literature sources to learn how to exhibit caring (e.g., Duffy, Hoskins, and Seifert, 2007; Ousey and Johnson, 2007). The case study by Como integrates the use of Watson with NANDA-I, NOC, and NIC (p. 100).

Another philosophical approach to nursing is that of working in partnership with people to support them in being as healthy as possible (Bidmead and Cowley, 2005; Hook, 2006; McCormack and McCance, 2006; Splaine Wiggins, 2008). Working in partnership means that the recipient of care and nurses are intimately involved in all aspects of the nursing process: assessment, diagnosis, planning, interventions, and evaluation of outcomes. Many case studies in this book illustrate a partnership process.

2. **In the context of the selected approach to nursing, conduct nursing assessments of the person to identify the problems, risk states, readiness for health promotion, and strengths that are appropriate to guide nursing care (*applying standards, information seeking, predicting*).** The goal in nursing assessment is to work in partnership with people to obtain data that support or reject nursing diagnoses to provide nursing interventions to achieve positive health outcomes. To obtain these data, an assessment framework that yields information about the person's responses to health problems and life processes is needed.

Assessment frameworks that are consistent with conceptual models of nursing are available. These can be used in conjunction with diagnostic reasoning to identify nursing diagnoses as demonstrated by Gigliotti (2002) using Neuman's systems model. If a nursing model or theory is used as an assessment framework, the broad categories of assessment are guided by the theory itself. For example, with use of Neuman's systems model, the nurse can assess the person using five broad variables: physiological, psychological, sociological, cultural, and spiritual (e.g., Gigliotti, 2002). With each category, the nurse identifies the current status with the person. After the assessment, the nurse and person together decide upon the diagnosis.

If there is no nursing-theory-based framework available, the functional health pattern framework (Gordon, 1994, 2008; deBarros, 2003; Higa, 2006; Murphy, 2006) was shown to be useful in generating the data needed for making nursing diagnoses (see Appendix B). In Gordon's functional health pattern framework (2008), for example, the nurse starts with broad nursing concepts to decide which category of diagnoses to consider, e.g., management of health, nutrition, elimination, activity, and sleep/rest. Within each of these categories, data are collected to be able to determine whether the person's health status is consistent with what is expected. After completing pattern assessment, the nurse and the person determine the appropriate diagnoses to guide nursing care.

The assessment frameworks used for data collection must represent a nursing model for practice because frameworks based on other models do not yield the necessary data. For example, using the biosystems framework yields data regarding structural and functional pathology of body systems but *does not* yield sufficient data to consider diagnoses of human responses.

3. **During assessments use the seven cognitive skills and 10 habits of mind of critical thinking (see Chapter 1 and Table 1.1) along with the thinking processes of the person receiving nursing care (*applying standards,* i.e., metacognition and partnering with consumers of care).** Assessment processes always yield data, but data are useless to nurses unless they lead to interpretations that are useful for providing nursing care. The purpose of data collection is data interpretation or diagnoses. Data interpretation is only possible, however, when there are sufficient data to decide whether specific relevant diagnoses are accurate or not, i.e., to rule in or rule out diagnoses. Sufficient data to support possible diagnoses are collected when the nurse thinks about possible data interpretations during the data collection process and conducts focused assessments to support or rule out possible diagnoses.

The goal is to know the other person well enough to diagnose, but human beings are unique and do not "know" each other (Munhall, 1993). Thus, it is important to integrate the thinking of the person who is the recipient of care with the nurses' own thinking while gathering data to support or reject nursing diagnoses.

4. **Conduct focused assessments to identify the specific responses that the person may be experiencing considering the situational context (*contextual perspective*).** Specific responses, such as *acute pain* or *disturbed body image*, are known to occur in specific situations. For example, there is a high risk of *disturbed body image* when a person's face or body changes through injury, surgery, or accident (Weaver, Resnick, Kokosa, and Etzel, 2007). Some of the contextual characteristics that can guide nurses to conduct focused assessments for specific diagnoses are health problems such as heart disease and cancer; life processes such as poverty, birth of a baby, and developmental stage; family medical history; and cultural background.

For example, if an individual has an identified chronic illness such as heart disease, the nurse should ask the individual about the therapeutic regimen that is being followed and, in partnership with the individual, determine whether self management is effective or not. If not, the nurse and individual can follow up by identifying factors that interfere with *effective self health management*.

Cultural assessments should be conducted to determine the relation of the person's cultural background to responses to health problems and life processes. Nurses need to strive for cultural competence so they can help people to integrate their cultural ways of life with health promotion, health protection, and health restoration.

5. **Obtain a sufficient amount of high and moderate relevance data to support or reject (rule in or rule out) the specific diagnoses being considered (*logical reasoning*).** Clinical judgment is required, and, when possible, nurses should work in partnership with the recipient of nursing care to know whether there are sufficient high and moderate relevance data to support specific diagnoses. To determine whether there are sufficient data, the nurse can compare the data from the person with the defining characteristics of the diagnosis as identified through research (NANDA-I, 2009).

For many diagnoses, one or two cues are insufficient to identify the existence of a problem diagnosis. For example, if a nurse notices that a person with high blood pressure is eating a cake that is high in sodium, this is insufficient evidence to say that the person's response is *ineffective self health management*. The diagnosis should not be made without further assessment. One or two cues indicating that the person might need some help from a nurse, however, could be used to identify a risk state or the opportunity for health promotion, e.g., the case study by Fairlie (p. 325).

With some problem diagnoses, one salient cue may be enough to make a diagnosis. For example, if a person says, "I am afraid," the diagnosis of *fear* should be selected; if the person says "I have a sharp pain," the diagnosis of *acute pain* is selected. The goal of evidence-based practice should serve as a guide to nurses when deciding how to make a diagnosis (Levin, Lunney, and Krainovich-Miller, 2005). With many diagnoses, however, the research bases are insufficient to provide an evidence-based protocol for decision making. In many cases, decisions of whether or not the cues are sufficient to select a diagnosis will be based on the nurse's clinical judgment, working in partnership with the consumer. In the future, when there are additional research bases to guide nurses' decision making, diagnostic decisions may be guided more often by evidenced-based protocols.

When deciding whether cues are sufficient it is also appropriate for nurses to determine whether the situation represents a problem, risk state, or need for health promotion. For many years, the NANDA-I classification was mainly focused on problems, so nurses were in the habit of only naming problems. Now there are many risk states and health promotion diagnoses on the NANDA-I approved list, so these should be considered as well. Generally, risk states and readiness for health promotion require fewer cues for naming a diagnosis than do problems. Even in acute care settings, there are many instances in which nurses should be identifying opportunities for addressing risks and providing health promotion services, rather than naming everything as problems, e.g., the case study by Amicucci (p. 321).

6.   **Compare the assessment data with the NANDA-I standardized nursing diagnoses, i.e., the labels, definitions, and defining characteristics (*applying standards*).** Knowledge is a necessary characteristic of diagnostic reasoning, which involves discernment of the best diagnosis to guide interventions and outcomes (*predicting*). The knowledge bases that are needed are the diagnostic phenomena that are nursing responsibilities, their meanings, and the processes by which these phenomena can be identified, e.g., the diagnoses approved by NANDA-I (2009). Additional knowledge bases to address diagnoses are available in recent research findings. Therefore, in order to ensure evidence-based practice, nurses must learn how to conduct literature searches for the latest research evidence (Cruz, Pimenta, and Lunney, 2006; Levin et al., 2005).

An additional consideration is that the NANDA-I classification is not complete. Sometimes a nursing diagnosis is identified that has not yet been developed and approved by NANDA-I, e.g., the case study by Mitchell (p. 286). When nurses identify a diagnosis that has not yet been approved by NANDA-I, they should use the diagnosis and consider a concept analysis and/or design a nursing research study to develop this new diagnosis for submission to NANDA-I (2009).

7.   **Consider other possible diagnoses as you collect data (cognitive skill of *analyzing*, habits of mind of *flexibility, inquisitiveness, open mindedness*).** When diagnosing, data from the person become the cues or evidence from which diagnoses are made (*analyzing, discriminating, logical reasoning, intuition*). In analyzing, the nurse considers the strength of specific cues in relation to possible diagnoses. For example,

the nurse decides the degree of importance of a person not taking a blood pressure medication every day as prescribed in relation to the diagnosis of self health management. In discriminating, the nurse decides whether the cue has more meaning in relation to one diagnosis versus other diagnoses. In logical reasoning, the nurse clusters the cues as a group to help determine which diagnosis best explains the data. Intuition can be used when the nurse has sufficient experience with a given type of situation (Banning, 2008; Lyneham, Parkinson, and Denholm, 2008).

A sufficient amount of evidence to support or reject diagnoses can only be accumulated if the diagnostician consciously decides to collect the data needed (*information seeking, applying standards, intellectual integrity, perseverance*). Using the example of pain assessment, the data needed include the location, degree, and type of pain, precipitating factors, methods of relief, and so forth. Diagnosis-focused assessments are essential to yield adequate data.

8.   **Whenever possible, considering the situational context, validate diagnostic impressions with the individual or family (cognitive skills of *logical reasoning, predicting*; habits of mind of *contextual perspective, confidence, flexibility*).** All diagnostic impressions should be validated, whenever possible, with the recipient of nursing care. Nurses should validate diagnostic impressions with all children and adults who are considered mentally competent and concerned about their own health. If individuals, families, or groups are not considered mentally competent, then nurses can validate diagnoses with their caregivers.

There may be instances when the consumer does not agree with the nurse's diagnosis; however, the nurse must record the diagnosis and use it for the safety of the consumer, e.g., the case study by Paradiso (pp. 151–156). There are other instances when the nurse does not work in partnership with the person because the person is too sick or has no interest, e.g., the case study by Fernandez–Roibas and Espinosa–Fresnedo (p. 220). In instances such as these, nurses use clinical judgment to do whatever they think is best to support the health of the person or family.

When people who are willing and able to work in partnership with nurses agree with diagnostic impressions, it provides additional data to support accuracy and a sound foundation for nursing interventions. When people disagree with diagnostic impressions, they may be inaccurate and/or nursing interventions will not be perceived as supportive. **Note:** *Except when the recipient of nursing care is unable to evaluate helpfulness, nursing interventions are only helpful when the person receiving nursing care perceives them as such.*

9.   **If there is more than one diagnosis, identify the priority diagnosis or diagnoses (*applying standards, discriminating, logical reasoning, flexibility, confidence*).** Identifying the priority nursing

diagnoses involves considerations of patient safety, the interactions of one diagnosis with other diagnoses, and the need for nursing interventions. When safety and survival are at stake and problem or risk level diagnoses require immediate and important interventions, they are a priority, e.g., a patient who is experiencing *impaired gas exchange* must be diagnosed and interventions provided as soon as possible. Risk states such as *risk of suicide*, e.g., the case study by A. Lunney (pp. 296–299), or *risk of falls*, e.g., the case study by Pilosoph (p. 87), must also be considered as priorities.

The responses or experiences in one category, e.g., coping and stress tolerance, are likely to interact with responses or experiences in other categories, e.g., nutrition, elimination, sleep. A very important issue is the relation of the diagnosis to interventions that are likely to be effective, e.g., if high anxiety is affecting sleep disturbances, then *anxiety* is the priority diagnosis to guide interventions.

Other times, the priority diagnosis is identified by the person or family receiving care. If the consumer believes that the most important response to address is one diagnosis but the nurse thinks it should be something different, the consumer is not likely to participate in the process of achieving positive outcomes unless his or her priority diagnosis is addressed. Examples are the case studies by Baumann (p. 176) and Cummings (p. 311). The women in these case studies preferred to focus on health promotion of coping, not long-term problems with coping.

If a response is identified as a priority by the nurse who knows pathophysiology and potential complications of disease states that the person or family may not know, the nurse must first ensure that the consumer understands why the diagnosis and interventions are a priority. For example, a mother may not be administering an antibiotic correctly to a child who has a Streptococcus infection of the throat. At that point a diagnosis of *ineffective family management of therapeutic regimen* would apply. Prior to this, the mother may not have understood the complications of strep throat but the nurse can explain the complications associated with incorrect administration of the antibiotic.

10. **Communicate, verbally and in writing, the selected priority diagnosis or diagnoses to others as a basis for planning outcomes and interventions (*predicting*).** One of the main reasons for using standardized nursing languages such as NANDA-I, NOC, and NIC is to communicate nurses' thinking to others. Communication is essential as a means of collaboration with consumers, other nurses, physicians, social workers, and so forth. The complexity of health and nursing care is such that very few responses to health problems and life processes can be addressed by one provider and at only one point in time. The diagnostic thinking of nurses must be communicated so that everyone can work together toward the same goals. Collaboration is the most

effective way to achieve outcomes because many people are working toward similar goals.

Sharing diagnoses that were carefully made with the person receiving care influences other providers to work toward the same outcomes or to disagree and ask for revision of the diagnoses. For example, a nurse might mistakenly diagnose a person who is not following a prescribed diet with *deficient knowledge*. By communicating this nursing diagnosis, another nurse or a nutritionist who is working with the same consumer can challenge the accuracy of the diagnosis to say that there is a different issue that should be addressed, e.g., poverty.

Nursing diagnoses need to be revised as indicated by the input of other providers and in partnership with the recipient of care. Revised diagnoses need to be documented in paper-based and electronic records because the purpose is to guide care.

Use of the NOC Outcomes

The nursing process has always included a planning phase, the first step of which was to select the most appropriate outcome expectations for the consumer (Wilkinson, 2007; Yura and Walsh, 1967). In the past, these outcome expectations were generally phrased as complete sentences that described what the consumer would do and the time frame in which it would be done, e.g., "Patients who have had abdominal surgery will be able to move from bed to chair within 24 hours after surgery." In the evaluation phase, the nurse would evaluate whether or not the expected outcomes were met. The problem with this method of stating outcomes was that there were too many different kinds of statements, and the statements were not standardized, so it was impossible to keep track of how many people actually achieved the expected outcomes. Knowing how well an individual person achieved an outcome was important for care of that person but also to determine the overall quality of care and compare quality from one agency to another. However, the data needed to be standardized so that nurse leaders could determine, for example, how many people who had abdominal surgery actually achieved mobility-related outcomes. In the past, the health outcomes that were sensitive to changes in the quality of nursing care could not be measured. The NOC outcomes are standardized measures that are sensitive to changes in nursing care quality. A tremendous advantage of using the NOC outcomes is that they are research-based. Development of NOC was partially supported with research funds from the National Institutes of Nursing Research.

The current NOC reference (Moorhead, Johnson, Maas, and Swanson, 2008) contains 385 outcome labels. For a more complete description of how to use the NOC outcomes, readers should consult the NOC reference book.

The NOC outcomes are neutral concepts, e.g., *coping* and *comfort status*, each of which is associated with a specific 5-point scale. There are 14 different 5-point scales; nurses using the NOC need to know which scale should be used with the specific NOC label being used. For example, the 5-point scale that is associated with *coping* is: 1 = never demonstrated, 2 = rarely demonstrated, 3 = sometimes demonstrated, 4 = often demonstrated, and 5 = consistently demonstrated. As with this scale for *coping*, the number 1 always refers to the worst outcome and the number 5 always refers to the best outcome.

To choose the best outcome for a specific diagnosis, four different methods can be used and combined: (1) the diagnostic and outcome concepts can be matched; (2) the NOC book or other books can be consulted for lists of possible outcomes to consider with specific diagnoses; (3) the definition and indicators of selected NOC labels should be compared with the expectations for the specific consumer being served, and (4) nurses in local agencies can conduct consensus validation studies to identify the outcomes that would be used with the common NANDA-I diagnoses for the people they serve. If the nursing diagnosis is *ineffective coping*, for example, it is logical that the *coping* outcome would be used. If the nursing diagnosis is *anxiety*, *anxiety level* is a logical outcome to use. There are 42 knowledge outcomes that would be considered for diagnoses of *deficient knowledge*.

The NOC book also contains a chart of the most commonly used outcomes with specific diagnoses (pp. 746–834). These lists were developed by nurse experts. Additionally, a book of NANDA-I, NOC, and NIC linkages was authored by members of the NOC and NIC research teams (Johnson et al., 2006)

When selecting outcomes, it is important to compare the outcome definition and indicators with the nurse's and consumer's interpretations of feasibility in the allotted time period and of the consumer data that are used to determine the ratings on the 5-point scale. The outcome indicators were selected with great care by the NOC research team and should be used to determine the consumer's baseline score and goal score, e.g., the indicators may show that the baseline score for *coping* is 2 (rarely demonstrated), and the goal score should be 3 (sometimes demonstrated). The goal score is determined by consumer and nurse expectations of what is possible to achieve in specific time frames, e.g., by discharge from the hospital.

Consensus validation studies are a means of identifying the specific diagnoses, outcomes, and interventions that are commonly relevant to the people served by nurses, as described by Carlson (2006). At the NANDA-I 2008 conference in Miami, Florida, consensus validation studies were reported by nurses in two agencies (McGuire, Endozo,

Waddy-McIntosh, and Lunney, 2008; Minthorn, Lunney, Skeegan, and Van DerWiele, 2008).

Use of the NIC Interventions to Achieve Positive Health Outcomes

Traditionally, nursing interventions were identified in the planning phase of the nursing process, which was followed by the implementation phase (Yura and Walsh, 1967). However, just like outcomes, the interventions were written as a broad array of phrases and sentences, e.g., "assist the patient to the bathroom," that were not standardized in any way that would allow them to be summarized and described. There were also so many descriptions of how nurses help people that it would be unlikely to include all of them in computerized systems. In developing the NIC classification, the NIC research team identified, summarized, and organized the existing literature, both practical and research–based (Bulechek, Butcher, and Dochterman, 2008). This 20-year research project was partially funded by the National Institutes of Nursing Research.

The 2008 version of the NIC contains 540 interventions, both direct care, e.g., *airway management*, and indirect care, e.g., *case management*. A major advantage of NIC is that these nursing interventions, summarized through nursing research methods, have been formally named, defined, and described. The intervention is the major concept, e.g., *coping enhancement*, and its definition. The activities listed under the intervention indicate how the intervention should be or was performed. This means that every detail of how an intervention was performed does not need to be documented; the description is available in the standardized description. In computerized systems, when an intervention is performed, the nurse may just have to click on the title of the intervention. When specific activities of an intervention should be consistently performed for a consumer, e.g., in the case of a specific type of wound care, nurses can identify those activities in the health record, but they do not have to list every single activity performed.

The comprehensive nature of the NIC intervention classification makes it possible to describe nursing care for complex clinical situations by choosing the many types of interventions that can be used for one or more diagnoses. For example, for a complex situation when the diagnosis is *ineffective self health management* and the outcomes are *acceptance: health status* and *diabetic self management*, the nurse can select the interventions of *active listening, presence, mutual goal setting, coping enhancement, teaching: disease process, emotional support, nutritional counseling, smoking cessation assistance, health literacy enhancement*, and *referral* among other interventions.

Similar to the NOC outcomes, nursing interventions can be selected using the same four methods: (1) logical comparison of intervention concepts with diagnosis and outcome concepts, (2) the NIC book or other books can be consulted for lists of possible interventions for specific diagnoses and outcomes, (3) nurses with clinical experience in the agency where the nurse works can conduct consensus validation studies to identify the interventions that would be used with the common NANDA-I diagnoses for the people they serve, and (4) the definition and description of the activities with the intervention labels should be compared with what the nurse believes to be useful for the specific consumer. Logical comparison is evident with a diagnosis such as *anxiety* that can be matched with the NOC outcome of *anxiety level* and the NIC intervention of *anxiety reduction*. Another example is the diagnosis of *risk of infection*, which can be matched with the NOC of *infection control* and the NIC of *infection protection*.

The NIC reference book (Bulechek et al., 2008) contains lists of interventions that were identified by research methods for nursing care in a variety of specialties. These lists were identified as important interventions for nurses to know how to implement in these specialties, e.g., chemical dependency nursing. The book that explains NANDA-I, NOC, and NIC linkages (Johnson et al., 2008) contains lists of interventions that apply to specific NANDA-I diagnoses and NOC outcomes.

Just as in identifying NOC outcomes, consensus validation studies can be used to identify the NIC interventions that are commonly used, as shown in the research design by Carlson (2006). Carlson's paper represents a standard approach to developing this type of study. In addition, the agency standards of care should be used as a guide.

Comparing the definition and description of the NIC interventions with what the nurse and, whenever possible, the consumer, thinks the consumer needs may be the most common way of selecting NIC interventions. Novice and advanced beginner nurses (Benner, 1984) can consult with more experienced nurses for guidance. Nurses who are at the competent level in working with people who experience specific types of responses, problems, risk states, and readiness for health promotion are likely to have the ability to make decisions about the NIC interventions.

Summary

This chapter provided 10 guiding principles for use of nursing diagnoses and NANDA-I and general instructions for use of NOC and NIC. The NANDA-I, NOC, and NIC books should be consulted for additional information about these systems.

References

Banning, M. (2008). A review of clinical decision making: Models and current research. *Journal of Clinical Nursing, 17,* 187–195.

Barrett E.A.M. (1990). A measure of power as knowing participation in change. In O. Strickland and C. Waltz (eds.), *Measurement of nursing outcomes: Volume four, measuring client self-care and coping skills* (pp. 159–180). New York: Springer.

Barrett, E.A.M. (2000). The theoretical matrix for a Rogerian nursing practice. *Theoria: Journal of Nursing Theory, 9*(4), 3–7.

Bidmead, C., and Cowley, S. (2005). A concept analysis of partnership with clients. *Community Practice, 78,* 203–208.

Bulechek, G.M., Butcher, H.K., and Dochterman, J.M. (2008). *Nursing interventions classification (NIC)* (5th ed.). St. Louis: Mosby.

Carlson, J. (2006). Abstract: Consensus validation process: A standardized research method to identify and link the relevant NANDA, NIC and NOC terms for local populations. *International Journal of Nursing Terminologies and Classification, 17,* 23–24.

Carlson-Catalano, J. (1998). Nursing diagnoses and interventions for post-acute phase battered women, *Nursing Diagnosis: Journal of Nursing Language and Classification, 9,* 101–110.

Carnevali, D.L., and Thomas, M. D. (1993). *Diagnostic reasoning and treatment decision making.* Philadelphia: Lippincott.

Cruz, D.A.L.M., Pimenta, C.A.M., and Lunney, M. (2006). Teaching accuracy of nurses' diagnoses and evidenced-based practice: Goes together like a horse and carriage. In R.F. Levin and H.R. Feldman (eds.), *Teaching and learning evidenced-based practice in nursing: A guide for educators.* New York: Springer.

deBarros, A. (2003). Transition, utilization, and psychometric properties of the Functional Health Pattern Assessment Screening tool with patients in Brazil. *International Journal of Nursing Terminologies and Classifications, 14*(4), Supplement 17.

Duffy, J.R., Hoskins, L., and Seifert, R. (2007). Dimensions of caring: Psychometric evaluation of the caring assessment tool. *ANS: Advances in Nursing Science, 30,* 235–245.

Gigliotti, E. (2002). A theory-based clinical nurse specialist practice exemplar using Neuman's systems model and nursing's taxonomies. *Clinical Nurse Specialist, 16*(1), 10–16.

Gordon, M. (1994). *Nursing diagnosis: Process and application* (3rd ed.). St. Louis: Mosby.

Gordon, M. (2008). *Manual of nursing diagnosis.* (12th ed.). New York: McGraw-Hill.

Higa, R. (2006). Specific nursing care for pregnant women with HIV/AIDS. *International Journal of Nursing Terminologies and Classifications, 17,* 37–38.

Hook, M.L. (2006). Partnering with patients—A concept ready for action. *Journal of Advanced Nursing, 56,* 133–143.

Johnson, M., Bulechek, G.M., Dochterman, J.M., Maas, M.L., Moorhead, S., Swanson, E., and Butcher, H. (2006). *NANDA, NOC and NIC linkages: Nursing diagnoses, outcomes and interventions* (2nd ed.). St. Louis: Mosby.

Leininger, M.M. and McFarland, M. (2006). *Culture care diversity and universality: A worldwide nursing theory* (2nd ed.). Boston: Jones and Bartlett.

Levin, R., Lunney, M., and Krainovich-Miller, B. (2005). Improving diagnostic accuracy using an evidenced-based nursing model. *International Journal of Nursing Terminologies and Classifications, 15,* 114–122.

Lyneham, J., Parkinson, C., and Denholm, C. (2008). Intuition in emergency room nursing: A phenomenological study. *International Journal of Nursing Practice, 14,* 101–108.

McCormack, B., and McCance, T.V. (2006). Development of a framework for person-centred nursing. *Journal of Advanced Nursing, 56,* 472–479.

McGuire, M., Endozo, N., Waddy-McIntosh, D., and Lunney, M. (2008). *Consensus validation results: NANDA, NIC and NOC categories for care of people with traumatic brain injuries in long term care.* Abstracts, NANDA International 2008 Conference, Miami Fl. Retrieved on September 1, 2008 from http://www.nanda.org.

Minthorn, C., Lunney, M., Skeegan, L., and Van DerWiele, D. (2008). *Participant action research with nurses to identify NANDA-I, NIC and NOC categories for care of people with diabetes and women in labor.* Abstracts, NANDA International 2008 Conference, Miami Fl. Retrieved on September 1, 2008 from http://www.nanda.org.

Moorhead, S., Johnson, M., Maas, M.L., and Swanson, E. (2008). *Nursing Outcomes Classification (NOC)* (4th ed.). St Louis: Mosby.

Munhall, P.L. (1993). "Unknowing": Toward another pattern of knowing in nursing. *Nursing Outlook, 41,* 125–128.

Murphy, F. (2006). Dialysis: A case study exploring a patient's non-compliance. *British Journal of Nursing, 15,* 773–776.

NANDA International. (2009). *Nursing diagnosis: Definitions and classification, 2009–2011.* Hoboken, NJ: Wiley-Blackwell.

Neuman, B., and Fawcett J. (2002). *The Neuman systems model* (4th ed.). Upper Saddle River, NJ: Prentice Hall.

Orem, D.E. (2001). *Nursing: Concepts of practice* (6th ed.). St. Louis: Mosby.

Ousey, K., and Johnson, M. (2007). Being a real nurse: Concepts of caring and culture in the clinical areas. *Nurse Education in Practice, 7,* 150–155.

Pender, N.J., Murdaugh, C.L., and Parsons, M.A. (2006). *Health promotion in nursing practice* (5th ed.). Upper Saddle River, NJ: Pearson Prentice Hall.

Rogers, M.E. (1992). Nursing science and the space age. *Nursing Science Quarterly, 5,* 27–34.

Roy Sr., C., and Andrews, H.A. (2009). *The Roy adaptation model.* (3rd ed.). Englewood Cliffs, NJ: Prentice Hall.

Splaine Wiggins, M. (2008). The partnership care delivery model: An examination of the core concept and the need for a new model of care. *Journal of Nursing Management, 16,* 629–638.

Watson, J. (2005). *Caring science as sacred science.* Philadelphia: F.A. Davis.

Weaver, T.L., Resnick, H.S., Kokoska, M.S., and Etzel, J.C. (2007.). Appearance-related residual injury, post-traumatic stress, and body image: Association within a sample of female victims of intimate partner violence. *Journal of Trauma and Stress, 20,* 999–1008.

Wilkinson, J.M. (2007). *Nursing process and critical thinking.* (4th ed.). Upper Saddle River, NJ: Prentice Hall.

Yura, H., and Walsh, M. (1967). *The nursing process.* Washington, DC: Catholic University Press.

Application of the Guiding Principles and Directions for Use of NANDA-I, NOC, and NIC

Margaret Lunney, RN, PhD

Chapter Objectives

By completion of this chapter, readers will be able to:

1. Apply the guidelines from Chapter 3 with four types of NANDA-I diagnoses:
   - Problem diagnoses
   - Risk diagnoses
   - Health promotion diagnoses
   - Wellness or strength diagnoses
2. Apply the directions in Chapter 3 for use of NOC and NIC with the four types of diagnoses.

There are four types of NANDA-I approved diagnoses: problem diagnoses, risk state daignoses, health promotion diagnoses, and wellness diagnoses, or strengths. In this book, wellness diagnoses are conceptualized as strengths. Problem diagnoses are discussed first because it is expected that nurses prioritize their care to help people with problems before addressing risk states or readiness for health promotion. The consumer's strengths are diagnosed and recorded so that they can be used as resources for health promotion and health protection and to save nurses the task of reassessing the same phenomena.

The diagnosis of responses to health problems and life processes is important because it represents society's most common view of the role of nurses. In fact, human responses to health problems was identified as a nursing scope of practice in many state-level nurse practice acts, e.g., the New York State (NYS) Nurse Practice Act. The NYS Nurse Practice Act (Office of the Professions, 2008) states:

> The practice of the profession of nursing as a registered professional nurse is defined as: diagnosing and treating human responses to actual or potential health problems through such services as case-finding, health teaching, health counseling, and provision of care supportive to or restorative of life and well-being, and executing medical regimens prescribed by a licensed or otherwise legally authorized physician or dentist. A nursing regimen shall be consistent with and shall not vary any existing medical regimen (Scope of Practice established by state law, 1972).

Use of the 10 Guidelines with Problem Diagnoses

When the NANDA-I classification began in 1973, the primary focus was on identifying problem responses that are the focus of nursing care (Gebbie, 1976). Diagnosing problem responses to health problems and life processes is a very important role of nurses because problem responses interfere with health status. Some examples are:

- *Ineffective breathing pattern*
- *Ineffective infant feeding pattern*
- *Imbalanced nutrition: less than body requirements*
- *Deficient fluid volume*
- *Impaired urinary elimination*
- *Impaired bed mobility*
- *Fear*
- *Anxiety*
- *Powerlessness*
- *Disturbed body image*

Applying the guidelines and directions from Chapter 3 to the diagnosis of problem responses will be explained using the problem diagnosis of *ineffective self health management* (NANDA-I, 2009). This diagnosis applies broadly to any health care setting where nurses work; its focus of care is helping people to manage their chronic illnesses. NANDA-I diagnoses related to this concept are available for individuals, families, and communities. The basis of this diagnostic concept is that nurses support and help people to self manage their illnesses. Currently, there is extensive research-based literature on self management of chronic illnesses. Examples of chronic illnesses are:

- Heart and lung diseases
- Cancers
- Diabetes and other endocrine problems

- Arthritis and other mobility problems
- Irritable bowel syndrome and other GI problems
- Overactive bladder and other urinary problems
- Multiple sclerosis and other neurological problems
- Chronic depression and other mental health problems

The rates of chronic illnesses are very high worldwide. In the U.S., it is estimated that chronic diseases are among the most prevalent, costly, and preventable of all health problems (U.S. Department of Health and Human Services, Centers for Disease Control and Prevention, 2007). Seven of every 10 Americans who die each year, or more than 1.7 million people, die of a chronic disease. The prolonged course of illness and disability from such chronic diseases as diabetes and arthritis results in extended pain and suffering and decreased quality of life for millions of Americans. Chronic, disabling conditions cause major limitations in activity for more than one of every 10 Americans, or 25 million people.

People with chronic illnesses also have therapeutic regimens involving nutrition, exercise, and medications that they must manage themselves. They must integrate these regimens into their daily living routines. This is difficult and complex, so those with chronic illnesses need nurses to help them with self management of their therapeutic regimens. It is unethical to expect individuals and families to self manage their chronic illnesses without adequate knowledge and support from health providers (Redman, 2005).

An assumption related to the diagnosis of self health management is that people know themselves better than nurses or other providers do (Munhall, 1993). With this perspective it is important for nurses to work in partnership with the recipients of care to help them manage their chronic illnesses. Assessment factors to identify are people's past habits and behaviors; their likes and dislikes; the support of family, friends, and others; the community resources that are available; and the perceived barriers and perceived benefits of managing the therapeutic regimen (Pender, Murdaugh, and Parsons, 2006).

Nurses who diagnose the effectiveness and ineffectiveness of people's self health management must:

- Ask the individual or family if they want help integrating the therapeutic regimen into daily living;
- If the individual or family says yes, review the state of their knowledge related to the chronic illness and its management. Knowledge is necessary but not sufficient for self management;
- Identify factors other than knowledge that support or interfere with optimum therapeutic regimen management. Two health care models that can be used to discern other factors that impact individual and family health behaviors are Pender's Model of Health Promotion and the Health Belief Model (Pender et al., 2006).

An Example Using the 10 Guidelines with a NANDA-I Problem Diagnosis

Guideline 1: Use one or more nursing theories to guide your philosophical and theoretical approaches to nursing care. Using the Functional Health Patterns as a nursing assessment framework (Gordon, 2007; see Appendix B) with Watson's theory of nursing (Rosenberg, 2006; Watson, 2005), the home health care (HHC) nurse, Marian Gonzalez, visited John P (see the box titled "Initial Home Care Visit, Health History Data from John P") as a routine post-hospitalization admission visit. Upon gaining admission to the home, the nurse showed caring by respectfully establishing relationships with John P and the family members who were present during the visit and reviewed with them the purpose and methods of the visit.

Initial Home Care Visit, Health History Data from John P

Age <u>64</u> Gender <u>M</u> Occupation <u>Retired Construction Laborer</u>

Health Perception-Health Management Pattern

Glad to be home, had a tough time in the hospital, didn't expect my respiratory status to get that bad. Guess my health status is not as good as I thought, will have to rethink my behaviors so I can stay out of the hospital.

   For most of my life, I did things in moderation, e.g., ate fairly healthy, exercised, and socially drank beer or cocktails. My big problem was smoking; I smoked from age 12 to 55, about two packs a day. I stopped at 55 because my doctor told me I had emphysema. About two years ago, I slipped on ice and fractured two ribs. Had to be hospitalized after getting pneumonia; my respiratory status really deteriorated after that.

   Have been seeing my MD regularly and follow her advice as well as possible, not sure how I got pneumonia again. I don't take my blood pressure and usually do not worry about it; no history of high blood pressure.

Medications

Aspirin, 325 mg, 1 daily
Multivitamin (senior), 1 daily
Co-Enzyme Q10, 1 daily
Vitamin C, 1,000 mg, 1 daily
Combivent, 2 inhalations every two hours

Atrovent nebulizer (500 micrograms/2.5 milliliter) solution (0.02%)—use in nebulizer every eight hours as needed for bronchospasm

I know how and when to correctly use the inhaler and nebulizer. I try not to overdo it because I want to stay as healthy as possible, especially because I am in bad shape for my age. Smoking for so long "did me in." Family hx includes colon cancer; have colonoscopy every five years; had to retire on medical leave; monthly income is adequate; wife is still working.

Nutrition-Metabolic Pattern

Eat small meals five to six times a day; generally follow the recommended intake of protein, fats, and carbohydrates. Will do a three-day diet history for next visit. Wife shops; I do a lot of the cooking; sometimes I don't have the energy. With the respiratory problems, I've lost weight so happy now with my weight. No special influences on food choices. When I get a respiratory infection, my appetite is poor.

Elimination Pattern

Urinate without problems, light yellow, no odor, no problems with flow, generally do not have to get up during the night. Bowel movements one time a day, brown, formed, no difficulties.

Activity-Exercise Pattern

Take short walks outdoors until I get tired, up and down the stairs during the day; no specific exercise pattern; was taught how to do rhythmic breathing with activity such as stair climbing but have not been doing it. When not short of breath (SOB), I do household chores, such as laundry. The pulmonologist wants me to go for pulmonary rehabilitation; thinking about it.

Sleep-Rest Pattern

Sleep rituals are to watch sports or a comedy show before bedtime; it helps me relax. I sit in a chair beside the bed to watch TV and go to bed about 11 pm. Sleep OK on two pillows, sometimes wake up SOB; have to sit up until it subsides. Of course, it is always worse when I have a respiratory infection. I don't take naps; rest by watching TV or reading.

Cognitive-Perceptual Pattern

High school graduate; took a few college courses but did not like it. As far as I know, my brain is fine, no problems yet. I read, do

Sudoku, play mind games on the computer (bridge, free cell). My comfort level is OK now; no pain. Before hospitalization I had feelings of pressure in my chest with shortness of breath.

Self Perception Self Concept Pattern

I generally feel good about myself. I was productive before I retired, made decent money and have always supported my family. I'm not happy to have my life limited by these respiratory problems, but it's better than the alternative, right?

Role-Relationship Pattern

Wife and I have a great relationship. Figured out ways to adapt our roles with me retired and her working. Many good friends, including couples with whom we play bridge and have some laughs.

Sexuality-Reproductive Pattern

No problems, no need to discuss further.

Coping-Stress Tolerance Pattern

Generally manage stress without difficulty, except when SOB. Read that breathing exercises help to relieve stress; sorry now that I did not pay attention to learn breathing exercises. Can you (nurse) help me with that? Thinking of doing yoga for relaxation.

Value-Belief Pattern

I am second generation Irish; we enjoy going to Irish concerts. Ethnicity does not really affect other things in my life; friends are from many other different ethnic groups. Middle class with no specific economic concerns. The things that are important to us are family, friends, and health. We go to church once in awhile but not all the time.

Guideline 2: In the context of the selected approach to nursing, conduct nursing assessments of the person to identify the problems, risk states, readiness for health promotion, and strengths that are appropriate to guide nursing care. A full assessment of John P had been conducted with his permission, using the Functional Health Patterns and standardized physical examination techniques (Weber and Kelley, 2006). During the physical examination, it was found that John P's resting respiratory rate was higher than normal when compared to other adults, so the nurse mentally considered the problem diagnosis of *ineffective breathing pattern*.

Guideline 3: During assessments, use the seven cognitive skills and 10 habits of mind of critical thinking (Chapter 1, Table 1.1) along with the thinking processes of the person who is the recipient of nursing care. The nurse used the cognitive skill of information seeking to identify whether John P's respiratory rate was abnormal for him. The nurse checked the chart for the respiratory rates provided on the referral form and asked John P whether his respiratory rate was higher than usual. John P said that he was having more difficulty than usual with his breathing and the nurse determined that his rate was about 10% higher than previous rates.

Guideline 4: Conduct focused assessments to identify the specific responses that the person may be experiencing, considering the situational context. Considering that John P has COPD, the nurse decided that, in addition to assessing for breathing pattern, she would determine whether there were any changes in sleep, rest, activity, nutrition, and coping. At this point, no other nursing diagnoses were indicated by the data.

Guideline 5: Obtain a sufficient amount of high and moderate relevance data to support or reject (rule in or rule out) the specific diagnoses being considered. The determination that John P's respiratory rate was relatively higher than his usual rate provided insufficient data to select the diagnosis of *ineffective breathing pattern*; therefore, the nurse continued assessing for cues to this specific diagnosis.

Guideline 6: Compare the person's data with the NANDA-I standardized nursing diagnoses, i.e., the labels, definitions, and defining characteristics. The nurse compared John P's status with the NANDA-I list of defining characteristics for the diagnosis of *ineffective breathing pattern*: depth of breathing, chest excursion, inspiratory and expiratory pressure, minute ventilation, vital capacity, dyspnea, anterior-posterior diameter, nasal flaring, possible orthopnea, prolonged expiration, pursed lip breathing, timing ratio, and use of accessory muscles.

Guideline 7: Consider other possible diagnoses as you collect data. While collecting data to confirm or rule out *ineffective breathing pattern* and other possible diagnoses, the nurse asked John P whether there were any changes in sleep, rest, appetite, and emotional status, and assessed his self health management. John P said there were minor changes in his sleep pattern and his appetite was slightly decreased. Assessment data on self health management revealed that John P was not doing regular deep breathing exercises as previously instructed, was not using specific patterned breathing while climbing stairs as learned in the hospital, and had been up and down the stairs about four times yesterday and today. With these data, the nurse considered that this was sufficient supporting data for the diagnosis of *ineffective breathing pattern*. Another respiratory diagnosis that the nurse considered was *impaired gas exchange*, but in this situation, the nurse did not have sufficient information about blood gases to make this diagnosis. It was also considered that it was not necessary to focus on sleep or nutrition since these patterns were probably influenced by his respiratory status.

Guideline 8: Whenever possible, considering the situational context, validate diagnostic impressions with the individual or family. The nurse discussed the proposed diagnosis with John P. He agreed that he needed help to improve his breathing pattern and that the sleep and appetite issues were probably influenced by his worsening respiratory status. He agreed that he could do better in self management of his therapeutic regimen and might have been climbing the stairs too many times per day without attending to the breathing pattern he had learned to use.

Guideline 9: If there is more than one diagnosis, identify the priority diagnosis or diagnoses. John P and the nurse decided that the problem diagnosis that needed to be addressed was *ineffective breathing pattern* and that the health promotion diagnosis of *readiness for enhanced self health management* should also be considered.

Guideline 10: Communicate, verbally and in writing, the selected priority diagnosis or diagnoses to others as a basis for planning outcomes and intervention. The HHC nurse charted the problem diagnosis of *ineffective breathing pattern* related to irregular use of deep breathing exercises at rest and with activity, and began to consider the NOC outcome and NIC interventions to use.

Use of NOC with the Problem Diagnosis

The nurse examined the overview of the NOC taxonomy (Moorhead, Johnson, Maas, and Swanson, 2008, pp. 125–143) to identify the most appropriate outcome for use with John P's diagnosis and considering John P's personal goals. John P said he was beginning to realize that he had to be effective in self management of his respiratory illness to prevent relapses and to optimize the quality of his life. Using the NOC taxonomy, the nurse decided that *Class Q, health behavior,* was the most likely to contain the most appropriate outcome for this clinical situation. Within *Class Q,* the outcome of *treatment behavior: illness or injury* was selected as a possible measure of John P's health outcome. The nurse read the outcome definition and examined the indicators to determine if it was a good fit with John P's situation, and it was.

Using the indicators, the nurse and John P agreed that his baseline score on the outcome was 3 (sometimes demonstrated). They discussed the target score and decided that it should be 5 (consistently demonstrated).

Use of NIC with NOC and the Problem Diagnosis

The nurse examined the overview of the NIC taxonomy (Bulechek, Butcher, and Dochterman, 2008, pp. 74–91) to identify possible interventions to support and help John P as needed to reach his target goal of consistent demonstration of treatment behaviors for his illness. The nurse looked for interventions in Class K, respiratory management, and in Class R, coping assistance. The interventions selected from Class K, respiratory management, were *chest physiotherapy, respiratory monitoring, cough enhancement,* and *oxygen therapy.* The nurse reviewed what John P had learned in the hospital about optimizing oxygenation through diaphragmatic breathing during exercises such as stair climbing, and reviewed the deep breathing exercises he was supposed to be doing on a regular basis. John P was advised that the nurse would request an evaluation visit by the respiratory therapist and would call John P's physician to provide information about John P's status. Other issues would be addressed at the next visit, e.g., teaching his wife how to conduct chest physiotherapy to prevent accumulation of secretions in the lower lobes. Oxygen therapy was discussed for use on an "as needed" basis. It was expected that over the next few weeks of regular visits, John P would reach the target outcomes.

The nurse also considered use of interventions in the coping assistance category because coping with chronic illness is known to be challenging and difficult (Larsen and Lubkin, 2009). Coping assistance strategies support people through coping difficulties so that coping problems do not have negative effects on health status. The interventions of *coping enhancement, emotional support,* and *self awareness enhancement* were selected to work with John P in the process of optimizing his quality of life, given the reality of having to live with this chronic illness. With vigilance in daily functioning and self health management, John P would be able to live as healthfully and happily as possible.

Example of Using the 10 Guidelines with a NANDA-I Risk Diagnosis

The NANDA-I risk diagnoses provide guidance for nursing care to reduce risks when significant risk factors are present that may lead to problem states. Because of John P's compromised respiratory status, he has significant risk factors for respiratory infection. John P, his family, and the nurses who provide his care must be aware of and attend to this risk in order to prevent the problem of a respiratory infection. The diagnosis of *risk for infection* is used when nursing interventions are needed to prevent risks from becoming realities. John P also has risk factors for *impaired gas exchange, imbalanced nutrition: less than body requirements,* and *ineffective coping.* The nurse needs to decide whether or not these risks are significant enough to require a nursing plan of care that includes outcomes and interventions.

Guideline 1: Use one or more nursing theories to guide your philosophical and theoretical approaches to nursing care. With the Functional Health Pattern framework and Watson's theory of nursing, the HHC nurse demonstrated use of Watson's Clinical Carative Processes by tactfully discussing possible risk states with John P. The nurse established a transpersonal relationship of trust in which the two of them would work together over the next few weeks to review how to manage these issues. With the overwhelming number of concerns that were possible for John P, many of which could be life threatening, the nurse's verbal and non-verbal approach needed to portray a loving concern for him as a person.

Guideline 2: In the context of the selected approach to nursing, conduct nursing assessments of the person to identify the problems, risk states, readiness for health promotion, and strengths that are appropriate to guide nursing care. Because assessment procedures had already been conducted to identify possible problems, the nurse had sufficient data to project John P's possible risk states. The nurse did not know, however, whether John P had sufficient knowledge of the various risk states associated with his compromised respiratory status.

Guideline 3: During assessments use the seven cognitive skills and 10 habits of mind of critical thinking (see Chapter 1 and Table 1.1) along with the thinking processes of the person who is the recipient of nursing care. The nurse used the cognitive skills of information seeking and applying standards to identify whether John P had a full understanding of his risk factors and their relation to possible negative health outcomes. The nurse explored John P's thinking in relation to managing the risk factors for infection.

Guideline 4: Conduct focused assessments to identify the specific responses that the person may be experiencing considering the situational context. John P said he knew that having COPD with the associated reduced-immunity put him at higher risk for infection than people without these risk factors, but he did not know how to improve his risk status. The nurse noticed that aspects of his home environment could be improved to reduce risk factors. Family members who had upper respiratory infections visited him, and his mother-in-law smoked when she visited. Studies show that second-hand smoke is a factor in recurrent respiratory infections (Odermarsky et al., 2008).

Guideline 5: Obtain a sufficient amount of high and moderate relevance data to support or reject (rule in or rule out) the specific diagnoses being considered. Because John P had COPD that had worsened to the point that he needed hospitalization for respiratory care, and there were home environmental factors that could be improved, the nurse validated that there were sufficient data to state the diagnosis, *risk for infection*.

Guideline 6: Compare the person's data with the NANDA-I standardized nursing diagnoses, i.e., the labels, definitions, and defining characteristics. Using the NANDA-I list of defining characteristics for the diagnosis of *risk for infection*, data from John P were found to be a good match with this diagnosis.

Guideline 7: Consider other possible diagnoses as you collect data. While collecting data to confirm or rule out *risk for infection*, the nurse also checked for data to support the other risk diagnoses of *risk for* *impaired airway clearance, risk for imbalanced nutrition*, and *risk for ineffective coping*. These were ruled out at this point in time.

Guideline 8: Whenever possible, considering the situational context, validate diagnostic impressions with the individual or family. The nurse discussed the proposed diagnosis of *risk for infection* with John P. He agreed that he needed help to improve his risk status. He said that if he reduces his risk for infection, it would probably reduce other risks as well.

Guideline 9: If there is more than one diagnosis, identify the priority diagnosis or diagnoses. John P and the nurse decided that *risk for infection* would be communicated in his chart to other providers and that the nurse would develop a plan of care, approved by John P, for this diagnosis.

Guideline 10: Communicate, verbally and in writing, the selected priority diagnosis or diagnoses to others as a basis for planning outcomes and intervention. The HHC nurse charted the risk diagnosis *risk for infection* and began to consider the associated NOC, and NIC.

Use of NOC with the Risk Diagnosis

The nurse and John P again examined the NOC taxonomy (Moorhead et al., 2008, pp. 125–143) to identify the appropriate desired outcome. The nurse first looked for the word "infection" (the NOCs are in alphabetical order) because often there are direct matches between the diagnostic concepts and the outcome concepts. The NOC that was selected was *infection severity*. The indicators associated with this outcome were designed to reveal the overall score of infection severity. In this case, John P had no infection so the baseline score was identified as 5 (none). The goal was to maintain a score of 5 on *infection severity*. With NOC outcomes associated with other risk states, e.g., *nutritional status*, John P might score a 4 (mildly compromised) and the goal would be to remain at 4 or improve to a score of 5. With risk states, it is expected that the outcome would not be scored lower than 4 because, in most cases, lower scores would indicate that the phenomena was a problem rather than a risk state.

Use of NIC with NOC and the Risk Diagnosis

The nursing approach to risk states is to reduce the risk factors as much as possible. This requires a focus on improving health status through good nutrition, adequate sleep and rest, exercise within the limits of the person's capabilities, developing positive coping strategies, and helping the person to attain adequate knowledge of how to achieve an optimum health state and manipulate the environment to be as healthful as possible. The nurse and John P selected the NIC interventions of *infection control, nutrition counseling, exercise promotion, self awareness enhancement, sleep enhancement, coping enhancement,* and *environmental management*. The nurse's focus in implementing these interventions was to help John P optimize his health status and subsequently improve his overall immunity to infection and mitigate the environment to reduce risk factors. Previously, it was thought that reducing the incidence of allergens such as dust mites would reduce the *risk for infection*, but a recent Cochrane review of 54 trials with 3,002 patients showed that there was inadequate research support for this claim (Getzsche and Jahnsen, 2008). Part of the reason for the lack of research support is that the research designs were not done carefully enough to draw conclusions. In the absence of good studies to say otherwise, nurses should still advise people to reduce the incidence of allergens such as dust mites by covering mattresses and pillows with dust mite–resistant covers and removing rugs from rooms where the person spends a lot of time, e.g., the bedroom.

Example of Using the 10 Guidelines with a NANDA-I Health Promotion Diagnosis

It is important to learn diagnostic reasoning with health promotion diagnoses because an increased focus by nurses on health promotion services helps to keep people healthy (Pender et al., 2006). Helping people at all stages of heath and illness to adopt health promotion behaviors is likely to reduce the number of risk states and problems that occur. This type of approach has been referred to as "upstream thinking" (Butterfield, 2002). Historically in the U.S., the major focus has been on downstream thinking. The analogy is that the focus in the U.S. has been on waiting downstream for people to fall in the river (as in getting sick) and then pulling them out one at a time (as in the U.S. focus on primary care of people who are already sick), instead of looking upstream and preventing them from falling in the river (as in primary health care, which focuses on health promotion and health protection, Stanhope and Lancaster, 2006).

The health and vital statistics of people in the U.S. indicate that upstream thinking is sorely needed. For example, the U.S. was 42nd in the world in life expectancy and 40th in the world in infant mortality rates (World Health Organization, 2007), two key indicators of the health of a society. Other countries that have stronger health promotion services, such as Norway, Sweden, Japan, and France, have much better health statistics than the U.S. The U.S. spends more than two times the money per capita on health care than any other country (United Nations Development Programme, 2006) and has poor health statistics to show for it. Nurses in the U.S. and other countries can contribute to improving the health of their country's people by increasing their focus on health promotion.

Most of the NANDA-I health promotion diagnoses are new to the NANDA-I taxonomy, so many nurses do not know how to use them. Some nurses incorrectly believe, for example, that health promotion diagnoses are only used when people are healthy or in a high state of wellness. However, individual and family readiness for health promotion needs to be considered at all stages of health and illness (Pender et al., 2006), even when a person is critically ill or dying, e.g., the case study by Germano and Terjesen (p. 268). All consumers of nursing services deserve the incorporation of health promotion in their care if it is diagnosed as needed and wanted. Health promotion requires clinical judgment (thus diagnosis) to decide whether or not a person is ready for health promotion services.

With insufficient evidence of problems or risk states, health promotion diagnoses may apply, e.g., when a nurse thinks that a person could use some help with coping or decision making and there are not enough data to say that the diagnosis should be *ineffective coping* or *decisional conflict*. And, with the assumption that people know themselves better than nurses know them, if the recipient of care prefers the qualifier *readiness for enhanced* to the qualifiers of *risk of* or *ineffective*, a health promotion diagnosis should be used.

Suggestions of when to use health promotion diagnoses are:

- When there are cues that a person needs help with health behaviors and the person agrees to accept the nurses' help;
- When the person states there is no clear problem or risk state;
- To avoid "blaming the victim" as in some instances when diagnoses such as *ineffective coping* and *chronic low self-esteem* are used, e.g., the case study by Cummings (p. 311).

With diagnoses such as *chronic low self-esteem* and *ineffective coping*, individuals and families may be more likely to agree to health promotion diagnoses for themselves than to problem diagnosis.

Guideline 1: Use one or more nursing theories to guide your philosophical and theoretical approaches to nursing care. In discussion with John P related to health promotion, the nurse continued to use Watson's 10 Clinical Carative Processes and maintained a transpersonal relationship with him.

Guideline 2: In the context of the selected approach to nursing, conduct nursing assessments of the person to identify the problems, risk states, readiness for health promotion, and strengths that are appropriate to guide nursing care. The nurse decided that no further assessment data were needed to support a health promotion diagnosis, other than what was already known.

Guideline 3: During assessments use the seven cognitive skills and 10 habits of mind of critical thinking along with the thinking processes of the person who is the recipient of nursing care. John P had said that he was ready to learn more about self health management.

Guideline 4: Conduct focused assessments to identify the specific responses that the person may be experiencing, considering the situational context. With John P, the situation was such that he needed to manage his chronic illness 24 hours a day and seven days a week. Health providers were only available to help him for short periods; the bulk of the responsibility and burden fell on him and his family. The nurse identified both his and his family's acceptance of this reality, and it was determined that they fully accepted this responsibility.

Guideline 5: Obtain a sufficient amount of high and moderate relevance data to support or reject (rule in or rule out) the specific diagnoses being considered. Because all consumers who are ready for health promotion should receive health promotion services if the nurse has the time and ability to do so, the HHC nurse planned to provide these services for John P. Health promotion is integral to HHC nursing, a specialization within community health nursing (Stanhope and Lancaster, 2006).

Guideline 6: Compare the person's data with the NANDA-I standardized nursing diagnoses, i.e., the labels, definitions, and defining characteristics. The data from John P were a good match with the NANDA-I diagnosis of *readiness for enhanced self health management.*

Guideline 7: Consider other possible diagnoses as you collect data. Over the next few weeks, when the HHC nurse visited John P and addressed the problem, risk state, and health promotion diagnoses, the nurse would continue to observe for other health promotion opportunities.

Guideline 8: Whenever possible, considering the situational context, validate diagnostic impressions with the individual or family. Because John P already agreed, the nurse informed him that the diagnosis of *readiness for enhanced self health management* would be recorded on his chart so that all providers would be able to collaborate in the process of helping him with self management.

Guideline 9: If there is more than one diagnosis, identify the priority diagnosis or diagnoses. The priority diagnoses of *ineffective breathing pattern* and *risk for infection* had been identified. This health promotion diagnosis would support his overall improvement in all related outcomes.

Guideline 10: Communicate, verbally and in writing, the selected priority diagnosis or diagnoses to others as a basis for planning outcomes and intervention. In John P's chart, the nurse recorded the health promotion diagnosis of *readiness for enhanced self health management,* along with the problem and risk state diagnoses.

Use of NOC with the Health Promotion Diagnosis

First, the nurse looked in the NOC book for the concept of health promotion and noted that there was a NOC *health promoting behavior.* After reading the definition and reviewing the indicators, the nurse and John P decided that this outcome was a good match with the selected health promotion diagnosis. They decided on a baseline score of 4 (often demonstrated) with a target score of 5 (consistently demonstrated). The indicators used to make this decision were: balances activity with rest, performs healthy behaviors routinely (the concept of healthful behaviors was interpreted in the context of him having COPD), maintains adequate sleep, uses financial resources to promote health, and uses social support resources to promote health.

Use of the NIC with the NOC and the Health Promotion Diagnosis

Many of the NIC interventions are appropriate for health promotion, as well as for treatment of problems or risk states. This includes the teaching interventions, interventions that include the word "enhancement," and others (see below).

The NIC interventions that were selected to enhance John P's *self health management* were *self awareness enhancement, multidisciplinary care conference, teaching: prescribed activity/exercise*, and *self efficacy enhancement*. The nurse assisted John P to enhance self awareness of attitudes, his attributes, behaviors, and motivation because understanding his own thoughts, feelings, and behaviors would guide his ongoing participation in self management of his chronic illness. Previous hospital-based teaching regarding how to successfully integrate activity and rest into his daily living were reinforced and clarified. The nurse, respiratory therapist, and John P met to discuss the various ways in which he could deliberately compensate for his compromised respiratory status. Self-efficacy was enhanced to strengthen his confidence in the ability to live healthfully in the context of this chronic illness.

Example of Using the 10 Guidelines with a Strength Diagnosis

Identification of strengths is generally part of any good nursing assessment but actually stating an individual or family's strengths as a nursing diagnosis may only be done selectively for specific reasons. Decisions about when and how often to state consumer strengths is an agency decision. For example, in long-term care, it is useful to routinely state the strengths of residents so that these strengths can serve as a foundation for interventions for other diagnoses. With people who live in long-term care settings, it is expected that there will be many routine diagnoses such as *self care deficit* and *impaired mobility*, so stating diagnoses such as *effective self care* may help to motivate both the resident and the staff members to optimize other aspects of the person's health status.

Another reason to identify strengths as diagnoses is to save nurses' time in assessment and diagnosis, e.g., if a woman has a mastectomy and all nurses who provide care expect the woman to have changes in body image but one of the nurses diagnoses *positive body image*, it would save other nurses the time of future assessment and interventions and save the woman from being asked repeatedly about body image.

Guideline 1: Use one or more nursing theories to guide your philosophical and theoretical approaches to nursing care. The nurse continued to use the functional health patterns as a framework for assessment and Watson's caring science to identify significant strengths of John P.

Guideline 2: In the context of the selected approach to nursing, conduct nursing assessments of the person to identify the problems, risk states, readiness for health promotion, and strengths that are appropriate to guide nursing care. From the previous assessment, the nurse noted that John P had no problems in some of the functional health patterns; these were cognitive/perception, role/relationships, coping/stress tolerance, and values/beliefs.

Guideline 3: During assessments use the seven cognitive skills and 10 habits of mind of critical thinking along with the thinking processes of the person who is the recipient of nursing care. The nurse asked John P what he considered to be his strengths. He said, "I effectively deal with whatever problems I have and I generally find ways to cope with problems, one way or the other."

Guideline 4: Conduct focused assessments to identify the specific responses that the person may be experiencing, considering the situational context. The nurse asked John P to give examples of what he meant. He described losing a job in the past and the strategies he used to find a new job and avoid letting it "get me down."

Guideline 5: Obtain a sufficient amount of high and moderate relevance data to support or reject (rule in or rule out) the specific diagnoses being considered. With the data that the nurse had obtained in the initial assessment of the coping pattern and this new information, the nurse decided that there were sufficient data to support *effective coping* as a strength diagnosis.

Guideline 6: Compare the person's data with the NANDA-I standardized nursing diagnoses, i.e., the labels, definitions, and defining characteristics. Checking the NANDA-I book, the nurse noted that *effective coping* was not an approved NANDA-I diagnosis, but with the multi-axial system of Taxonomy II, Axis 3 included the word "effective" as a qualifier that could be used with the NANDA-I concepts to describe the nurses' clinical judgment. The nurse compared the cues from John P with the cues for *ineffective coping* and determined that his positive behaviors represented *effective coping*.

Guideline 7: Consider other possible diagnoses as you collect data. At this time, the data did not reveal any other existing issues or concerns.

Guideline 8: Whenever possible, considering the situational context, validate diagnostic impressions with the individual or family. The nurse said to John P, "Would you say that *effective coping* was a personal strength of yours?" John P said "Yes."

Guideline 9: If there is more than one diagnosis, identify the priority diagnosis or diagnoses. Priority diagnoses had already been identified.

Guideline 10: Communicate, verbally and in writing, the selected priority diagnosis or diagnoses to others as a basis for planning outcomes and intervention. The nurse decided that it would be important to record the strength diagnosis of *effective coping* because when other nurses and providers visited John P, they would be able to use this strength as a resource to address other issues.

Use of NOC with the Strength Diagnosis

The NOC that was selected was *coping*. Because John P's *coping* was a strength, it was expected that his baseline score was 5 (consistently demonstrated) and it was. The target score was to remain at 5.

Use of NIC with NOC and the Strength Diagnosis

With John P's target score on *coping* to remain at 5, the nurse selected the NIC interventions of *coping enhancement*, *active listening*, and *emotional support*. This meant that nurses and other health professionals would continue to support and enhance his coping abilities. *Active listening* enabled them to identify whether there were any changes in coping over time. *Emotional support* was used as continued support for positive coping strategies.

Evaluation

The outcomes that had been selected for all diagnoses were evaluated at the time of John P's discharge from HHC services. The evaluation decisions made by John P and the nurse were that the target scores were met. John P knew that if he needed help in the future he could ask his physician to request reevaluation by the HHC nurse to see if he qualified for additional at-home services.

Conclusions

The examples provided in this chapter illustrate how to use the guidelines and directions from Chapter 3 with the four types of NANDA-I diagnoses and the associated NOCs and NICs. These examples show that these languages can easily be used to represent nursing practice. The words and phrases of these languages represent the similarities among nursing situations, not the differences (Hayakawa and Haykawa, 1990). There are many differences among nursing situations that cannot be captured using these or any other languages.

The experience of clinical situations in nursing will always be more complex and diverse than can be captured with the words and phrases of languages such as NANDA-I, NOC, and NIC. But the effort to capture at least the similarities among nursing situations enables nurses to communicate with each other and with others in the health care system. Standardization of the meanings of words and phrases that represent nursing care are essntial to advance nursing science (Hayakawa and Hayakawa, 1990).

References

Butterfield, P.G. (2002). Upstream reflections on environmental health: An abbreviated history and framework for action. *ANS: Advances in Nursing Science*, *25*, 32–49.

Gebbie, K.M. (1976). *Summary of the second national conference: Classification of nursing daignoses*. St. Louis: National Group for Classification of Nursing Diagnoses.

Getzsche, P.C., and Johansen, H.K. (2008). House dust mite control measures for asthma. *Cochrane Database of Systematic Reviews*, Issue 3, Number CDCD001187.

Gordon, M. (2007). *Manual of nursing diagnosis* (11th ed.). Boston: Jones and Bartlett.

Larsen, P.D. and Lubkin, I.M. (2009). *Chronic illness: Impact and interventions* (7th ed.). Sudbury, Mass.: Jones and Bartlett.

Munhall, P.L. (1993). "Unknowing": Toward another pattern of knowing in nursing. *Nursing Outlook*, *41*, 125–128.

Odermarsky, M., Anderson, S., Pesonen, E., Sjoblad, S., Yia-Herttuala, S., and Liuba, P. (2008). Respiratory infection recurrence and passive smoking in early atherosclerosis in children and adolescents with type 1 diabetes. *European Journal of Clinical Investigation*, *38*, 381–388.

Office of the Professions, New York State Education. (2008). *Definition of Nursing Practice*. Retrieved on September 20, 2008 from http://www.op.nysed.gov/article139.htm.

Pender, N.J., Murdaugh, C.L., and Parsons, M.A. (2006). *Health promotion in nursing practice* (5th ed). Upper Saddle River, NJ: Pearson Prentice Hall.

Redman, B.K. (2005). The ethics of self-management preparation for chronic illness. *Nursing Ethics*, *12*, 360–369.

Rosenberg, S. (2006). Utilizing the language of Jean Watson's caring theory within a computerized clinical documentation system. *CIN: Computers, Informatics, Nursing*, *24*, 53–56.

Stanhope, M., and Lancaster, J. (2006). *Foundations of nursing in the community: Community oriented approach* (2nd ed.). St. Louis: Mosby.

U.S. Department of Health and Human Services, Centers for Disease Control and Prevention. (2007). The state of aging and health in America, 2007. Retrieved on March 7, 2009 from http://www.cdc.gov/aging/pdf/saha_2007.pdf

Watson, J. (2005). *Caring science as sacred science*. Philadelphia, PA: F.A. Davis Company.

Weber, J.R., and Kelley, J. (2006). *Health assessment in nursing* (3rd ed.). Philadelphia: Lippincott, Williams and Wilkins.

World Health Organization. (2007). Global health status. Retrieved on September 9, 2008 from http://www.who.int/global/atlas/

Case Study Application of Strategies

Part II consists of case studies in each of four categories: problem diagnoses, risk diagnoses, health promotion diagnoses, and wellness/strength diagnoses. Cases with more than one type of diagnosis are categorized by the primary diagnosis. The primary references below were used for each and every case study. These references are not cited with the case studies because it would be redundant.

References

Bulechek, G.M., Butcher, H.K., and Dochterman, J.M. (2008). *Nursing Outcomes Classification (NOC)* (4th ed.). St. Louis, MO: Mosby.

Moorhead, S., Johnson, M., Maas, M.L., and Swanson, E. (2008). *Nursing Interventions Classification (NIC)* (5th ed.). St Louis, MO: Mosby.

NANDA International. (2009). *Nursing diagnosis: Definitions and classification, 2009–2011.* Hoboken, NJ: Wiley-Blackwell.

Use of Critical Thinking with Each Case Study

One way to engage with the case studies for learning is to read the cases, formulate analyses, and compare your analyses with the authors' analyses. It is important to accept that your analyses and those of the authors may not be the same because the author was present with the person or family and may have had additional information that was not identified and recorded. In addition, the words of a case study can never fully represent the complexity of a real person or family or the context of the situation. Written case studies are valuable for learning (Lunney, 2008), but to make the best decision, you have to be there. Accepting the complexity of diagnosis in nursing indicates the personal strength of tolerance for ambiguity.

When you see this icon, do the following:

- After listing the possible diagnoses identified in the case (use flexibility, intuition, and open-mindedness), select the diagnoses with the strongest evidence (use logical reasoning, discriminating, analyzing, information seeking, and/or applying standards).
- Considering the person or family's story, identify the most likely priority issue or concern (use contextual perspective).
- Considering the type of setting (e.g., hospital, home), identify the nurse's likely priority concerns (use contextual perspective and applying standards).
- From the most likely diagnoses, consider possible outcomes (use predicting and transforming knowledge) and select the best outcome (or outcomes) for the diagnosis and this consumer (use analyzing, applying standards, discriminating, information seeking, and/or predicting).
- List the nursing interventions that you would select to address the identified outcomes (analyzing, applying standards, flexibility, contextual perspective, confidence, creativity)
- Compare your selections of diagnoses, outcomes, and interventions with those of the author (use applying standards, logical reasoning, predicting, transforming knowledge, flexibility, inquisitiveness, intellectual integrity, open-mindedness, perseverance, and/or reflection).
- Reflect upon the areas of congruence and incongruence between the author's selections and your own (use discriminating, transforming knowledge, open-mindedness, and reflection).
- Accept that in each case, the author had the best clinical judgment because he or she was present with the consumer and experienced more data than he or she was able to include in the written case study.

Reference

Lunney, M. (2008). Current knowledge related to intelligence and thinking with implications for the development and use of case studies. *International Journal of Nursing Terminologies and Classifications, 19,* 158–162.

Abbreviations Used in the Case Studies

ABG	Arterial blood gases
am	Before noon
BID	Two times a day
BP	Blood pressure
BMI	Body mass index
CBC	Complete blood count
CHF	Congestive heart failure
cm	Centimeters
CNS	Clinical nurse specialist
CT	Computerized tomography
D	Dextrose
dl	Deciliter
ED	Emergency department
EKG	Electrocardiogram
F	Fahrenheit
gm	Gram
Hgb	Hemoglobin
Hct	Hematocrit
hg	Mercury
HR	Heart rate
IV	Intravenous
K	Kilograms
L	Left
lb	Pound
m	Minute
mcg	Microgram
mg	Milligram
ml	Milliliter
MRI	Magnetic resonance imaging
mm	Millimeter
mm^3	Millimeter to third degree
NS	Normal saline
pm	After noon
QD	Every day
R	Right
RR	Respiratory rate
SaO_2	Saturated oxygen
T	Temperature
WNL	Within normal limits

Case Studies with a Primary Focus on Problem Diagnoses and Associated Outcomes and Interventions

5.1. Woman Admitted for Diagnostic Testing of a Lung Nodule

Fabiana Gonçalves de Oliveira Azevedo Matos and
Diná de Almeida Lopes Monteiro da Cruz

Ms. AL, a 72-year-old female, was admitted to a Brazilian hospital for diagnosis of an R lung nodule. Ms. AL is single, has no children, and is a retired nurse.

The admitting nurse conducted an assessment using the eleven functional health patterns (Gordon, 1994). Interviewing and examining Ms. AL, the nurse identified possible problems in six different patterns: (1) nutritional-metabolic (lost 8 Kg last year, BMI = 17.5), (2) elimination (for two months has had constipation), (3) sleep-rest (complained that she awakened during the night and got up tired in the morning), (4) activity-exercise (she took walks but stopped in the middle for tiredness, felt tired all day, was afraid of falling while taking a shower, and had an unsteady gait), (5) perceptive-cognitive (felt pain in the legs for about one year, currently hospitalized for pain in chest and shoulder), and (6) coping-stress tolerance (uncomfortable with the uncertainty of the lung problem and pain, "tired" of going to a number of physicians with no diagnoses, family worried about her physical and emotional condition, and smoked to relieve tension).

The nurse thought it was very likely Ms. AL was worried that her problem was lung cancer. Ms. AL had worked for 30 years in a radiological setting, and would be familiar with situations like the one she was living as a patient. The nurse thought that Ms. AL not mentioning this concern could be a sign of a coping problem. Ms. AL also exhibited signs of anxiety.

In extending the pain assessment, the nurse learned that Ms. AL was treating the chronic pain in her legs for three months with opiates. It was after starting the use of opiates that her intestinal problems began. Ms. AL reported that her last bowel movement was the day before hospitalization and she had no abdominal discomfort.

At present, her leg pain was reported as 7 on the 10-point scale and Ms. AL's facial expression was tense and contracted. Ms. AL told Sofia that when she started pain treatment for the leg pain, she also started sleeping better, and pain was not disturbing her sleep anymore, but when the lung problem appeared she started awakening during the night again and was keeping herself awake thinking about the problem. Concomitantly, the leg pain also became worse.

The nurse asked Ms. Al what her most important problem was. Ms. AL said "this pain ... waiting for this exam ... this doubt ... I am very worried and distressed about everything ... I hope it finishes soon."

STOP. THINK. Which diagnoses, outcomes, and interventions would you select?

Submitter's Analysis and Use of NANDA-I, NOC, and NIC

Interpreting Ms. AL's data to arrive at accurate and priority diagnoses required analysis of the situational context and consideration of the length of time that Ms. AL would be under nursing care in the current event. Although Ms. AL presented with many possible health problems, her hospital stay for diagnostic testing would likely be short, one or two days. In an ideally integrated health system, nursing care in acute care settings would be addressed as an adjustment of the working nursing care plan established in the ambulatory care setting, but this was not the case with Ms. AL.

The nurse noted relevant cues for the nursing diagnoses of *anxiety, pain, constipation, impaired walking, risk for falls, fatigue, imbalanced nutrition*, and *insomnia*, and considered that some of these diagnostic hypotheses were associated with each other. The diagnoses of *impaired walking, constipation, fatigue, insomnia*, and *imbalanced nutrition* were excluded.

Impaired walking was ruled out because interventions for this diagnosis were not appropriate for this hospitalization. The major concern with Ms. AL's walking problems in the hospital would be her safety. *Constipation* was ruled out because it was related to taking opiates for leg pain and, as a nurse, Ms. AL knew how to manage this. *Imbalanced nutrition* was ruled out because it was not a priority in Ms. AL circumstance. After the current medical problem was diagnosed and medical treatment started, a complete nursing reassessment would be required to identify Ms. AL's nutritional and other needs.

The nurse encouraged Ms. AL to talk about her worries and at the same time validate the priority diagnoses of *acute pain* and *anxiety*. The pain level of 7 was important and had to be managed for Ms. Al's comfort, so *acute pain related to ineffective control of chronic pain* was accepted as a nursing diagnosis to guide care. Also, the diagnosis of *anxiety* was selected, with rumination, facial tension, insomnia, fatigue, diminished productivity, apprehension, and anorexia as the defining characteristics (Young, Polzin, Todd, and Simuncak, 2002). Ms. AL agreed with the nurse that relieving *pain* and *anxiety* could positively impact her sleep and fatigue. *Risk for falls* was the third diagnosis to be addressed because of Ms. AL's tiredness, muscle weakness, and unsteady gait.

Studies have shown that people who are hospitalized for testing related to a potentially life-threatening illness are likely to develop a higher level of psychological distress than the general population (Fantini, Pedinielli, and Manouvrier, 2007). Ms. AL was probably anticipating a lung cancer diagnosis as a result of the biopsy. Distress and fear of cancer and death were found the major negative aspects of subjects who received screening tests for cancer (McGovern, Gross, Krueger, Engelhard, Cordes, and Church, 2004).

NOC Outcomes

The NOC outcomes that were selected for Ms. AL were *anxiety level*, *pain level*, and *fall prevention behavior*. For *anxiety level*, the baseline score was determined as 2 (substantial) and the target score was set as 3 (moderate). For *pain level*, the baseline score was determined as 2 (substantial) and the target score was set as 4 (mild). For *fall prevention behavior*, the baseline score was identified as 5 (consistently demonstrated) and the goal was to maintain a level of 5.

NIC Interventions

The interventions that were selected to achieve these outcomes and address the nursing diagnoses were *anxiety reduction*, *pain management*, and *fall prevention*. The nurse informed Ms. AL of the intervention focus and Ms. AL agreed with the plan. The nurse obtained information about Ms. AL's pain medications taken at home and her usual reactions to them, and shared this information with her physician. The physician and nurse collaborated on a different analgesic treatment, including medication on an as needed basis. The nurse administered the analgesic, and told Ms. AL to rest and she would return. She also asked Ms. AL to call a nurse as needed using the bell, particularly to get out of bed. The nurse told Ms. AL how to use the bell and left it near her, and also explained to her that the bedrail must be kept elevated to keep her safe.

Thirty minutes later, the nurse returned to Ms. AL who was sleeping. The nurse thought Ms. AL's pain had decreased; this was later confirmed by Ms. AL who said she slept deeply for forty minutes after the medication and scored her pain as 3.

While Ms. AL was sleeping, the nurse found out that Ms. AL's biopsy was scheduled for the next day at 11:00 am. The nurse gave this information to Ms. AL, who agreed to discuss how to manage the expectation until the procedure time. The nurse discussed anxiety with Ms. AL to identify the personal resources that would help her to deal with this stressful situation, and also to give her an opportunity to express her feelings and threats (Fishel, 1998). The nurse listened attentively to Ms. AL, and learned that she was nervous about having lung cancer; that she would like to know the diagnosis as soon as possible, because she had many things to arrange before things got worse. The nurse told Ms. AL she could imagine how difficult it was to deal with the uncertainty and asked her opinion about trying a relaxation technique (Conrad and Roth, 2007). Ms. AL said that when she was young, she practiced progressive relaxation and accepted the nurse's guidance in remembering how to perform it. Ms. AL asked to be left alone to practice the relaxation technique. The nurse accompanied Ms. AL to the toilet, helped her to return to bed, confirmed that light and noise were acceptable, and left Ms. AL alone. The nurse discussed Ms. AL's responses with her physician, who decided to consider an anxiety reducing medication in Ms. AL's prescription after assessing relaxation outcome.

Evaluation

Before shift report, Ms. AL rang the bell and asked for help to position herself for lunch. The nurse noticed that Ms. AL was less tense, and Ms. AL said that she was more comfortable after the relaxation exercise. Ms. AL commented on the details of the relaxation technique and that, in the past, she was able to get better results from relaxation, and that this "was good for body and soul." As Ms. AL showed interest in the technique, the nurse encouraged her to repeat it in the afternoon, assuring her that retraining would improve the results. Ms. AL agreed to repeat the relaxation techniques but said she was not sure that it could completely relieve her tension.

The nurse also evaluated that Ms. AL was free of pain—her *pain level score* was 5 (none)—and that Ms. AL consistently demonstrated *fall prevention behavior* (score = 5). The nurse scored *anxiety level* at 3 (moderate).

References

Conrad, A., and Roth, W.T. (2007). Muscle relaxation therapy for anxiety disorders: It works but how? *Journal of Anxiety Disorders, 21*, 243–64.

Fantini, C., Pedinielli, J.L., and Manouvrier, S. (2007). Psychological distress in applicants for genetic screening for colorectal cancer. *Encephale, 33*, 117–123.

Fishel, A.H. (1998). Nursing management of anxiety and panic. *Nursing Clinics of North America, 33*, 135–151.

Gordon, M. (1994). *Nursing diagnosis: Process and application* (3rd ed.). St. Louis: Mosby.

McGovern, P.M., Gross, C.R., Krueger, R.A., Engelhard, D.A., Cordes, J.E., and Church, T.R. (2004). False-positive cancer screens and health-related quality of life. *Cancer Nursing, 27,* 347–352.

Young, L.K., Polzin, J., Todd, S., and Simuncak, S.L. (2002). Validation of the nursing diagnosis anxiety in adult patients undergoing bone marrow transplant. *International Journal of Nursing Terminologies and Classification, 13,* 88–100.

5.2. Adaptation to the Pain of a Fractured Hip

Alsacia Pacsi, RN, MS, FNP, CEN, CCRN

Teresa S. is a 55-year-old Hispanic woman who was admitted to the ED following a motor vehicle accident. In the ED, an X-ray revealed a hip fracture involving the intracapsular region of the L femur. She was scheduled for an open reduction and internal fixation the same day. She complained of severe pain.

Her vital signs were: BP 130/88, T 98 °F; P 126 and regular; RR 32/m. Teresa was alert and oriented and verbalized appropriate responses to all questions. Breath sounds were clear bilaterally, respirations were even and unlabored. Peripheral pulses presented at 2+ except for the L pedal pulse, which was +1 (weak and thready), and her capillary refill response was five seconds on the L side. The L leg was shorter than the R leg and external rotation was noted. She had "no known allergies."

Teresa was crying and fiddling with her fingers during the assessment. She stated that she had never been hospitalized but confided that she had spent a lot of time at the hospital last year when her husband died of cancer. No significant health history was noted. Teresa said that she usually takes one multivitamin a day and no medications.

Based on the nurse's observation about Teresa's increased agitation, moaning, grimacing, and crying, the nurse decided that she needed to assess the effects of Teresa's current situation. She asked, "Teresa, how do you feel about being hospitalized and having surgery?" Teresa stated that the pain she was experiencing to her L hip and groin area, particularly when she attempted to move it, was unbearable and that it was making her very anxious. Teresa's face was flushed and she stated she was overwhelmed with the severe pain.

The nurse initially asked Teresa to verbally rate her pain using the numeric scale from 0 (no pain) to 10 (the worst possible pain), but she was not able to assign a number to her pain. The nurse then used the Faces Pain Scale—Revised to determine the intensity of Teresa's pain (Hicks, VonBaeyer, Spafford, Korlaar, and Goodenough, 2001). Teresa was able to easily select a face that reflected her pain.

The results confirmed, along with the physiological parameters, that Teresa was in severe pain. The face she selected was the equivalent of a 10 on the 10-point scale. By using the Faces research-based pain assessment tool, in conjunction with obtaining a complete health history and performing a physical examination, the nurse was able to more accurately assess the intensity of the pain.

 STOP. THINK. Which diagnoses, outcomes, and interventions would you select?

Submitter's Analysis and Use of NANDA-I, NOC, and NIC

Using Roy's adaptation model, the nurse viewed Teresa's hip fracture as an event that activated Teresa's adaptation processes (Roy and Andrews, 2008). Teresa's responses to this injury were examples of *regulator subsystem* activity. The regulator subsystem is the adaptive process for physiological stimuli with physiological outcomes and occurs without conscious awareness. First, during the injury process, internal stimuli, both chemical and neural, started endocrine and central nervous system activity to generate physiological responses to the fracture, e.g., local swelling and delayed capillary refill to the affected extremity, tachycardia, tachypnea, and increased blood pressure. External stimuli, e.g., the nurse positioning the affected leg to prevent adduction, also affected her regulator subsystem activity and her body's response to the pain (Roy and Andrews, 2008). The regulator subsystems are interrelated and are actively involved in adaptation processes (Roy and Andrews, 2008).

The second key adaptation process is referred to as the *cognator subsystem*, which occurs with conscious awareness (Roy and Andrews, 2008). This subsystem reacts through four cognitive-emotive channels: perceptual and information processing, learning, judgment, and emotion (Roy and Andrews, 2008). In Teresa's case, dealing with the pain of the fracture resulted in physical, psychological, and social changes. The interpretation that Teresa gave to these stressors influenced her coping processes and fostered adaptation.

The perceptual–psychomotor process linked the cognator subsystem with the regulator subsystem (Roy and Andrews, 2008). Teresa's accident was the external stimulus and the control process was neural and not within conscious control. The stimulus and the nursing diagnosis was *acute pain related to fractured hip*.

Teresa's awareness of the pain was within conscious perception. This perception, which links the cognator and the regulator subsystems, may be altered through past experiences. This process fosters unification of the person to create a biopsychosocial whole.

NOC Outcomes

The NOC outcome that was selected for Teresa was *pain level* because she said that the discomfort in her left leg was unbearable. The baseline score on pain level was 1 (severe) and the goal score was 4 (mild).

NIC Interventions

The NIC interventions selected to address the pain outcome were *pain management, analgesic administration, emotional support*, and *active listening*. The nurse's primary goal was to relieve pain and the secondary goal was to help Teresa develop adaptation processes. The nurse provided physiological support by intravenously administering morphine (4 mg). Parenteral opioid analgesics such as morphine may be given pre-operatively for acute pain control in people with hip fractures (Beaupre, Jones, Saunders, Johnston, Buckingham, and Majumdar, 2005). Morphine relieves pain without causing loss of consciousness, has a rapid onset, peaks in 20 minutes, and lasts for four to five hours. Another reason why morphine was the drug of choice for Teresa was because it decreased the cardiac preload and afterload, having positive results on Teresa's blood pressure, pulse rate, and respirations. Morphine changes the brain's perception of pain, which fosters effective adaptive responses in the cognator and regulator coping subsystems.

The nurse provided emotional support by using touch and empathetic nursing communication, both verbal and nonverbal, to encourage Teresa to verbalize her fears. She maintained a calm, supportive, competent manner when interacting with her. The nurse also used active listening to anticipate Teresa's needs and address her concerns regarding pain management and impending surgery. She provided information centered on the present needs of the patient at a level that was easily understood and encouraged questions and clarification of information given.

Shortly thereafter, pre-operative blood was drawn and sent to the laboratory. The surgeon obtained consent from Teresa for the surgery, the pre-operative checklist was completed, and a report was given to the operating room nurse informing her that morphine IV (4 mg) was given for pain.

While Teresa was in the ED, the nurse continued to use the Faces scale to measure changes in pain level because studies found that older adults and Hispanics favored the Faces scale when attempting to quantify their pain level (Ware, Epps, Herr, and Packard, 2006). This was important because pain may be underestimated in aging adults, so nurses and health care providers need to use pain rating scales that facilitate accurate assessment, diagnosis, and the development of a pain management plan that meets the person's individual needs (Flaherty, 2008).

Evaluation

Using the NOC rating system, Teresa's target score on the outcome of *pain level* went from 1 (severe) to 4 (mild). Her vital signs were BP 120/72, P 82, RR 18 and T 98.6 °F by mouth. As a result of the interventions, Teresa was able to integrate physiological, psychological, social, and interdependence responses to adapt to the situation (Roy and Andrews, 2008).

References

Beaupre, L., Jones, A., Saunders, L. Johnston, D., Buckingham, J. and Majumdar, A. (2005). Best practices for elderly hip fracture patients: A systematic overview of the evidence. *Journal of Internal Medicine*, *20*,1019–1025.

Flaherty, E. (2008). Using pain–rating scales with older adults: The numeric rating scales, verbal descriptor scale and Faces Pain Scale–Revised. *American Journal of Nursing*, *108* (6), 40–47.

Hicks C., von Baeyer C., Spafford P., van Korlaar, I., and Goodenough B. (2001). The *Faces Pain Scale* CT: *Revised*. Retrieved July 24, 2008, from www.painsourcebook.ca

Roy, C. and Andrews, H. (2008). *The adaptation model* (3rd ed.). Norwalk, CT: Appleton-Lange.

Ware, J., Epps, C., Herr, K. and Packard, A. (2006). Evaluation of the Revised Faces Pain Scale, Verbal Descriptor Scale, Numeric Rating Scale, and Iowa Pain Thermometer in older minority adults. *Pain Management Nursing*, *7*, 117–125.

5.3. Acute Presentation of an Elderly Woman with Cancer

Mary Pilossoph, RN, MA, NP

Mrs. D is an 80-year-old woman of Irish descent who is quite proud of her heritage. For example, she said, "We are eligible for the Daughters of the American Revolution, we go back so far." She presented to the breast cancer clinic with mobility-limiting pain of the L hip and midback rated as 10 by Mrs. D, in spite of using analgesics that had previously given her relief. An MRI was positive for "metastatic lesions of the L ischium and T12 spine." Ten years ago, she had a bilateral mastectomy for breast cancer, followed by five years of Tamoxifen for estrogen receptor and progesterone receptor positive (ER/PR+) disease. Since then, there has been no evidence of disease.

Approximately five months ago, Mrs. D developed L hip and thigh pain that was diagnosed as sciatica based on a negative lumbar-sacral X-ray and clinical presentation of back pain radiating down the L leg. She received PT during that time, but has suffered increased pain in the last two months. An MRI was ordered of the spine and hips one week ago, with results provided yesterday to Mrs. D. Mrs. D's daughter scheduled an appointment with this office based on Mrs. D's history of breast cancer.

She has three adult children, two daughters and one son, who live near her and are involved in her care. One of her daughters was in attendance at the time of the initial evaluation, providing physical and emotional support. Mrs. D expressed that she sees herself as "lucky that all my diseases so far have been fixable" and stated, "I have a high tolerance for stress." She feels that she puts things in perspective, has faith in God, and relies on this faith in times of trouble, which "gives me peace." When asked if she was surprised or concerned that the cancer had come back, she stated she was glad that at long last they figured out the source of the pain.

Mrs. D's other medical history includes Schizo-affective disorder for 50 years that is well managed with Stelazine (10 mg) daily. She was hospitalized for a psychotic episode two years ago, one year after her physician cancelled her anti-psychotic medication after 50 years of use because she was stable. Reinstitution of medications resolved her symptoms, but resulted in a change of living situation from senior housing to assisted living placement. Mrs. D has been treated for hypertension for 12 years.

At the breast cancer clinic, the NP's physical examination revealed atrophy of the L quadriceps and tightening of the L hamstring. The remainder of the data was non-contributory. She could not bear weight on the L leg. Based on her history of ER/PR+ breast cancer she was presumptively diagnosed with metastatic breast cancer to the bone. Mrs. D. was given a fentanyl patch in the lowest dose of 25 mcg in 72 hours, a slow-release opioid narcotic. An intravenous bisphosphanate was administered, and arrangements were made to admit Mrs. D to the hospital for evaluation by radiation oncology. She was started on an aromatase inhibitor, in light of her history of ER/PR+ breast cancer to presumptively treat metastatic lesions to the bone and decrease the risk of further metastasis. A full work-up was planned to rule out other metastatic sites.

Upon admission to the inpatient unit, Mrs. D revealed to the nurse her concern about relieving her leg pain; she was hoping that now that they knew the source of the pain they would have better success at controlling it. Mrs. D had a pain score on admission of 9 on movement, 7 at rest. She was also concerned about wanting to get up and go to the bathroom independently while in the hospital, she felt "insecure" on her feet with the pain and weakness in her L leg but she didn't want to "bother" the nurses.

STOP. THINK. Which diagnoses, outcomes, and interventions would you select?

Submitter's Analysis and Use of NANDA-I, NOC, and NIC

The following two top priority nursing diagnoses were developed with Mrs. D: *acute pain* related to metastatic lesions and nerve compression in T12 spine and L ischium at insertion of acetabulum, and *risk for falls* related to weakness and pain in L leg, unfamiliarity with hospital surroundings, and reluctance to call staff for help. Characteristics of Mrs. D that contributed to her risk of falls were her age, having cancer, and having pain that needed to be treated with drugs (Close, 2005; Holley, 2002). Managing Mrs. D's pain began prior to admission, but initiation of a narcotic for a woman who is receiving anti-psychotic medication warrants close monitoring for dose adjustment and increased risk for falls related to possible change in mental status.

NOC Outcomes

The nursing outcome of *pain level* was scored as 1 (severe) and the goal was set as 3 (moderate). On the 10-point pain scale, the goals were 4 to 5 on movement and 0 at rest. The outcome related to her fall risk was *falls occurrence* with a baseline score of 5 and a goal of 5, i.e., no (0) falls while in the hospital.

NIC Interventions

Nursing interventions to achieve acute pain relief were discussed with Mrs. D and her family. The agreed-upon intervention for acute pain relief was *pain management*. This included immediate application of a Fentanyl patch, and use of Actiq, a short-acting narcotic, for break-through pain when movement was necessary. Another activity was monitoring every 30 minutes during the first 12 hours for untoward side effects, especially changes in mental status. Proactive prevention of constipation was initiated with Senokot (two tablets twice a day), so as not to obscure the signs and symptoms of possible impending spinal cord compression (*constipation*).

Mrs. D and her family collaborated with the nurses in the discussion of her fall risk and participated in the planning. The NIC intervention of *fall prevention* was initiated with Mrs. D being placed on the hospital's high risk fall protocol. This included rounding by nurses and ancillary staff every 30 minutes and documentation of this on the fall prevention log, every half hour mental status assessment, every two hour assessment of Mrs. D's ability to use the call bell, and every half hour assessment of Mrs. D's understanding of the requirement to use the call bell. In a review of research studies, it was determined that falls can be prevented with older people when there is sufficient attention given to fall prevention protocols (Close, 2005). It was decided that it was not appropriate at this point in time for Mrs. D to be able to inde-pendently get out of bed (OOB). The nurses continued to assess her understanding of this, as well as her ability to locate and press the call bell.

Evaluation

Eight hours later an evaluation of Mrs. D's status revealed a score on the 10-point pain scale of 8 on movement and 0 at rest. The Actiq helped to reduce the pain when getting out of bed. Mrs. D had no falls while in the hospital, and she continued to communicate her under-standing of the need to call for assistance and demonstrated ability to do so on regular assessments of nursing staff. She said to the staff, "you must really mean it; you keep asking me about this!" There were no episodes of attempts to get OOB without assistance. Mrs. D reported that assistance was available when she needed to get OOB to the bathroom and used the call bell. Mrs. D's pain score continued on a downward trend without untoward effect on her mental status or bowel regimen. The plan was continued, as deemed effective, to maintain her 0 falls status and until pain outcomes were achieved.

Mrs. D. received inpatient radiation until her improved symptoms allowed her to be discharged from the hospital and radiation continued from an inpatient rehabilitation setting, from which she returned to her assisted living arrangements with only minor additional assistance in housekeeping. Mrs. D. returned to the clinic one month post discharge and a CT of the thoracic spine and L hip revealed healing post radiation with no evidence of disease present; the metastatic lesions were gone and her breast cancer tumor marker level had returned to a normal level. Mrs. D. was ambulating independently with a walker for support and stated she was pain free. Mrs. D. was a very different woman upon return to the clinic and many of the nursing staff did not recognize her, and were certainly thrilled with her great outcome.

References

Close, J.C.T. (2005). Prevention of falls in older people. *Disability and Rehabilitation*, 27, 1061–1071.

Holley, S. (2002). A look at the problem of falls among people with cancer. *Clinical Journal of Oncology Nursing*, 6, 193–197.

5.4. Substance Abuse Crisis Associated with Stress Overload

Sondra A. Rivera, RN, MSN-Ed

LAR is a 48-year-old Hispanic male admitted to the ED by ambulance. In the initial assessment, he was confused, lethargic, and anxious when responding to questions. He was oriented to person, but was unable to identify place or time. The police and paramedics reported finding him naked with an unidentified white substance. LAR is a hotel manager who resides in a suite at the hotel. He was able to report at that time that he took a drug and immediately felt uneasy. He said that he thought the drug he purchased was cocaine. Later, the toxicology results revealed the substance was angel dust. LAR stated the time of ingestion was approximately 11 pm on Friday. LAR was found semi-conscious on Saturday about 5 pm. LAR was able to provide information on who to contact in his family.

When LAR arrived on the medical unit, initial assessment was performed using the functional health pattern framework (Gordon, 2008). Upon admission to the unit, LAR was fluent in conversation when alert, but transient between alert and stupor. He became agitated when recalling the events of his ingestion of a substance he believed was cocaine. Nevertheless, he was eager to talk about what happened. He said that when he was unable to move following ingestion of the drug, he saw and heard a battle between what he believed was God and the Devil.

LAR reported having severe pain rated at 10+ in his R lower extremity with limited movement. Unable to move, LAR was found in his hotel suite lying on his right side. The timeline estimation was approximately 16 hours.

LAR is divorced and has had many long- and short-term relationships. He has one adult son, 27 years old, who resides in Germany. Currently he is not in a relationship, but he has had multiple sex partners of the opposite sex. LAR stated, "I am glad that my son and former women friends are not here to see me in this condition." He verbalized sadness and shame about the trouble he caused his siblings.

LAR stated he usually eats frequently during the day and does not follow a particular diet. His usual diet consists of starches, red meat, and sweetened ice tea. He usually has daily protein drinks to enhance his physical appearance. His admission diet was clear liquids with fluid restriction of 1,000 ml a day with strict intake and output monitoring.

LAR denied any pain, discomfort, or loss of continence prior to admission. The admission report, however, noted he was incontinent of urine. An indwelling Foley catheter and a 24-hour urine collection were initiated. The results of the urine collection led to the medical diagnosis of early stages of acute renal failure indicated by increased blood levels of creatinine and blood urea nitrogen, as well as decreased urine output. The concluding medical diagnosis was rhabdomyolysis—the release of myoglobin from skeletal muscles into the bloodstream. LAR's muscle injury was a result of his prolonged 16-hour immobility. Urine specimens were obtained to analyze acidity and alkaline (pH) levels, which is one indicator for acute renal failure as a sequelae to rhabdomyolysis. LAR stated that he usually engages in anaerobic and aerobic exercises daily and takes vitamin supplements. LAR was on bed rest until the medical diagnosis was decided.

LAR stated that he usually slept four to six hours when working the night shift and six to eight hours when working the day shift. Since the "hallucination" about God and the Devil, he fears sleeping.

LAR verbalized the emotions of isolation and despair since he relocated for employment. Prior to relocating, he lived near his two siblings, who visited at various times in his hospitalization.

He displayed increased nervousness when he discussed his substance abuse and his unknown health status. LAR stated a "terrifying feeling" and "weird discomfort . . ." regarding ". . . God won the battle for my soul." LAR expressed feelings of shame and embarrassment about drugs and being found naked.

LAR said he was sexually active with multiple partners of the opposite sex and he used condoms for protection. He agreed to tests for human immunodeficiency virus (HIV) and sexually transmitted disease (STD); the results were negative.

LAR admitted to functioning in high stress work situations. He said that, with the distance from his family, he has not adjusted well. LAR spoke about having an "uneasy feeling" when purchasing this substance from a street dealer, and admitted to having poor judgment and regret. LAR expressed fear regarding his immobility and its possible effect on his independence.

LAR stated that he has a strong spiritual belief system and, prior to relocating for employment, he attended church with his family on a weekly basis. LAR asked to see a chaplain and to visit the hospital chapel. He prayed daily with his family and the nursing staff.

STOP. THINK. Which diagnoses, outcomes, and interventions would you select?

Submitter's Analysis and Use of NANDA-I, NOC, and NIC

Two diagnoses that were initially considered but ruled out as priority diagnoses were *impaired urinary elimination* and *risk for falls*. His elimination problems at this time were caused by his altered consciousness and were not due to an underlying etiology, and they were expected to resolve with time; there was no need for nursing interventions other than following the medical plan of care for rhabdomyolysis. The nursing diagnosis of *impaired urinary elimination* would not add more information for nurses to help LAR with his health status. *Risk for falls* was a potential risk, not an actual occurrence, and because LAR was on strict bed rest and closely monitored, the risk was reduced and less of an immediate priority.

The two diagnoses that were derived from the data and validated with LAR to guide nursing care were *acute pain* and *ineffective coping* related to stress overload and use of ineffective coping strategies. The selection of *acute pain* as a priority diagnosis was based on the cues that his pain was rated as 10+ on the 10-point scale and he had limited movement of his right lower extremity. When assessing and discussing the current situation with LAR, including his substance abuse, he agreed with the second diagnosis of *ineffective coping*. He confirmed that he experienced stress overload from the job relocation, the challenges of the job, lack of sleep, the absence of social supports, and a sense of isolation.

NOC Outcomes

The NOC outcome selected with LAR for the *acute pain* diagnosis was *pain level*. His overall baseline score was 1 (severe) and the target score for the first day was 3 (moderate) and a subsequent goal was set as 5 (none).

The NOC outcome selected for the *ineffective coping* diagnosis was *coping*. The baseline score was determined to be 3 (sometimes demonstrated) and the target score was 4 (often demonstrated). It was planned that the two other outcomes that would be tracked while he was hospitalized were *psychosocial adjustment* and *risk control: alcohol and drug use*. His baseline scores on these outcomes were 3 (sometimes demonstrated) and the target scores were 5 (consistently demonstrated).

NIC Interventions

The NIC interventions for *acute pain* were *medication management, guided imagery,* and *meditation facilitation.* Medication administration provided pain relief by bringing his pain down from 10+ to 3, 4, and 5. Initially, morphine intramuscular (IM) was administered for LAR's acute pain. With his addiction history, however, it was important to wean him off potential habit-forming medication before it became a primary focus for LAR. The change from morphine IM to methadone by mouth (PO) was effective in facilitating LAR's collaboration in his treatment, including *guided imagery.* When his pain levels were tolerable or below 5 on the 10-point scale, *guided imagery* was used to direct his attention away from the pain. For both *guided imagery* and *mediation facilitation,* he was assisted to perform deep breathing. Both medication and meditation gave LAR a sense of control and enhanced his perception and ability to focus on a positive approach to coping strategies for *acute pain* as well as the stressors he had been experiencing. The *medication administration* and *meditation facilitation* enabled him to participate in active and passive ranges of motion while on bedrest and engage in physical therapy. In studies of both acute and chronic pain, meditation was shown to reduce pain and have positive effects on the quality of life (Morone, Lynch, Greco, Tindle, and Weiner, 2008; Praissman, 2008; Teixeira, 2008).

LAR articulated his situation with blunt honesty, and he was receptive to the nurses' interventions for *ineffective coping.* The NIC interventions used were *emotional support, counseling, meditation facilitation,* and *spiritual support.*

Emotional support was implemented by actively listening to LAR while he openly discussed his actions and fears and expressed hope that he would not resume taking illegal drugs when he felt stress overload. *Emotional support* also included praying with LAR and allowing him the opportunity to feel heard as he vented feelings and questioned his actions.

For *spiritual support,* the nurse arranged a visit by the chaplain and prayed with LAR. Theoretical models of nursing and research studies have substantiated that *spiritual support* is an important nursing responsibility and was shown to be connected with the illness experience (Burkhart and Hogan, 2008; van Leeuwen, Tiesinga, Jochemsen, and Post, 2007). Referrals were made to Alcoholics Anonymous and the nurse contacted the Veterans Administration to identify support groups for him and opportunities for rehabilitation. LAR had strong family support and all discussions included the family.

Evaluation

At the time of discharge planning on the 21st day after admission, the outcome of *pain level* was rated as 4 (mild) and the outcome of *coping* was rated as 4 (often demonstrated).

LAR's acute renal failure and rhabdomyolysis reversed without medical intervention. Physical therapy was therapeutic in ambulating LAR with the use of a cane and then independently. LAR reported pain had decreased below 3 on the 10-point scale. He openly conversed about his history of drug use with his family, chaplain, physicians, nurses, and psychiatrist. LAR decided to terminate his current employment and return to his hometown with his family to seek other employment.

References

Burkhart, L., and Hogan, N. (2008). An experiential theory of spiritual care in nursing practice. *Qualitative Health Research, 18*, 928–938.

Gordon, M. (2008). *Manual of nursing diagnosis*. (12th ed.). New York: McGraw Hill.

Morone, N.E., Lynch, C.S., Greco, C.M., Tindle, H.A., and Weiner, D.K. (2008). "I feel like a new person." The effects of mindfulness meditation on older adults with chronic pain: Qualitative narrative analysis of diary entries. *Journal of Pain, 9*, 841–848.

Praissman, S. (2008). Mindfulness-based stress reduction: A literature review and clinician's guide. *Journal of American Academy of Nurse Practitioners, 20*, 212–216.

Teixeira, M.E. (2008). Meditation as an intervention for chronic pain: An integrative review. *Holistic Nursing Practice, 22*, 225–234.

van Leeuwen, R., Tiesinga, L.J., Jochemsen, H., and Post, D. (2007). Aspects of spirituality concerning illness. *Scandinavian Journal of Caring Science, 21*, 482–489.

5.5. Communication of Perceptions and Mechanical Ventilation

Catherine Paradiso, RN, MS, APRN, BC

Mrs. M is a 55-year-old woman with acutely exacerbated chronic obstructive pulmonary disease (COPD) admitted to the medical ICU. She is a Mexican immigrant who speaks English. She works as a cashier in a local delicatessen and is a single woman with three children ages 35, 30, and 20. Her daughters reported that she had a cold for several weeks, but did not seek medical attention because she has no health insurance and the clinic hours interfere with her work hours. As she continued to go to work, she became increasingly ill, had an episode of severe shortness of breath, and was rushed to the ED. There, she was placed on mechanical ventilation, with settings of volume control 10, tidal volume 700, and fraction of inspired oxygen 40%.

Although Mrs. M had some recent EKG changes, she was sleeping peacefully when a resident physician visited. He examined her while asleep, and then awakened her suddenly. She began to stir and tried to communicate with him by moving her lips. He did not respond, but she remained calm at that point.

The physician looked directly at her and said, "I am going to put a catheter in your heart." Then, he exited the room and asked the nurse to prepare for a Swan-Ganz insertion because he suspected that the EKG changes were related to an impending MI. She had a history of CHF so early hemodynamic monitoring would benefit the diagnostic process.

The nurse entered the room and found Mrs. M trying to talk and the ventilator alarms blaring. The nurse gave her a pad and pencil and Mrs. M wrote down "hurt," touched her chest, and began to shake her head. The entire time she tried to speak in a way that moved air from her lungs against the ventilator air moving into her airway, causing the ventilator alarm to constantly ring.

The physician re-entered the room and said "She is very nervous, give her a valium to calm her down." With this, she started waving her arms widely. Mrs. M wrote on the blackboard that she previously had a "bad" reaction to a sedating drug.

Health History

Mrs. M is an undocumented person with a 10th grade education who came to America five years ago; her children are also undocumented. There was no reliable history provided from her early years, but, as a patient of the clinic, there was a history of cigarette smoking (two packages a day), asthma, chronic obstructive pulmonary disease, and past episode of CHF.

STOP. THINK. Which diagnoses, outcomes, and interventions would you select?

Submitter's Analysis and Use of NANDA–I, NOC, and NIC

The physician's request that Mrs. M be given valium was based on an assumption that Mrs. M was experiencing *anxiety*. The nurse questioned the advisability of giving this drug because she believed that this was an incorrect assumption. The possibility of an inaccurate diagnosis of *anxiety* was checked by the nurse before administering the drug. With Mrs. M being intubated, verbal statements related to anxiety could not be established, but the nurse was able to assess for the objective defining characteristics of *anxiety*, which are very similar to those of *fear* (Bay and Algase, 1999; Schulz, 2006).

Mrs. M first mentioned "hurt," so the nurse thought she was afraid of pain. Second, she became increasingly more agitated at the mention of valium. These two cues revealed that Mrs. M knew what was making her agitated and was trying to tell the nurse.

Instead of *anxiety*, the nurse explored the diagnosis of *fear of pain* associated with placing a catheter in the heart. When the nurse asked Mrs. M to validate the diagnosis of *fear* and gave Mrs. M the blackboard to write her answer, Mrs. M responded that this was correct. Also, because of Mrs. M's exaggerated response to the suggestion of a sedating drug, the nurse asked about this response as well. Mrs. M's behavior produced further stress because Mrs. M had been sedated in the past and had a "bad" experience. While valium may not produce the same reaction, she perceived that it would, creating another source of *fear*. The resulting agitation led to increased myocardial oxygen consumption, worsened by the actions of trying to talk above the ventilator, which further reduced her oxygen intake. With these data, the nurse made a diagnosis of *fear of* pain associated with the Swan-Ganz procedure and perceptions of sedation.

Based on Sullivan's theory of anxiety versus fear, with fear the object can be identified, whereas with anxiety the source is "obscure and infinitely varied" (Schulz, 2006, p. 111). With the similarity in objective characteristics of the two diagnoses, identifying the source of the feeling enabled the nurse to differentiate the diagnosis of *fear* from *anxiety*. The interventions for these diagnoses are different, so accuracy was important. For *anxiety*, the interventions focus on helping the person to relax. For *fear*, the interventions focus on mitigating or removing the source of the fear. The nurse did not give the valium and informed the physician so that another medication, or possibly no medication, could be substituted.

With mechanical ventilation there were some diagnoses that the nurse routinely implemented to meet the unit-based standards of care. These were *risk of infection, impaired bed mobility, impaired verbal communication, powerlessness, risk for constipation, self-care deficit,* and *feeding self care deficit*. The outcomes and interventions for these diagnoses were standardized in this setting and the nurse applied them for routine care of Mrs. M.

NOC Outcomes

The NOC outcome that was selected for the diagnosis of *fear* was *fear level* with a baseline score of 3 (moderate) and a target score of 5 (none). Airway patency is always a priority, and the case describes how Mrs. M opposed air entry in her excitement, and reduced the response of mechanical ventilation, making the outcome of *respiratory status* a concern beyond the routine application of this outcome. For this outcome, the baseline score was determined as 2 (substantial deviation from normal range) and a target score was set as 5 (no deviation from normal range). A third outcome of *mechanical ventilation response: adult* was applied with baseline score of 4 (mild deviation from normal range) and a target score of 5 (no deviation).

NIC Interventions

The NIC interventions to address Mrs. M's *fear level* were *emotional support, environmental management, family presence facilitation,* and *preparatory sensory information*. The activities described in these interventions somewhat overlap; all activities were focused on the reduction of fear. For *emotional support*, the nurse used soft, calm touch. Then supportively, slowly, and patiently, the nurse explained to Mrs. M what would happen with the insertion of the catheter, that it would not hurt, and the valium would not be given.

The interventions of *environmental management* and *family presence facilitation* were accomplished by asking Mrs. M if she wanted a family member to be with her during the procedure. Mrs. M nodded her head for "yes," so the nurse called the daughter at home to ask her to come as soon as possible. When the daughter arrived, the nurse explained the situation to her slowly and calmly.

Preparatory sensory information was carried out by describing in concrete terms exactly what was going to happen and how she would feel during the Swan-Ganz insertion. Mrs. M was assured that the nurse would be with her throughout the procedure. During the procedure, the nurse used distraction and encouraged deep breathing to help Mrs. M focus on other things besides the procedure taking place.

The NIC intervention that was used to meet the outcome of *mechanical ventilation response: adult* was *mechanical ventilation*. In collaboration with the physician and the respiratory therapist, the nurse managed the mechanical ventilation so that Mrs. M would obtain maximum benefits from this intervention.

Evaluation

With the correct diagnoses to guide care, all outcomes met the target score of 5 (no deviation from normal range). With *emotional support, preparatory sensory information,* and the presence of nurse and daughter during catheter insertion, Mrs. M was able to easily move through the procedure.

References

Bay, E.J., and Algase, D.L. (1999). Fear and anxiety: A simultaneous concept analysis. *Nursing Diagnosis: The Journal of Nursing Language and Classification, 10,* 103–111.

Schulz, C.G. (2006). Applying Sullivan's theory of anxiety versus fear. *Psychiatry, 69,* 110–112.

5.6. Preparing for Orthopedic Surgery with Other Health Problems

June M. Como, RN, MSA, MS, CCRN, CCNS

Mrs. Y is a well-groomed, 79-year-old married woman who was discharged from the coronary care unit of a local hospital. She had been undergoing medical clearance for L total hip replacement when it was discovered that her coronary artery stent had occluded by 90%. She underwent immediate placement of two coronary stents and then transferred to the coronary care unit. She experienced mild cardiac decompensation related to a reperfusion dysrhythmia, which was controlled pharmacologically with beta-blockers during her three-day stay. Her previous history was significant for angioplasty with stent, osteoarthritis for 21 years, and previous R total hip replacement. She was referred to home care for follow up, pain management, and teaching.

Mrs. Y was alert and oriented to her surroundings, scoring 30 (within normal limits) on the mini-mental health screening tool (Souder and O'Sullivan, 2000). She had bibasilar fine crackles, rate of 22/m, and mild exertional dyspnea. Mrs. Y shared that she had been feeling better the last two days. Medications included furosemide (20 mg QD), atenolol (50 mg BID), and aspirin 81 mg QD. Cardiac assessment was unremarkable with no dependant edema, and heart sounds S1 and S2. Blood pressure was 126/76, no orthostatic changes, regular HR of 72, and capillary refill less than 3 seconds. Bowel sounds were normal. At 5'4" she weighed 196 lbs with a BMI of 34. The genitourinary system was unremarkable. Musculoskeletal system problems included altered joint mobility and pain ranging on a scale from 5/10 to 10/10, limiting her ability to be active.

The quality of pain was described as "grating, sending hot, searing pain through my whole body and shoots down my leg." Any form of movement initiated the pain but she tried to bear it and stated, "I have had this pain for over a year now." She used a quad cane when ambulating. She relied heavily on the quad cane with strain evident on her face as facial grimacing. Walking up steps "was impossible" and limited her desire to leave the apartment. Relief of pain occurred by "not moving" or by taking "the medicine the doctor prescribed (hydroco-done) when I can no longer bear it." Effects of the pain were anxiety, anticipation of the pain, difficulty in resting, irritability "with my husband and family" and crying when it was "a 10." Postponement of hip surgery led to Mrs. Y's great concern and disappointment because she had "mentally prepared" herself for the surgery and then became unsure of whether to proceed with hip surgery or not. She stated that she had three grown children who helped her whenever needed.

STOP. THINK. Which diagnoses, outcomes, and interventions would you select?

Submitter's Analysis and Use of NANDA-I, NOC, and NIC

The home health care (HHC) nurse used Watson's model of caring to implement a transpersonal relationship with Mrs. Y (Watson, 1985, 2005). Mrs. Y, her family, and the HHC nurse worked together so that the care plan would be based on both the symptomatology and Mrs. Y's health experiences, chronic illness, previous hospitalization, and impending hip surgery. The use of various established tools, e.g., a family assessment tool, comprised the technical processes needed for diagnosis.

Mrs. Y had just been released from the hospital post cardiac stent placement with mild decompensated heart failure; however, the HHC nurse's physical assessment revealed that she was stable and had more pressing issues. The nurse conducted a family assessment involving her husband and initiated a phone conference with her children to support and facilitate a family-centered approach to care.

Understanding the interrelatedness of chronic pain, stress, and the psychophysiologic impact it had on mobility, weight management, sleep patterns, family interactions, anxiety levels, and cardiac status, the nurse and Mrs. Y decided on *chronic pain* as the nursing diagnosis priority (Chapman, Tuckett, and Song, 2008; Hwang, Kim, Kim, Park, and Kim, 2008; Larsen and Lubkin, 2009).

Imbalanced nutrition: more than body requirements was also selected because weight control measures would be important in both her cardiac and perioperative care. Her weight was 20% above normal with a BMI of 34. Weight loss would positively impact pain levels, mobility, and the perioperative progress once she was cleared for hip surgery.

The diagnosis of *impaired physical mobility* was also selected because improvements in mobility would enhance Mrs. Y's ability to control her weight and improve cardiovascular status through motion. Mrs. Y's *impaired physical mobility* was related to pain from severe osteo-arthritis and fatigue with mild dyspnea from her cardiac status. Participation in activities of daily living and ability to do aerobic and strengthening activities of the upper body were impaired and Mrs. Y felt that she would feel much better if she were able to participate in these activities. She often felt that it was a burden to her family that she could not participate in family activities related to her "problems." The negative consequences of immobility affect every body system and social interaction abilities.

NOC Outcomes

Pain control was chosen as the most important nursing outcome. Mrs. Y's overall rating was 2 (rarely demonstrated). The nurse and Mrs. Y set the target rating as 4 (often demonstrated).

The second nursing outcome that they decided upon was *weight loss behavior*. Mrs. Y's baseline rating was 2 (rarely demonstrated). The target rating was set as 4 (often demonstrated) with a target weekly weight loss of 0.5 lb.

In addition, the outcome of *mobility* was selected. Her baseline score was 2 (substantially compromised), with only the indicator of walking being used. They decided that the goal score was 3 (moderately compromised).

NIC Interventions

Professional caring, characterized by the nature of the interpersonal encounter that took place between Mrs. Y and the HHC nurse, was implemented throughout this case (Watson, 1985, 2005) and illustrated through documentation using NANDA-I, NOC, and NIC (Rosenberg, 2006). Transpersonal caring sought to connect Mrs. Y with the nurse through the process of caring during caring moments. Caring moments occurred whenever the nurse and Mrs. Y came together with their own life stories, phenomenal fields, and emic views that supported the groundwork for movement to a higher state of wellness. The nurse shared her phenomenal field with Mrs. Y through caring processes such as assessment, collaborative planning with her and her family, and evaluation of the outcomes of care. Outcomes were optimized when Mrs. Y's characteristics and the nurse's competencies matched through an active mixing of knowledge, skills, experience, and attitudes needed to meet her needs (Curley, 1998). Mrs. Y sometimes felt that she was able to cope with the stressors in her life but that the chronic pain interfered with her social life, exercise, and participation in family activities. Interventions to address chronic pain would improve her ability to mobilize, socialize, and manage her nutritional balance.

The interventions of *pain management* and *analgesic administration* were implemented first. The primary care physician, pain management specialist, and nurse discussed the *pain management* regimen. A comprehensive regimen was instituted, including a slow release narcotic patch with rescue oral pain relievers when needed. The following interventions were slowly incorporated into the ongoing plan of care: *active listening, heat/cold application, humor, music therapy, progressive muscle relaxation, massage, guided imagery,* and *relaxation therapy.*

Weight reduction assistance was initiated with a goal of 0.5 lb loss a week to address the outcome of *weight loss behavior.* Fruit and vegetable consumption was low; she never ate 5 to 6 servings of fruit and vegetables a day. The nutritional program included a low salt/low fat diet, a heavy reliance on the use of fruits and vegetables, provision of daily fiber, and vitamins for the metabolic function and healing needed to prepare for surgery (Dudek, 2006).

Energy management was implemented to address fatigue from her recent hospitalization and from chronic pain. This involved correction of physiologic deficits, selection of interventions to improve energy, and ensuring adequate nutritional intake. Physical activity was made possible by alternating rest periods. The nurse explored Mrs. Y's prior exercise experiences and her progress with exercise was monitored weekly. After consulting with a physical therapist for assistance in planning the exercise regimen, *exercise therapy: ambulation* resulted in more independence through the use of a walker.

Telephone follow-up was important so the nurse could answer any questions or concerns that Mrs. Y and her family had. A continuing relationship with Mrs. Y was established that helped her maintain her medication, exercise, and dietary regimens.

Evaluation

Pain control was achieved; Mrs. Y reached her overall target of 4. Nursing interventions geared toward chronic pain reduction proved helpful for Mrs. Y as evidenced by her statement "I can now lay down in the afternoon and really rest. I close my eyes and think of something pleasant while my husband gently rubs my hip and I sleep!" Mrs. Y was able to be pain free (level of 3/10) with the new regimen and started to participate in more social activities, which eventually had a positive impact on weight reduction.

The overall score on *weight loss behavior* was rated as 4 at the six-week follow-up. Mrs. Y was able to achieve a loss of 2 lbs by the third week. This was related to her dietary control and improved mobility but also to a new cardiac regimen. At six weeks she had lost 6 lbs, exceeding the goal of 0.5 lb a week.

The *mobility* outcome went from a baseline score of 2 to a rating of 4, which exceeded the target of 3. Mrs. Y was now using a walker, which provided her with more confidence in walking than with the quad cane. Her pain management regimen had substantially reduced her pain so that she was more mobile and she reengaged in important activities of daily living.

Restoration of Mrs. Y to an optimum level of wellness defined by herself was the desired outcome that was attained through the transpersonal relationship. Validation of feelings and experiences through the transpersonal caring relationship using clinical carative processes helped Mrs. Y move toward positive outcomes. Although Mrs. Y was not able to have the hip surgery as soon as she had wanted, her motivation in remaining with the prescribed plan resulted in medical clearance and surgery two years post re-stent.

References

Chapman, C., Tuckett, R., and Song, C. (2008). Pain and stress in a systems perspective: Reciprocal neural, endocrine, and immune interactions. *Journal of Pain, 9*, 122–145.

Curley, M.A.Q. (1998). Patient-nurse synergy: Optimizing patients' outcomes. *American Journal of Critical Care, 7*, 64–72.

Dudek, S.G. (2006). *Nutrition essentials for nursing practice* (4th ed.). Philadelphia: Lippincott.

Hwang, G., Kim, S., Kim, H., Park, S., and Kim, S. (2008). Influence of psychological stress on physical pain. *Stress and Health: Journal of the International Society for the Investigation of Stress, 24*, 159–164.

Larsen, P.D. and Lubkin, I.M. (2009). *Chronic illness: Impact and interventions* (7th ed.). Sudbury, Mass.: Jones and Bartlett.

Rosenberg, S. (2006). Utilizing the language of Jean Watson's caring theory within a computerized clinical documentation system. *CIN: Computers, Informatics, Nursing, 24*, 53–56.

Souder, E. and O'Sullivan, P. (2000). Nursing documentation versus standardized assessment of cognitive status in hospitalized medical patients. *Applied Nursing Research, 13*, 29–36

Watson, J. (1985). *Nursing: The philosophy and science of caring*. Niwot, CO: University Press of Colorado.

Watson, J. (2005). *Caring science as sacred science*. Philadelphia, PA: F.A. Davis Company.

5.7. Helping a School Child with Asthma

Roberta Cavendish, PhD, RN, CPN

The gym teacher brought Craig C, a 10-year-old fifth grader, to the school health office early one January morning. This was Craig's third asthmatic episode that the school nurse (SN) had observed this month.

Craig was a pale, slim boy of average height with sandy colored, curly hair. He had dark circles under his eyes, and looked like he was about to cry. He had a non-productive, hacking cough, and said that he "couldn't breathe right." His breathing was labored and he had slight nasal flaring. The teacher brought Craig to the nurse because he was coughing and having difficulty breathing. This was after he was seen racing other students across the gym. While trying to hold back tears, Craig said, "I can never have any fun." He started to cry and his breathing became more irregular between spasms of coughing. The SN noted an audible wheeze.

The SN checked Craig's health record and noted that he had a written asthma management plan. This plan guided prescribed medications and devices, i.e., peak flow meter to measure ease of breathing, metered dose inhaler, nebulizer that delivers medication in mist form, dry inhaler, and spacer that attached to inhaler, and identified symptoms that indicated the need for more comprehensive interventions. Craig had been put on restricted gymnastic activities. Other written instructions that had been developed with the parents' permission were: (a) give the rescue medication of albuterol as prescribed to treat acute symptoms, using a metered dose-inhaler, and (b) notify parents immediately of illness episodes. Craig had a metered-dose inhaler (adrenergic drug) for school use but the nurse noted that he was not using it correctly and he did not use a spacer. He said, "It's hard to breathe and I'm itchy and sweaty all over!"

STOP. THINK. Which diagnoses, outcomes, and interventions would you select?

Submitter's Analysis and Use of NANDA-I, NOC, and NIC

If Craig did not have a history of asthma, the sudden onset of coughing, chest pain, dyspnea, and unexplained wheezing could be symptoms of several respiratory conditions. Foreign body aspiration is a common occurrence in school-aged children. This possibility, however, can be ruled out when the wheezing responds to a bronchodilator.

Several cues related to adaptation, self care, and developmental transitions suggested a host of nursing diagnoses such as: *anxiety, risk for injury, risk for disproportionate growth, risk for delayed development,* and *activity intolerance.* Lunney's Scale for Degrees of Accuracy (Appendix C) was applied to determine the accuracy of these diagnoses.

The diagnosis of *anxiety* was suggested early in the case study by the breathing difficulty, facial expression, crying, and verbal response. This was a +2 level of accuracy since the cues were present but *anxiety* was not as high a priority as the two physiologic diagnoses that were identified as highly accurate (see below). After the immediate interventions, there were few to no cues to support the diagnosis of *anxiety,* supporting the decision not to consider it as a diagnosis. After the event, *anxiety* might be considered as a −1 level of accuracy.

The diagnosis *risk for injury: medication toxicity/overdose* was suggested by the medications that Craig was taking and the fact that he did not improve with the first use of the inhaler. If Craig was in a school without a SN, he might have taken higher amounts of the prescribed medication when the drug that was supposed to relieve symptoms did not do so. However, there was an SN available to provide the medications and oversee Craig's use of the metered-dose inhaler and spacer, so there was little risk of medication toxicity or overdose from inappropriate use of the medications. Because Craig's school health plan included specific guidelines on the medication dosages, the SN followed the plan. This diagnosis would be assigned a value of +1 on the accuracy scale because it was suggested by the cues but there were insufficient cues to support the diagnosis.

Craig's statement, "I can never have any fun" and his attempts to be as active as the other children despite a prescription for restricted gym activities could be an indication that he felt different from his peers and may be at *risk for situational low self-esteem.* There was also insufficient data to support this diagnosis. This diagnosis should be explored further by the SN at a later point in time. Other diagnoses that should be explored further are *risk for disproportionate growth* and *risk for delayed development.* These diagnoses were suggested by the chronic illness, and Craig's personal characteristics of pale and slim and being unable to engage in peer-related sports.

Other diagnoses that were only suggested by the cues and therefore would be scored as +1 on the seven-point accuracy scale were *activity intolerance* and *deficient knowledge*. *Activity intolerance* was secondary to cooling and drying airways, and the depletion of chemical mediators, which triggered bronchospasm. *Deficient knowledge* was only suggested by the fact that Craig did not correctly use the metered-dose inhaler.

The two diagnoses that were identified as the highest accuracy diagnoses to guide the initial nursing interventions for Craig were physiologic responses secondary to chronic asthma (Casale, 2008; Randolph, 2008). These were: (a) *ineffective breathing pattern* related to increased airway resistance, hyperinflation of alveoli, and forced expiration through narrowed lumen, and (b) *ineffective airway clearance* related to gas trapping, increased airway resistance, and decreased efficiency of respiratory muscles. These diagnoses were high priorities, classically illustrated, and supported by relevant cues. The teacher's prompt action regarding Craig's difficulty with breathing demonstrated the effectiveness of the team approach when used to meet the special needs of a chronically ill school child (Coffman, Cabana, Halpen, and Yelin, 2008).

The nursing diagnosis that guided the SN's interactions with Craig, his mother, and the school team after the asthmatic episode was *readiness for enhanced self health management*. This health promotion diagnosis summarized a cluster of cues in the case study, was congruent with all of the cues, and was considered as the highest level of accuracy or +5 (see Appendix). The diagnosis of *ineffective self health management* was not used because Craig and his mother were generally managing his asthma quite well but just needed reinforcement and review. The cues that were considered highly relevant to make this diagnosis were Craig's need to self manage his chronic illness, inhaler used incorrectly by Craig, and family recently moved to a new apartment. Other cues that support this diagnosis were Mrs. C's willingness to address therapeutic regimen management.

Craig's situation portrayed a chronically ill child in a community setting, which is a scenario experienced with increased frequency by SNs (Ducharme and Bhogal, 2008). School nurses assume a major role in the health supervision, health counseling, and health education of chronically ill children such as Craig. School nurses need to be aware that low accuracy interpretation of the cues is possible and that nursing interventions, including *referrals*, are based on interpretations of cues. School nurses, just as other diagnosticians in nursing, medicine, and other disciplines, have the potential to misinterpret these and other cues. Awareness of the potential for low accuracy will help SN's to continually work toward higher levels of accuracy.

NOC Outcomes

The NOC outcome that was selected for the diagnosis of *ineffective breathing pattern* was *respiratory status: ventilation*. The overall baseline score for this outcome was 2 (substantial deviation from normal range) and the target score was 5 (no deviation from normal range).

For the diagnosis of *ineffective airway clearance*, the outcome selected was *anxiety level*. The overall baseline score was 2 (substantial) and the target score was set as 5 (none).

NIC Interventions

The immediate NIC interventions used by the SN were *airway management, respiratory monitoring,* and *emotional support*. The activities used were positioning Craig, providing fluids, providing reassurance, monitoring respiratory rate, administering prescribed medication, and teaching. Craig was encouraged to sit on a chair next to the SN's desk and lean forward for maximum ventilatory effect. *Emotional support and reassurance* provided by the SN helped him to relax as noted by a less tense body posture. He sat forward and listened attentively as the nurse reviewed how to use the metered-dose inhaler and the spacer, because the first dose was not effective. After the demonstration Craig correctly self-administered the medication. He drank sips of water from a cup that the nurse had given him. He responded to the medication and the water that helped to loosen the secretions. He was able to control his breathing, and improved his ventilatory capacity. He smiled and said he felt better.

Subsequent NIC interventions with Craig and his mother were *health education, health screening guidance, learning facilitation, learning readiness enhancement,* and *risk identification*. The nurse notified Craig's mother by phone, who said she would be at school within a half hour to take him home. During the SN's discussion with Craig, she learned that Craig's family had recently moved into a new apartment. When his mother arrived at the office, the SN proposed that the previous plan of care be re-evaluated with Craig, his family, and his physician. Because of the three recent attacks, it was recommended that the physician re-evaluate Craig's medications. A home visit was suggested to assess environmental factors in the new apartment. Although Craig's respiratory effort had decreased and he was breathing more easily, the SN suggested that Mrs. C take him home to rest. An appointment was made for a home visit and for Mrs. C to return to participate in a possible revision of Craig's plan of care.

Evaluation

The outcome goals were met. Craig had improved ventilatory effort and wheezing subsided. His breathing pattern and respiratory rate were within normal limits. Correct use of the inhaler was demonstrated by Craig. His facial expression and body language demonstrated absence of distress. Craig's mother responded promptly to the call from the SN, accepted the idea of reevaluating the current plan of care, and scheduled a home visit and follow-up meeting. When the SN visited the home, she reassessed the environmental, physiologic, psychosocial, and developmental factors that impacted on Craig's *self health management* for asthma.

References

Casale, T. (2008). Guidelines for the treatment of asthma. *JAMA, 299*, 2855–2862.

Coffman, J., Cabana, M., Halpin, H., and Yelin, E. (2008). Effects of asthma education on children's use of acute care services: A meta analysis. *Pediatrics, 121*, 575–86.

Ducharme, F. and Bhogal, S. (2008). The role of written action plans in childhood asthma. *Current Opinions in Allergy Clinical Immunology, 8*, 177–88.

Randolph, C. (2008). Exercise–induced bronchospasm in children. *Clinical Review of Allergy Immunology, 34*, 205–16.

5.8. Birth of a 25-week Neonate

Menay Drake, RN, MS, IBCLC

Infant girl N was born at 25 weeks gestation and weighed 720 gm. She was born by emergency cesarean (C) section to a 32-year-old female, Mrs. HN. The infant's mother was admitted for hypertension. She developed preeclampsia and was treated with magnesium sulfate, but then had a seizure or eclampsia. Her physicians preformed an emergency C-section to remove the infant from the mother. Mrs. HN was given betamethasone 24 hours prior to delivery of her infant to prevent respiratory distress syndrome in the neonate.

The neonatal intensive care unit (NICU) team was at the delivery of Baby N. Her Apgar score at delivery was 7 at one minute, color pink, RR 50, HR 140, muscle tone was good, with transparent skin. Infant resuscitation was immediately started in the labor and delivery room. The infant was dried, stimulated, and positioned. Her airway was opened using the "sniffing" position. A blanket roll was placed under the neck and shoulders of Baby N to maintain this position, and oxygen was set at 5 liters.

Mrs. HN was unable to see the infant because she was sedated. Mr. HN viewed the infant and touched her.

Baby N was transferred to the NICU in a warmed incubator. She was admitted to the NICU and placed in the radiant warmer with a skin temperature probe in place. Fluids were administered by an IV line. Blood was drawn for CBC, Hgb, Hct, type and cross match, immunoassays, cytogenetic, and immunology tests.

At two hours of age, Baby N's RR increased to 75, with intercostal substernal retractions, expiratory grunting, and poor air entry heard on auscultation with generalized cyanosis. Her HR increased to 180.

She was placed on continuous positive airway pressure (CPAP), and umbilical, arterial, and venous lines were inserted. At 15 hours of age,

Baby N's vital signs remained the same with intercostal, substernal retractions. The chest X-rays showed respiratory distress syndrome. Baby N was intubated with an endotracheal tube and placed on mechanical ventilation.

 STOP. THINK. Which diagnoses, outcomes, and interventions would you select?

Submitter's Analysis and Use of NANDA, NIC, and NOC

With the seriousness of this situation, the survival of Baby N was at risk. The nursing care indicated by her physiological condition was very complex. The highest priority nursing diagnosis, however, was *ineffective breathing pattern* related to immaturity. This was supported by her high respirations with substernal, intercostal retractions, and high HR. Premature birth at such a low birth weight indicates many other possible diagnoses that nurses must identify and provide interventions for (see the box titled "Additional Common Nursing Diagnoses with Premature Infants"). In NICU units, these diagnoses and the associated outcomes and interventions are basic standards of care.

Additional Common Nursing Diagnoses with Premature Infants

Impaired gas exchange
Impaired nutrition balance
Deficient fluid volume
Hypothermia
Hyperthermia
Ineffective thermoregulation
Parental role conflict
Impaired skin integrity
Risk for infection (immature immunity)
Risk for delayed growth and development
Risk for disorganized infant behavior

This case study addresses the priority problem diagnosis of *ineffective breathing pattern* and the two risk diagnoses of *risk for infection* (Baby N) and *risk for impaired parenting* (family). Infants with respiratory distress syndrome improve slowly and progressively if they can be kept infection free. Some infants can be discharged with oxygen supplementation. Some infants have recurrent pulmonary infections and growth restrictions.

The family is at *risk for impaired parenting* because parent-infant bonding is more difficult based on the prematurity of the infant. Parents often express feelings of anxiety, grief, and disappointment. This is not the normal path taken by parents of a full-term infant. The parents may have bonding and attachment problems related to the uncertainty of the outcomes.

NOC Outcomes

The NOC outcomes selected to address the immediate problem of *ineffective breathing pattern* were *respiratory status and tissue perfusion: cardiac*, and *tissue perfusion: cerebral*. On the *respiratory status* outcome, her baseline score was 1 (severe deviation from normal range) and the target score was 5 (no deviation from normal range). On the *tissue perfusion* outcomes, her baseline scores were 3 (moderate deviation from normal range) and the target scores were 5 (no deviation from normal range).

The NOC outcome selected for *risk for infection* was *infection severity*. The baseline score was 5 (none) and the target score was 5.

The NOC outcome selected for *risk for impaired parenting* was *parent-infant attachment*. The baseline score was identified as 5 (consistently demonstrated) and the target score was 5.

NIC Interventions

The NIC interventions that were selected to maintain and improve respiratory status were *oxygen therapy, respiratory monitoring, ventilation assistance, airway management, aspiration precautions, documentation*, and *surveillance*. The oxygen therapy was monitored by pulse oximetry. The nurse continuously ensured that oxygen administration remained warm at 70% and humidified. Vital signs were monitored every hour for changes in HR, RR, BP, and T, and included auscultation of breath sounds (Merenstein and Gaardner, 2006).

With Baby N on CPAP, the nurses secured prongs in her nostrils, removed them every four hours to check for redness and exudates, and cleaned and dried the nostrils and prongs. When Baby N was intubated, the nurses noted the depth of the tube at the lip line and posted this information at the bedside. The nurses secured the endotracheal tube (ETT) with Neo-Bar or tape to the upper lip of Baby N's mouth. The nurses observed for signs of extubation when performing care and suctioned the ETT with in-line suction devices to decrease risk for infection (Mattson and Smith, 2004). Suctioning of the ETT was performed when: (a) secretions were audible; (b) there were changes in vital signs, and (c) changes in oxygenation were indicated by Baby N's behavior, e.g., restlessness. The nurses aspirated the orogastric tube to decrease abdominal distention and secretions (Mattson and Smith, 2004).

Any changes in vital signs and Baby N's behavior were documented on the flow sheet. With accurate and frequent documentation, patterns of change could be noticed quickly, so that nursing care could be modified as needed and referrals could be made for immediate medical care.

Surveillance was implemented in that the nurses continuously observed Baby N for changes in physiological status and overall behavior. To conserve energy and help to maximize the use of available oxygen, nursing care was kept to a minimum and essential care activities were clustered in short periods.

To address the *risk for infection*, the nurses implemented the NIC intervention of *infection protection*. This included monitoring Baby N's temperature, and use of standard precautions, such as frequent hand washing and teaching the parents and visitors how to wash their hands before and after touching Baby N. For changing IV tubes and administering antibiotics, a central catheter bundle/closed drug-delivery system was used. This decreases the incidence of nosocomial and catheter-related bloodstream infections (Merenstein and Gaardner, 2006).

The NIC interventions to support *parent-infant attachment* were *emotional support, counseling, kangaroo care*, and *breastfeeding assistance*. The nurses provided support by assessing the parents' responses to their infant and facilitating their acquaintance and attachment processes with the infant. The nurses explained the equipment and Baby N's condition and answered questions. During each parent visit with the infant, nurses provided emotional support. The nurses encouraged the parents to visit Baby N and to call at any time of the day to ask about her condition. The parents were asked to stroke, touch, and talk to their infant and to take a picture. When able to assist the parents with holding their infant, the nurses facilitated *kangaroo care* as soon as possible. Mrs. HN was assisted to pump her breast milk for Baby N. Providing breast milk for her infant fostered a feeling of connection with the baby because she was the only person capable of providing this for her infant. Also, breast milk helped Baby N's immune system to combat infection and reduced the risk of necrotizing enterocolities (NEC) (Walker, 2002).

The parents visited and had interactions with Baby N and demonstrated warmth toward their infant. Their anxiety levels were moderate to high when aware of the changes in condition of their infant. They named the infant.

Evaluation

The NOC outcomes related to respiratory status, infection severity, and parent-infant attachment were all met. Baby N was extubated in five days. She was fed breast milk through the orogastric tube for several days. She did not have any other respiratory problems or develop necrotizing enterocolities. Her mother and father held her and were able to do *Kangaroo Care* with her. She was discharged at four months of age. Mrs. HN was able to breastfeed Baby N before discharge and at home. When she was nine months old, the parents sent pictures of Baby N to the NICU staff. The staff members celebrated this success story. Baby N was progressing developmentally as expected for her age.

References

Mattson, S., and Smith, J.E. (2004). *Core curriculum for maternal-newborn nursing* (3rd ed.). Philadelphia: Saunders.

Merenstein, G.B., and Gaardner, S.L. (2006). *Handbook of neonatal intensive care* (6th ed.). St. Louis: Mosby.

Walker, M. (Ed.) (2002). *Core curriculum for lactation consultant practice.* Sudbury, MA: Jones and Bartlett.

5.9. Emergency Care for a Seriously Burned Man

Marie Giordano, MS, RN

NC is a 52-year-old man who was admitted to the burn unit after sustaining 50% partial and full thickness burns to his lower extremities, hands, arms, and trunk. This injury was the result of an oil burner explosion in a basement. The accident occurred while he was repairing the burner. He did not lose consciousness and was able to escape the room without inhaling any smoke. He has no past medical history.

The physical examination revealed no carbonaceous sputum or soot in nares or mouth. Lab values for carbon monoxide were 2.9 and blood gases were within normal limits. The burns to his legs and trunk were not circumferential. His forearm and hands, however, were completely burned. He had generalized edema, which continued to be a problem. His peripheral pulses were thready in his lower extremities and only heard using a Doppler in his upper extremity. His lungs were clear bilaterally. Vital signs were as follows: BP 100/45, apical and radial pulses 125, RR 36, T 36 °C. Bowel sounds were absent. A Foley catheter was inserted and his urine output was between 25 and 29 ml an hour. A central venous catheter was inserted and an X-ray confirmed placement without incident. Lactated Ringer's solution was started to replace the fluid volume loss that occurred from third spacing.

NC was shivering and in "a lot of pain." He said that he was anxious related to the uncertainty of his situation. He was also worried about a co-worker who was in the explosion with him. His wife and family were on their way to the hospital but they did not know the extent of his injury and what they were about to see.

STOP. THINK. Which diagnoses, outcomes, and interventions would you select?

Submitter's Analysis and Use of NANDA-I, NOC, and NIC

With a major burn, every organ system is compromised. Further deterioration of the person occurs as the compromised organ system affects the other systems, creating a "domino effect" (Supple, 2004). The nurses used Roy's adaptation model in caring for NC, which helped to maintain a whole person perspective on his experience of being burned. The assumptions of Roy's model are rooted in systems and adaptation theories (Roy and Andrews, 2009). Humans are adaptive systems with inputs (stimuli) and outputs (behaviors) affecting the whole person through interactive processes. NC's burn trauma (stimulus) was having a systemic effect (behavior) on his condition, so the nurse continuously assessed NC's responses.

In this case, NC was in the acute phase of the injury. Although *acute pain, anxiety, imbalanced nutrition* and *impaired skin integrity* were all problems to be addressed, airway, breathing, and circulation were the primary focus in this acute phase of the trauma. Three nursing diagnoses that were considered important to address at this point were *impaired gas exchange, deficient fluid volume,* and *ineffective tissue perfusion: peripheral.*

Inhalation injury is common when a fire injury occurs in an enclosed space, as with NC. With the risk of pulmonary injury or smoke inhalation, the nurse assessed NC for evidence of smoke inhalation that would affect gas exchange. In addition, in the case of a burn victim with inhalation injury, high carbon monoxide levels, singed nasal hairs, and carbonaceous sputum are indications of an inhalation injury. NC did not exhibit any of these defining characteristics; therefore, at this point, *impaired gas exchange* was ruled out.

Fluid resuscitation was based on weight and percent burn (Herndon, 2007). The nurse obtained a "dry" weight of 80 kg upon admission. With third spacing of fluids in the acute phase, large volumes of lactated Ringer's solution were needed to maintain vascular homeostasis (Herndon, 2007). The nurse administered pain medication, with careful attention to the dosage because of hemodynamic instability. NC's weight was expected to increase from edema, but the increase in weight was not used to calculate fluids, medications, or nutritional requirements at any time throughout the hospitalization. The BP, HR, and urine output indicated that the diagnosis of *deficient fluid volume* was accurate.

Ineffective tissue perfusion: peripheral occurred in relation to hypovolemia in the acute phase of the burn and edema formation from third spacing of fluids. NC was hemodynamically stable; however, the edema in his burned extremities was compromising blood flow to his tissues. Compounding this problem was the distribution of burns on his upper extremities. Third-degree burns present as leathery, non-elastic eschar, which prevents expansion from edema. As the interstitial space in his arms increased from edema, the burn compressed the tissue, even further increasing pressure. NC was beginning to show signs of increased pressure from edema. The thready pulse in his lower extremities and nonpalpable pulses in his upper extremities were signs of *ineffective tissue perfusion: peripheral.*

In this acute stage of the burn injury, the nurse focused on physiological processes that were life-threatening. The nurse also considered the psychological and emotional coping processes that contributed to NC's adaptive process (Roy and Andrews, 2009). *Risk for anxiety* and *fear* were diagnoses that were accurate but they are not the primary focus of this case study description.

NOC Outcomes

The NOC outcome for NC for the diagnosis of *deficient fluid volume* was *fluid balance*. At baseline, the NOC score was 2 (substantially compromised) and the target score was 4 (mildly compromised). During this acute phase the nurses continuously monitored the indicators of BP, HR, hourly urine output, and signs of hypovolemia related to third spacing of fluid. The NOC outcome selected for *ineffective tissue perfusion: peripheral* was *tissue perfusion: peripheral*. The baseline score was 2 (substantially compromised) and the target score was 5 (not compromised).

NIC Interventions

The NIC interventions that were selected for fluid balance were *intravenous therapy, fluid management, surveillance,* and *vital signs monitoring*. The stimulus of *deficient fluid volume* was addressed by these interventions that were aimed at correcting the deficit (Roy and Andrews, 2009). The effort to maintain intravascular fluid volume during the acute phase of the burn injury was a major priority and a challenge that required exquisite vigilance in nursing care. Using the Parkland Formula (4 cc/kg/% burn), the nurse calculated NC's needs as 8,000 ml (1,000 ml per hour) in the first eight hours, then 8,000 ml or 500 ml per hour over the next 16 hours (Blumetti, Hunt, Arnoldo, Parks, and Purdue, 2008). Although this formula provided a baseline for fluid needs, it was not exclusively used during the acute phase of the injury. In cases of severe inhalation injury, calculation of internal burns is not included in the formula, so fluid needs may be even greater. The nurse increased the fluids accordingly and continued to assess for outcomes. Over the next hour, the nurse observed an increase in BP, decrease in HR, and increase in urine output to greater than 30 ml/hour. NC continued to stabilize. Using the Roy adaptation model, these were considered to be adaptive responses and outcomes relating to the physical domain (Roy and Andrews, 2009).

The NIC interventions that were selected for the *tissue perfusion: peripheral outcome* were *fluid management, circulatory care* (arterial and venous insufficiency), *circulatory precautions, positioning, surveillance,* and *vital signs monitoring*. These interventions were aimed at re-establishing and maintaining blood flow to the peripheral tissues. The nurse elevated NC's extremities and continued to monitor his pulses. Escharotomies, or longitudinal incisions into the eschar, were performed by the physician to release the pressure of the edema. NC's pulses returned in the upper extremities and were palpable in the lower extremities. *Surveillance* until the third day post burn was critical because capillary "leaks" from the injury cedes and fluid shifts occur.

During the acute phase of the burn injury, the nurse considered NC's emotional and cognitive processes, including the stimulus of pain, as they related to his adaptive responses (Roy and Andrews, 2009). Continued assessment of NC's pain and timely administration of analgesics contributed to favorable adaptation. The nurse was attentive to NC's emotional needs at all times, listened to his expressions of fear, and explained all procedures. One important communication was to assure him of the efforts and expertise of the burn team in providing the best care possible. The nurse promised NC that his family would be able to visit and that he would not be alone.

Evaluation

After the acute phase of the burn injury, the target outcomes of *fluid balance* and *tissue perfusion* were met. The nurse continued to monitor fluid volume because of the shift from fluid in the interstitial space back into the intravascular system.

The interventions for effective tissue perfusion facilitated circulation and pulses were maintained in all extremities. Edema decreased because of the positioning and the fluid shift. NC was stabilized and entered the next phase of burn injury treatment. In the next phase, the focus was wound care, infection control, nutrition, psychological and social issues, and continued pain management.

References

Blumetti, J., Hunt, J., Arnoldo, B., Parks, J., Purdue, G., (2008). The Parkland Formula under fire: Is the criticism justified? *Journal of Burn Care and Research. 29*, 180–186.

Herndon, D. (2007). *Total burn care* (3rd ed.). Philadelphia: Saunders.

Roy, C., Andrews, H. (2009). *Roy Adaptation Model* (2nd ed.). Stamford, CT: Appleton and Lange.

Supple, K. (2004). Physiologic response to burn injury. *Critical Care Nursing Clinics of North America, 16*, 119–126.

5.10. Dilemma of Addressing Overlapping Diagnoses in Acute Care

June Como, RN, MSA, MS, CCRN, CCNS, and
Gloria Just, PhD, RN

Mr. W, a 55-year-old single male, was admitted to the telemetry unit with a diagnosis of cardiomyopathy with CHF. He had a history of hypertension and had been unemployed with a cardiac disability for three years.

For approximately three days prior to this admission, Mr. W was feeling "worse and worse." His breathing had become more labored, he developed a dry, hacking cough, and his legs became more swollen. He delayed calling his physician because he thought the symptoms would go away if he "took it easy." Instead, he was admitted to the hospital by ambulance at 3 am in respiratory distress. He was treated with IV lasix, morphine, oxygen, and dobutrex (Trupp, 2005) and was transferred to the telemetry unit at 7 am.

During the morning assessment, the nurse found Mr. W to be orthopneic; his respiratory rate was 35 and he was using accessory muscles to breathe. He responded to questions with short, choppy phrases because he was dyspneic. Crackles were heard throughout his lung fields on both inspiration and expiration. His X-ray revealed marked pulmonary congestion with cardiomegaly. He was receiving nasal oxygen at 2 liters/m by nasal cannula. Mr. W was listless, fatigued, and unable to perform even simple acts of self care. He refused to eat and could only drink sips of fluid with difficulty.

His cardiac monitor displayed a rhythm of sinus tachycardia, HR 118/m, with occasional premature ventricular contractions. His blood pressure was 90/58 (his normal was 134/78) and his skin was cool and clammy. Upon auscultation of his chest, an S_3 heart sound was heard. His legs were edematous with 2+ and 3+ edema from feet to thighs. He is 6 feet tall and his weight was recorded at 210 pounds. He reported that this was 10 pounds heavier than last week.

STOP. THINK. Which diagnoses, outcomes, and interventions would you select?

Submitter's Analysis and Use of NANDA-I, NOC, and NIC

Arriving at a priority diagnosis for Mr. W presented an intriguing dilemma. He had multiple problems and the nurse could easily have selected cues from the assessment and clustered them to support nursing diagnoses such as *activity intolerance, impaired gas exchange, ineffective breathing pattern, decreased cardiac output, fatigue, excess fluid volume, ineffective health maintenance, imbalanced nutrition: more than body requirements, ineffective tissue perfusion,* and *self-care deficit.* The nurse decided, however, that the highest priority diagnosis at this time was *decreased cardiac output* related to impaired cardiac function and *ineffective self health management* related to deficient knowledge regarding symptom identification and management. The defining characteristics of hypotension, tachycardia, S_3 heart sound, dyspnea, rales, dry hacking cough, cold clammy skin, dysrhythmia, fatigue, edema, and verbal statements of lack of knowledge were highly relevant cues for the selection of these diagnoses to guide nursing interventions.

In considering the etiologies for *decreased cardiac output (DCO),* the nurse was aware that this response can arise from mechanical or structural factors and combined cardiac abnormalities (Moser, Riegel, Paul, Lennie, and Kirkwood, 2009). A decision that Mr. W's *DCO* was related to a mechanical factor, i.e., inotropic changes in the heart associated with congestive (dilated) cardiomyopathy, provided specific direction for nursing interventions. His inability to recognize symptoms of *DCO* and take action to prevent cardiac crises were precipitating factors that, when stated in the diagnosis, reminded nurses to address this phenomenon before Mr. W was discharged.

Selecting a rather broad or encompassing diagnosis such as *DCO* had some advantages over selecting multiple nursing diagnoses to reflect Mr. W's problems. First, it was an efficient way to incorporate many of the assessment cues into a single diagnosis, rather than trying to deal with multiple diagnoses that might become unwieldy in planning the continuity of nursing care. Second, it saved the time and effort that would be needed to prioritize multiple nursing diagnoses. Third, this diagnosis was the most accurate one because it reflected Mr. W's major problem, a heart malfunction, while the other diagnoses were secondary to *DCO.* None of the other diagnoses captured or explained as many of the cues as *DCO.*

In Mr. W's case, the diagnosis of *DCO* provided a focus for extensive nursing care that addressed the multiple dimensions of this phenomenon. Nurses intervened for this complex phenomenon through documentation of *DCO* and its etiologies, instead of using multiple related diagnoses. This single diagnosis provided a focus for the comprehensive nursing interventions that helped Mr. W to recover and return home quickly.

NOC Outcomes

In the acute phase the priority was stabilization and improvement of the cardiac pump to effectively maintain perfusion to all body organs. The NOC outcome of *cardiac pump effectiveness* was selected and an overall baseline score of 2 (substantial deviation from normal range) was obtained. The outcome target score was set as 3 (moderate deviation from normal range). For people with co-morbidities and CHF, setting a target rating at 5 (no deviation from normal) is unrealistic based on the chronic nature of the disease processes. For Mr. W a target range of 3 would move him toward improved cardiac pump effectiveness.

The NOC outcome of *cardiac disease self-management* was also selected. The overall baseline rating was 3 (sometimes demonstrated) and the target score was set as 4 (often demonstrated).

NIC Interventions

Based on the outcome of *cardiac pump effectiveness*, a prioritized list of interventions was developed, some of which required close collaboration with the physician and other health care providers. The primary focus for nursing interventions was to assist Mr. W in regaining *cardiac pump effectiveness*. The NIC interventions of *cardiac care: acute* and *shock prevention* were immediately implemented to stabilize Mr. W. With these interventions, numerous activities were incorporated into the plan of care, e.g., monitoring cardiac rate and rhythm, auscultation of breath sounds, monitoring various blood values and hemodynamic status, anxiety reduction, medication administration, monitoring daily weights, and maintenance of airway and perfusion.

Oxygen therapy had been started in the ED at 2 liters/m by nasal cannula and was subsequently increased to 4 liters/m after pulse oximetry indicated a SaO_2 of 88%. Bed rest was implemented to assist Mr. W in adapting to decreased cardiac function and reducing cardiac workload. He was given a commode to facilitate urination and bowel movements. The Valsalva maneuver was explained to Mr. W and a prescription was obtained for a stool softener. He was given every opportunity to rest, especially after eating or performing activities associated with diagnostic testing. He was assisted to a high Fowler's position, and supported with pillows to facilitate optimum gas exchange.

To reduce energy expenditure, anxiety was reduced through the NIC interventions of *emotional support* and *calming technique*. He was encouraged to express and clarify his concerns and was given information and assurance that the nurse would be there to assist him. The nurse collaborated with the dietician and the physician on *nutrition management* so Mr. W could receive a low sodium, soft diet of six small meals to increase his nutritional intake.

Medications were administered based on discussion with the acute care nurse practitioner, including the use of the inotropic medication (dobutamine) to improve his myocardial contractility and stroke volume. The nurse carefully monitored for the efficacy of the inotrope and possible side effects. Frequent monitoring of vital signs and EKGs were done to note any changes from baseline. Afterload was reduced through the initial use of nipride and Mr. W was switched to vasotec, an antihypertensive. Mr. W's blood pressure was closely observed for hypotension.

Finally, lab results were analyzed for his electrolyte status because alterations in potassium from lasix administration and magnesium can cause dysrhythmias. Mr. W's input and output were carefully monitored as was his low sodium diet. He was weighed daily to assess his fluid balance status. His IV fluids were administered by pump to control the flow rate.

When Mr. W was feeling better his nurse began to plan interventions to meet the outcome of *cardiac disease self-management*. The nurse was able to determine Mr. W's readiness for learning when he began to ask questions about how he could prevent this from happening again. The interventions of *teaching: disease process, teaching: prescribed activity/ exercise, teaching: prescribed diet*, and *teaching: prescribed medication* were selected (Heo, Doering, Widener, and Moser, 2008). Teaching activities included information on how Mr. W could adapt his behaviors for his decreased cardiac function, improve cardiac pump performance, and reduce cardiac workload. Dietary tips to control salt and water retention were reviewed, including the need for daily weights and when to contact his health care provider. Medication management information included side effects and how to take a pulse and blood pressure.

Evaluation

Mr. W's condition gradually improved over approximately three days until he returned to his usual baseline. The *cardiac pump effectiveness* score was 3, as set on admission. Initial medications were still being administered and he was told he would be "worked-up" to see if he was a candidate for a heart transplant.

His *cardiac disease self-management* score improved from the initial score of 2 to 4. The nurse had taught him methods of adapting his lifestyle at home to his decreased cardiac function, of being aware of the symptoms of decreased cardiac output for early notification of his physician or nurse, and how to monitor his pulse and blood pressure.

References

Heo, S. Doering, L., Widener, J., and Moser, D. (2008). Predictors and effects of physical symptom status on health-related quality of life in patients with heart failure. *American Journal of Critical Care*, 17, 124–132.

Moser, D., Reigel, B., Paul, S., Lennie, T., and Kirkwood, P. (2009). Heart failure. In K. Carlson, *AACN advanced critical care nursing* (pp. 237–275). Philadelphia: Saunders.

Trupp, R. (2005). Optimal therapy delivery in acute heart failure. *AACN News* (September), 6–13.

5.11. The Hypermetabolic State

Nora Maloney, RN, MS, and Joyce Dungan, RN, EdD

Mrs. C is a 72-year-old Chinese-Hawaiian female admitted to the hospital in congestive heart failure. She spoke broken English but was able to give a complete health history. Two weeks ago, she was treated by her physician for an upper respiratory infection. Recently, she lost weight, and experienced dyspnea, fatigue, and ankle edema. She complained of anorexia, and some episodes of vomiting. She also said she felt "bloated" and could not eat. Mrs. C is 5 feet 2 inches tall and weighs 160 pounds.

She described feeling very "nervous" and said she felt as if "something terrible was going to happen to me." She said that sometimes she breaks out sweating and felt "hot all over." Her T was 99.2 °F, HR was 130 and irregular, BP was 150/60, and RR was 26. Laboratory values of interest included serum glucose 200 milligrams per deciliter (mg/dl), albumin 1.82 grams(g)/dl, serum transferrin 132 mg/dl, hemoglobin 12.5 g/dl, hematocrit (hct) 35%, white blood cells (wbc) of 5,600/mm^3, and red blood cell count (rbc) of 3.5 million/mm^3.

Auscultation of the chest revealed diminished breath sounds and fine rales at the base of both lungs. She had a moist cough. Mrs. C complained she had difficulty sleeping at night. She used two pillows, which usually worked well, but lately she had been waking up about 2 am. Last night, she "heard everything that happened in the hospital."

Mrs. C was married for 35 years, and now she is a widow, living alone in Hawaii. She had a daughter in San Francisco who was very concerned, but who could not get away from work to care for her mother. Other family members live on another island and are not available to help with Mrs. C's care. Mrs. C says she has many good friends, but does not want to bother them.

STOP. THINK. Which diagnoses, outcomes, and interventions would you select?

Submitter's Analysis and Use of NANDA-I, NOC, and NIC

Mrs. C's case is an example of a hypermetabolic state that is seen in acutely ill people. The cluster of defining characteristics that supported this impression were irregular heart rate of 130, BP 150/60, widened pulse pressure, respirations of 26/m, increased skin temperature, sweating, weight loss, and fatigue. Infection was considered even though her temperature was only moderately elevated and the white blood count was WNL because these symptoms are masked in the elderly.

Two nursing diagnoses were made that relate to the increased metabolic demand, *decreased cardiac output* and *imbalanced nutrition: less than body requirements*. The warm skin temperature indicated that this condition was associated with high output failure. Another etiology of *decreased cardiac output* was impaired cardiac function as evidenced by the diminished breath sounds, rales at the bottom of both lungs, and systemic edema of left- and right-sided failure. The excess demand imposed by the hypermetabolic state probably led to increased output at first until cardiac reserve was exceeded and acute failure occurred.

The diagnosis of *imbalanced nutrition: less than body requirements* was also related to decreased intake of nutrients secondary to anorexia, nausea, episodes of vomiting, and the subjective symptom of feeling "bloated." The laboratory findings of low albumin and a serum albumin level of less than 3.5 was considered an indicator of poor nutritional status. The serum glucose of 200 mg/dl, low serum transferrin, and borderline low Hgb and Hct suggest poor protein synthesis. This diagnosis was made despite the fact that Mrs. C is overweight by normative standards for her height. The overweight problem represents a diagnosis that can be considered after the present illness episode abates.

Other actual diagnoses were *impaired gas exchange* related to pulmonary edema, *ineffective tissue perfusion* related to decreased cardiac output, *and excess fluid volume* related to low serum albumin and sodium retention. To confound the problem, the low Hgb and Hct interfered with oxygen delivery. *Disturbed sleep pattern* related to *anxiety* and *fear* was also a problem. The major defining characteristic of this diagnosis was Mrs. C's statement about not being able to sleep at night. Sleeping with two pillows confirmed *orthopnea* as an etiological factor. The complaints of feeling nervous and having a sense that "something terrible is going to happen to me" suggested *anxiety* and *fear*.

Four high risk diagnoses were identified: *Risk for impaired physical mobility, risk for impaired skin integrity, risk for ineffective breathing pattern,* and *risk for ineffective self health management.* Risk factors for *ineffective self health management* were change in health status, lack of social support, and impaired energy level.

People such as Mrs. C present a unique challenge to nurses who must make clinical judgments in the face of relative uncertainties. This situation reflected the reality that data are seldom at hand to make definitive nursing diagnoses, yet the cluster of evidence (pattern of cues) leads to nursing actions that are often life saving. This case shows that understanding people's health experiences requires noticing patterns of relationships and using lateral and parallel thinking (DeBono, 1970, 2008). Nurses need to use holistic approaches such as this to select accurate diagnoses. Linear thinking and looking for mutually exclusive defining characteristics for discrete nursing diagnoses does not work well enough for nursing. Simultaneous processing of multiple cues is needed; this method of "knowing" is acquired as a result of substantial and growing knowledge in an area of expertise, along with using reflective practice.

NOC Outcomes

The first NOC outcome selected was *cardiopulmonary status.* Mrs. C's baseline score was 2 (substantial deviation from normal range) and the target score by discharge was set as 4 (mild deviation from normal range). The second outcome selected was *nutrition status: biochemical measures.* Her baseline score was 1 (severe deviation from normal range) and the target score was set as 4. The third outcome selected was *cardiac disease self management.* Her baseline score was 2 (rarely demonstrated) and the target score was set as 4 (often demonstrated).

NIC Interventions

The NIC interventions that the nurse used for the outcome of cardiopulmonary status were *cardiac care: acute, shock prevention, oxygen therapy, medication administration, surveillance, emotional support, calming technique,* and *anxiety reduction* (Moser, Reigel, Paul, Lennie, and Kirkwood, 2009). The nurse began by raising the head of the bed to facilitate oxygen exchange, administered oxygen by nasal cannula at 4 liters/m until her pulse oximetry increased to a minimum of 94% SaO_2, inserted an IV line, administered IV 5% dextrose and water, and administered the prescribed diuretic and cardiac inotropic drug. A portable bedside chest X-ray was obtained. Surveillance was initiated and carefully implemented until her cardiopulmonary and anxiety status stabilized. Emotional support, calming technique, and anxiety reduction were immediately provided because fear and anxiety increased oxygen consumption and her oxygen consumption was already compromised.

The nurse monitored many different aspects of Mrs. C's physiological condition, including cardiac rate and rhythm, blood pressure, input and output, respiratory rate and lung sounds, neurological status, and changes in behavior such restlessness. Vital signs were monitored every two hours. The nurse interpreted the results of diagnostic testing as the results became available in order to contact the physician as indicated for possible changes in the medical treatment regimen.

For the outcome of *nutrition status*, the nurse selected the NIC intervention of *nutrition therapy*. A nutritionist was consulted for the number and types of nutrients that would be needed. Because Mrs. C's albumin and serum transferrin levels were so low, the nutritionist recommended a high protein, high calorie diet until Mrs. C stabilized. Small frequent meals were offered and liquid intake was limited to 1,000 ml a day.

For the outcome of *cardiac disease self management*, the nurse selected the NIC interventions of *case management* and *discharge planning*. The nurse spoke with the daughter and Mrs. C and discussed possible post-hospital disposition. The nurse case manager and Mrs. C also discussed the discharge options of home versus skilled nursing facility. Mrs. C had Medicare and a supplemental insurance policy so the case manager followed up on the adequacy of coverage for acute care rehabilitation. The Medicare DRG (diagnosis related group) for heart failure length of stay was only four days, and it was expected that Mrs. C would not be able to adequately understand *cardiac disease self management* in that short time period. The nurses, Mrs. C, and her daughter agreed that the discharge plan should be rehabilitation in a skilled nursing facility. In the skilled nursing facility it would be decided whether or not she understood cardiac disease self management well enough for discharge to home.

Evaluation

In the four-day length of stay, Mrs. C was ready for discharge to the skilled nursing facility. Mrs. C's scores on *cardiopulmonary* and *nutrition status* were rated as 3 (moderate deviation from normal range), which was an improvement but not as much as needed for safe discharge to home. The *cardiac disease self management* score was also 3 (sometimes demonstrated). All of the NOC outcomes selected for Mrs. C were communicated to nurses in the skilled nursing facility to guide the acute care cardiac rehabilitation program.

References

DeBono, E. (1970). *Lateral thinking: Creativity step by step*. New York: Harper and Row.

DeBono, E. (2008) The on-line effective thinking course starts a new session: Now with commentary by Edward de Bono on each lesson. Retrieved on September 20, 2008 from http://www.edwdebono.com/index.html

Moser, D., Riegel, B., Paul, S., Lennie, T., and Kirkwood, P. (2009). Heart failure. In K. Carlson, *AACN advanced critical care nursing* (pp. 237–275). Philadelphia: Saunders.

5.12. Low Accuracy Nursing and Medical Diagnoses Can Lead to Harm

Catherine Paradiso, RN, MS, APRN, BC

Mr. J is a 46-year-old carpenter who fell from a scaffold and sustained multiple injuries, including a T5 fracture with paralysis of the upper extremities. He was intubated in the ED and is now in the surgical intensive care unit.

During the first morning, a nurse who had no experience working with people who had a spinal cord injury noticed that the skin on his face and arms was cold and clammy, but he also had splotches on his face. The arterial line revealed a BP of 200/110. The reading was found to be accurate by checking with a cuff pressure. He became bradycardic and mouthed the words "chest pain."

The nurse noticed that there was no urine in the Foley bag and diagnosed *decreased cardiac output*. An immediate 12 lead EKG was ordered, IV fluids were decreased, and a nitroglycerine tablet was placed under his tongue.

The resident physician arrived on the scene, was told by the nurse what was occurring, and thought that Mr. J was having a myocardial infarction (MI). The physician ordered morphine (5 mg) IV and a dobutrex drip. The BP subsequently became 220/130, which meant that he was at risk for cardiovascular complications, such as MI or cerebral vascular accident.

Hearing the commotion, the critical care nurse manager of 20 years entered the room. The staff nurse explained to the manager that Mr. J was experiencing *decreased cardiac output*. The manager examined Mr. J and checked the Foley catheter, which was kinked, and corrected the catheter position. Urine immediately began to flow. She stayed with Mr. J and evaluated his cardiovascular status until the blood pressure gradually declined, the Dobutrex was eventually discontinued, and the blood pressure gradually returned to normal.

129

STOP. THINK. Which diagnoses, outcomes, and interventions would you select?

Submitter's Analysis and Use of NANDA-I, NOC, and NIC

This was a very critical situation in which an accurate nursing diagnosis must be quickly made. In this case the nurse diagnosed and treated the nursing diagnosis of *decreased cardiac output* (DCO) and the physician diagnosed and treated MI, but both of them should have considered the possible diagnosis of *autonomic dysreflexia*, which was the accurate diagnosis identified by the nurse manager.

A person with a spinal cord injury at T6 or above is at risk of autonomic dysreflexia (AD) with any autonomic stimuli below the injury, such as full bladder, abdominal discomfort, fecal impaction, pain, pressure ulcers, or kidney stones (Elliot and Krassioukov, 2006; Vacca, 2007). Because stimuli cannot ascend the spinal cord, there is a mass reflex of the sympathetic nerves below the injury. The vagus nerve stimulates bradycardia and vasodilation.

In contrast, DCO is inadequate blood pumped by the heart to meet the metabolic demands. Table 5.1 shows how difficult it is to discern

Table 5.1. Similarities of defining characteristics: dysreflexia and decreased cardiac output.

Dysreflexia	Decreased Cardiac Output
Paroxysmal hypertension	Variation in blood pressure
Severe headache	Fatigue
Possible decreased urine output	Oliguria
Profuse diaphoresis above injury; chilling	Cold, clammy skin
Pallor below injury; facial erythema	Skin color changes
Chest pain	Chest pain (if angina or MI)
Bradycardia	Decreased pulses
Anxiety	Anxiety
Conjunctival congestion Blurred vision Paresthesia Pilomotor reflex (goosebumps) Nasal congestion	Jugular vein distention Rales Dyspnea, tachypnea, orthopnea, cough Restlessness Confusion Anorexia

the accuracy of these diagnoses because some of the defining characteristics are almost identical. With spinal cord injury, when a Foley tube is kinked and the bladder becomes full, it stimulates autonomic fibers in the bladder, which can lead to AD. An empty Foley bag might also be present when a person has DCO because DCO leads to poor renal perfusion and low urine output.

NOC Outcomes

The first priority was to meet the physiologic need for oxygen, so the NOC outcome was *circulation status*. The baseline score was 1 (severe deviation from normal) and the target score was set as 5 (no deviation from normal). The second outcome selected was *neurologic status: autonomic*. The baseline score was identified as 3 (moderately compromised) and the target score was set as 5 (not compromised).

The nurse also identified *comfort status* as an important concern, because Mr. J was experiencing chest pain. His baseline score was identified as 2 (substantially compromised) and the target score was set as 5 (not compromised).

NIC Interventions

The primary NIC interventions selected were *dysreflexia management* and *pain management*, as well as other interventions listed in Table 5.2. The nurse removed the offending stimulus (the kinked Foley catheter) and monitored for and identified signs of AD. The nurse continued to monitor Mr. J every three to five minutes, administered IV antihypertensives, and instructed Mr. J, his family, and the staff, about the causes, symptoms, treatment and prevention of AD.

Mr. J will always be at *risk for autonomic dysrelexia*, including with ejaculation (Elliot and Krassioukov, 2006). Nursing interventions must focus on prevention of this complication.

The nursing activities for *dysreflexia management* were implemented, which was first to remove the cause and give antihypertensives. The nurse manager assured that these activities would continue to be employed. The interventions in Table 5.2 focused on prevention of AD and sustaining his comfort.

Table 5.2. Standard NIC interventions to prevent and treat autonomic dysreflexia.

• Airway management	• Positioning
• Anxiety reduction	• Skin surveillance
• Bowel management	• Temperature regulation
• Fluid management	• Urinary elimination
• Fluid monitoring	• Vital signs monitoring

The serious condition of a T5 fracture is tragedy enough, but it would be even more tragic if autonomic dysreflexia was not prevented and/or immediately corrected.

Evaluation

Once the stimulation was removed, Mr. J recovered from the event without further complication. The nurse manager placed written alerts in the chart and in the room. She also held mandatory staff meetings to be certain that the nurses understood autonomic dysreflexia and how to prevent it. The nursing diagnosis, outcomes and prevention strategies were included on the care plan.

References

Elliot, S., and Krassioukov, A, (2006). Case report: Malignant autonomic dysre-flexia in spinal cord injured men. *Spinal Cord*, *44*, 386–392.

Vacca, V.M. Jr. (2007). Action stat: Autonomic dysreflexia. *Nursing*, *37* (9), 72.

5.13. Cardiac Disease and Self Management

Juliana de Lima Lopes, RN, MS, and Alba Lucia Bottura Leite de Barros, RN, MS, PhD

Mr. MF is a 55-year-old, divorced automobile mechanic who was admitted to the ED with chest pain of deep intensity. The pain occurred at rest, lasted 30 minutes, radiated to the jaw, and was coupled with diaphoresis.

He expressed extreme anxiety during the physical assessment, with a feeling of impending death. He was dyspneic with crackles in both lung fields. His BP was 190/100 mm hg and HR was 115. His health history revealed obesity, arterial hypertension, a two pack per day smoking history, and a myocardial infarction (MI) and angioplasty three months earlier.

Prior to the acute event, Mr. MF had mild chest pain at work that lasted a few hours; the pain "got better" with rest. He was unable to afford his cardiac medications and was currently not taking them. In addition, his concern of lost income contributed to his decision to remain at work with chest pain, and thus delayed his seeking medical attention.

A 12-lead EKG showed elevated ST segments in the anteroseptal and lateral wall leads. The medical diagnosis was acute myocardial infarction.

 STOP. THINK. Which diagnoses, outcomes, and interventions would you select?

Submitter's Analysis and Use of NANDA-I, NOC, and NIC

Based on Mr. MF's clinical status, the medical diagnosis, and information about the risk factors for *ineffective self management* of his illness, the nurses considered two nursing diagnoses to guide nursing care: *ineffective tissue perfusion: cardiopulmonary* related to interruption of arterial flow, and *risk for ineffective self health management*, with the risk factors of deficient knowledge and economic difficulties.

The highly relevant data that were clustered for these diagnoses were: chest pain, dyspnea, a sense of "impending doom," choices of daily living did not meet the goals of a treatment program, verbalized that he did not take actions to include treatment regimens in daily routines, and verbalized that he did not take action to reduce risk factors for progression of illness and sequelae.

Other nursing diagnoses such as *anxiety* and *ineffective breathing pattern* were considered by the nurses, but they were not used because they were considered secondary to *ineffective tissue perfusion: cardiopulmonary.*

NOC Outcomes

The nurse foresaw some outcomes by having two phases in mind: the acute phase and the recovery or instruction phase. In the acute phase the priority was stabilization, with a focus on increasing blood flow to the coronaries to improve heart oxygenation, thus preventing myocardial necrosis and deterioration of its function as a pump. In order to achieve this goal, two NOC outcomes were selected for this phase: *tissue perfusion: cardiac*, and *cardiac pump effectiveness.* The baseline scores were identified as 2 (substantially compromised) and the goal scores were 5 (not compromised).

In the recovery and instruction phase the aim was to help Mr. MF adopt effective self health management strategies by improving understanding of his condition and the importance of the medications. The NOC outcome that was selected for this phase was *cardiac disease self management*. The baseline score for *Cardiac disease self management* was 3 (sometimes demonstrated) and his target score was 4 (often demonstrated).

The American Heart Association (AHA) estimated that 500,000 people undergo recurrent infarction (AHA, 2005) and based on these data, it is essential that Mr. MF correctly self manage his disease and its treatment.

NIC Interventions

Based on a decrease in oxygen supply to the coronary arteries, the implemented intervention for Mr. MF in the acute phase was *cardiac care: acute.* The nurse implemented the activities of this intervention, including evaluation of chest pain, cardiac rate and rhythm, heart and lung sounds, and neurological status. He was reassured by his nurse about various aspects of the acute care environment. Oxygen therapy was started at 4 liters/m, and a venous access line was placed for blood tests.

The bed position was chosen according to Mr. MF's tolerance. The nurse explained that absolute rest was needed to decrease cardiac workload and oxygen consumption.

The prescribed drugs were given according to protocols for the treatment of acute myocardial infarction, i.e., sublingual nitroglycerin (SL nitro), ace inhibitor, aspirin, clopidogrel, and heparin (Piegas et al., 2004). Chest pain was assessed every 15 minutes, as well as vital signs and EKG, so the nurse would know whether there were any changes from baseline while the cardiac catheterization room was being prepared. Even after the use of SL nitro, Mr. MF still had chest pain with some restlessness, so morphine and an IV vasodilator were initiated.

When the cardiac catheterization room was ready, Mr. MF was transferred and subsequently underwent an angioplasty with stent placement in the left anterior descending artery. He was then transferred to the coronary care unit (CCU).

In the CCU, Mr. MF was calm, hemodynamically stable, and pain-free, and his HR was 76 with a BP of 130/92 mm Hg. There was resolution of the ST segment elevation on the 12-lead EKG. After Mr. MF was hemodynamically stable and he became familiar with the CCU equipment and health care team, the recovery and instruction plan was implemented. The CCU team focused on the instructions for Mr. MF to effectively self manage his cardiac disease.

The NIC interventions selected to address the risk factors of *risk for ineffective self health management* were *behavior modification, counseling, financial resource assistance*, and *teaching: disease process.* In the acute phase, the nurse had already established a relationship with Mr. MF that was based on empathy, confidentiality, and trust. At this point, the nurse asked about Mr. MF's daily life and habits, thus helping Mr. MF to identify his strengths and weaknesses. Mr. MF reported that in the past he enjoyed physical exercise, but recently he did not have enough time to exercise. He also said that he relied on "fast foods" because they were practical to prepare; he was divorced and lived alone.

The nurse encouraged Mr. MF to conduct a life self-analysis. After this analysis of his previous life habits, Mr. MF was willing to change his habits; he also started asking questions about his disease and its treatment. A bond formed between the nurse and Mr. MF that provided an opportunity for instruction and support related to treatment of his cardiac disease. A qualitative study of the medication-taking practices of 10 people with coronary artery disease over a three-month period showed that professional and social support was an important dimension of regularly taking the prescribed medications (Lehane, McCarthy, Collender, and Deasy, 2008).

The nurse identified Mr. MF's current knowledge and noticed that he knew little about the disease, its treatment, and the risk factors for an acute episode. The nurse described the anatomy and physiology of the heart and circulation, disease signs and symptoms, risk factors, and disease complications. The need to take the prescribed cardiac medications was reinforced, and the function of each drug was described. The need for pertinent lifestyle changes were addressed, such as changes in eating habits, physical activity, and smoking cessation. After each instruction the nurse asked MF to explain what he understood about each topic. In collaboration with the nutritionist, the nurse explained the recommended diet and its importance in disease management. Mr. MF was informed about services available through state and federal programs and he was enrolled in a medication assistance program.

Evaluation

On discharge the patient showed improved hemodynamics and no chest pain. The outcome of *tissue perfusion* was scored as 5, even though the EKG showed an inverted T wave, as expected, in the V1, V2, V3, and V4 leads.

On discharge, Mr. MF's behavior change and knowledge about *self management* of his cardiac disease were remarkably improved, going from a score of 3 to 5. At the first follow-up appointment two months after discharge, MF was 10 pounds leaner. He had been following his diet and had incorporated regular physical exercise in his daily routines. He walked after work, felt better, and was able to carry out his daily activities. He proudly showed the nurse a graph of how well he was doing. He was still smoking but he wanted to quit, so he was admitted to a smoking cessation program. Six months later he stopped smoking.

References

American Heart Association. (2005). Cardiovascular disease statistics. Retrieved on September 2, 2008 from http://www.americanheart.org/presenter.jhtml?identifier=4478.

Lehane, E., McCarthy, G., Collender, V., and Deasy, A. (2008). Medication-taking for coronary artery disease-patients' perspective. *European Journal of Cardiovascular Nursing, 70*, 133–139.

Piegas, L.S., Timerman, A., Nicolau, J.C., Mattos, L.A., Rossi Neto, J.M., Feitosa, G.S., Avezum, A., Carvalho, A.C.C., Mansur, A.P., Timerman, A., et al. (2004). III Diretriz sobre tratamento do infarto agudo do miocérdio (III Guidelines for the treatment of acute myocardial infarction). *Arquivos Brasileiros de Cardiologia, 83*(suppl.4), 1–86.

5.14. Woman with a Neurological Problem

Rick Jepson, RN

WS is a 75-year-old woman who woke up at home at 3:30 am to use the bathroom and fell to the ground as she tried to get out of bed. Both her left arm and left leg were weak and she was not able to get back up on her own. Her husband rushed her to the emergency department (ED), but by the time she arrived 30 minutes later, her weakness had subsided. She was, however, a bit confused and had some drooping on the left side of her face.

In the ED, WS said that she felt fine and was adamant about returning home, but the physician insisted on a basic evaluation and radiography of her brain. A CT angiogram of her brain showed no acute changes. But shortly after completing the CT test, WS became more confused and again developed left-sided weakness in both limbs. A neurologist was consulted, who recommended an MRI of the brain with and without contrast. The MRI showed an infarction of the posterior right thalamus and internal capsule.

WS was started on heparin, but, because of the time lapsed since her initial fall, she was not considered a candidate for thrombolytics. She was transferred to a medical floor with telemetry and regular neurological checks. Although her left hemiparesis and facial drooping persisted throughout the day, WS said she "felt fine," denied any physical or neurological deficit, demanded to go home, and tried repeatedly to get out of bed. She also babbled at times, repeated statements she heard, and had considerable mood swings.

Most notable was her preference toward her right side. Her head and eyes were turned constantly to the right. She ignored staff members when they addressed her from her left side. And she disdainfully referred to her flaccid left arm as "that thing." WS tried to read the nurse's nametag, but only read words on the right half of the tag.

STOP. THINK. Which diagnoses, outcomes, and interventions would you select?

Submitter's Analysis and Use of NANDA-I, NOC, and NIC

The nurse considered the nursing diagnosis of *unilateral neglect* as an explanation for WS's rightward preference and to guide the plan of care. *Unilateral neglect* is a response in which people with brain damage behave as if half their world, the half that is contralateral to the brain damage, has become unimportant or ceased to exist at all (Danckert and Ferber, 2006). People who are affected with *unilateral neglect* become inattentive to one side of their world and overly attentive to the other; they can seem drawn, almost magnetically, to the side of their world that is ipsilateral to their brain damage.

Unilateral neglect is a response to damage to the parietal and temporal lobes or to the thalamus, and can occur with damage to either hemisphere of the brain. *Unilateral neglect* from right brain damage is more common, severe, and permanent than left-sided damage (Ringman, Saver, Woolson, Clark, and Adams, 2004).

People with *unilateral neglect* from right hemisphere damage may ignore food on the left side of their trays, bump into leftward obstacles, ignore or deny ownership of their left limbs, fail to groom, position, or protect the left side of their body, and ignore people, objects, or sounds from the left side (Jepson, Despain, and Keller, 2008). WS demonstrated these types of behaviors by gazing always to the right, by treating her left arm as if it was an inanimate nuisance, and by reading only the right side of the nurse's nametag.

Nonetheless, the nurse was still uncertain about the diagnosis of *unilateral neglect* because this problem can be confused with *homonymous hemianopia (HH)*, or blindness in the same side of each eye. Also, people can have both *unilateral neglect* and *HH*, making it difficult to dissociate one from the other. A person with a right hemisphere stroke might have a damaged right optic radiation and, thus, blindness in the left field of each eye. This might lead to abnormal behavior such as missing leftward objects or just focusing on the right side.

There are, however, some distinguishing features between pure *unilateral neglect* and pure *HH* (Polanowska and Seniów, 2005). *HH* is a sensory problem, while *unilateral neglect* is a problem of searching, responding, or exploring. Because of this, a person with pure *HH* tends to be aware of the visual deficit and tries to compensate for it by scanning leftward. A person with pure *unilateral neglect*, on the other hand, tends to be unaware of the deficit and deny it, and does not try to compensate for it.

WS was clearly not aware of her rightward preference or, for that matter, of any other deficits. She was not attempting to compensate and acted as if things on the left side did not exist. She could also, when cued, briefly overcome her rightward preference. This amelioration was transient, but it lasted long enough to test her field of vision; her visual field was intact.

Another alternative diagnosis considered for WS was *unilateral extinction*. This response is much like *unilateral neglect*, except that it presents only when a person has simultaneous stimulation from both the right and left sides or tries to simultaneously use both left and right limbs (Mattingly, 2002). For example, if both hands were being tapped, a person with *unilateral extinction* would feel the tapping on only one hand.

There is no consensus regarding whether *unilateral extinction* should be considered part of a broad diagnosis of *unilateral neglect* or if it is a unique problem (Becker and Karnath, 2007). It is significant that *unilateral extinction* depends on the distraction of simultaneous stimulation and that it is not usually apparent in spontaneous behavior. But WS's neglect of things leftward, even of her own left arm, was quite apparent. And when she was tested specifically for *unilateral extinction*, she did not exhibit signs and symptoms.

WS's nurse decided to further investigate the possibility of *unilateral neglect* as the principal nursing diagnosis. The nurse wrote two words on a piece of paper and asked WS to read them: HOTPLATE and BASEBALL. People with *unilateral neglect* often fail to read whole words and instead start at the far right of a word and work backwards until they find something sensible. WS read "ate" and "all."

The nurse gave WS a copy of a line cancellation test, which consists of a sheet of paper with 30 randomly-placed lines for the person to cross through with a pen. When WS attempted the test, she only crossed through the five most rightward lines on the page (Figure 5.1). The nurse also gave WS a modified version of the baking tray task. WS was presented with a tray that had 12 peanut butter cups piled together in the center. She was then asked to spread the cups evenly around the tray as if they were cookies on a baking sheet. WS again demonstrated *unilateral neglect*; although she arranged the cups evenly in rows, all of the rows were on the right half of the tray (Figure 5.2). The results of these tests confirmed the diagnosis of *unilateral neglect*.

NOC Outcomes

The NOC outcomes set by the nurse and discussed with WS and her family were focused on restoring function and learning to compensate for functions that were not regained. The nurse planned to help WS become heedful of her left side and to have coordinated movements and corrected body positions, especially of her head and eyes. The

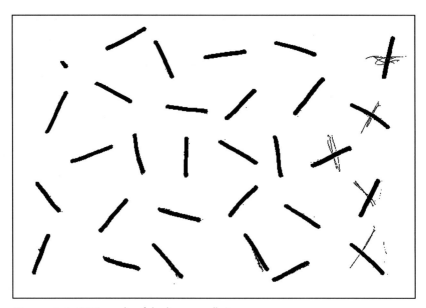

Figure 5.1. WS's results of the line cancellation test.

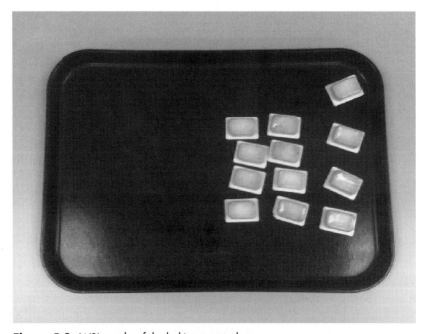

Figure 5.2. WS's results of the baking tray task.

NOC outcomes that were identified were *fall prevention behavior*, *balance*, *transfer performance*, and *personal safety behavior*. The baseline score for *fall prevention behavior* was 1 (never demonstrated) and the goal score was 3 (sometimes demonstrated). The baseline score for *balance* was 1 (severely compromised), with a goal score of 3 (moderately compromised). The baseline score for *transfer performance* was 1 (severely compromised) and the goal score was 4 (mildly compromised). The baseline score for *personal safety behavior* was 1 (never demonstrated) with a goal score of 4 (often demonstrated).

NIC Interventions

It was once thought that the best way to rehabilitate people with *unilateral neglect* was to force the person to engage with the contralesional world by doing things like positioning them in corners or putting their water and call light on the neglected side. This treatment method was too stressful and did not have therapeutic results (Harwood, Huwez, and Good, 2005).

The current activities provided in the NIC intervention of *unilateral neglect management* are more sensible and effective. They focus on safely reintegrating the patient toward the neglected half of the world while maintaining safety and comfort. Recommended measures include placing food, beverages, family members, and caregivers all on the patient's unaffected side. Then attention can be drawn gradually to the neglected side with touch, focused stimulation, and training the person to scan. As the person improves, people and items in the room can be incrementally shifted toward the affected side.

WS also needed to be kept safe after her stroke. The nurse helped to keep her left limbs protected and positioned, kept the left bedrail raised, and helped WS with balance and transfers.

Evaluation

Three days after her inpatient admission, WS was transferred to an inpatient rehabilitation center. Prior to discharge, the scores that were achieved on the NOC outcomes were 3 on *fall prevention behavior*, 4 on *balance*, 3 on *transfer behavior*, and 3 on *personal safety behavior*. Apparently, a few of the goal scores were set too high for achievement in a few days, but the scores showed that WS had significant improvement.

While at the rehabilitation center, WS showed further improvements. She still needed some cueing and reminding, but her gaze and head position were no longer drawn magnetically to the right. She responded to and interacted with people and items on her left side. After two weeks, she was discharged home with a continuing regimen of outpatient therapy.

WS benefited from the nurse's early recognition of her *unilateral neglect*. She was kept safe and comfortable, and nursing interventions were immediately begun. The entire rehabilitation team was better able to treat WS and set specific outcome goals because of the detailed nursing assessment performed on WS's first inpatient day.

References

Becker, E., and Karnath, H.-O. (2007). Incidence of visual extinction after left versus right hemisphere stroke. *Stroke, 38*, 3172–3174.

Danckert, J., and Ferber, S. (2006). Revisiting unilateral neglect. *Neuropsychologia, 44*, 987–1006.

Harwood, R., Huwez, F., and Good, D. (2005). *Stroke care: A practical manual.* Oxford: Oxford University Press.

Jepson, R., Despain, K., and Keller, D.C. (2008). Unilateral neglect: Assessment in nursing practice. *Journal of Neuroscience Nursing, 40*(3), 142–149.

Mattingly, J.B. (2002). Spatial extinction and its relation to mechanisms of normal attention. In H.-O. Karnath, D. Milner, and G. Vallar (eds.), *The cognitive and neural bases of spatial neglect* (pp. 289–309). New York: Oxford University.

Polanowska, K.E., and Seniów, J.B. (2005). Clinical picture and diagnostics of unilateral neglect syndrome. *Medical Rehabilitation, 9*(3), 3–12.

Ringman, J.M., Saver, J.L., Woolson, R.F., Clarke, W.R., and Adams, H.P. (2004). Frequency, risk factors, anatomy, and course of unilateral neglect in acute stroke cohort. *Neurology, 63*, 468–474.

5.15. Orthopedic Care of a Woman with Total Hip Replacement

Miriam de Abreu Almeida, RN, PhD; Amália de Fátima Lucena, RN, PhD; Deborah Hein Seganfredo, RN, BS

Mrs. IS is a 72-year-old white female, married with three children, who came to a Brazilian university hospital for total hip replacement surgery of the R hip to be conducted the next day. She was accompanied by her husband. She had suffered with osteoarthritis of the hip for four years.

Her medical history stated that she had hypertension for 10 years and she was overweight (BMI = 29.5). She takes antihypertensive medications daily.

During her interview with a nurse prior to surgery, Mrs. IS related that she was hopeful about the surgical procedure. With increased pain related to osteoarthritis, she had difficulty achieving everyday activities, including self-care. With limited functional abilities, her quality of life was low. The pain medication was no longer working well enough.

Mrs. IS's surgery took longer than usual because the surgeon had some difficulty with placement of the prosthesis. After surgery and after spending the night in the recovery room, Mrs. IS rated her pain intensity when moving in bed as 4 on the 10-point scale. She related having difficulty moving and manifested a clear will of taking a bath, although she could not independently do this.

Mrs. IS was admitted to the orthopedic unit with peripheral venous catheter in the R arm through which she received 5% D. After eating a good breakfast, the glucose solution was discontinued and normal saline was used to keep the vein open for administration of antibiotics.

Mrs. IS's surgical wound was covered with an occlusive dressing. A port-vac drain was in place with a small quantity of sanguineous drainage. She kept ice on the wound for 20 minutes every two hours. In bed she kept an abduction cushion in place to keep the hip correctly positioned. Elastic stockings helped to maintain optimum leg circulation.

The nurse conducted a nursing assessment using the human basic needs theory (Horta, 1979). Horta divided needs in the three hierarchic levels of psychobiological, psychosocial, and psycho-spiritual, with three subgroups in each. In psychobiological assessment, the nurse clustered the data as: level 4 pain, presence of venous peripheral access, prolonged surgery time, surgical wound with sutures and port vac drain, need for abduction pillow, cold compresses on the wound, difficulty moving, and need of help for hygiene.

 STOP. THINK. Which diagnoses, outcomes, and interventions would you select?

Submitter's Analysis and Use of NANDA-I, NOC, and NIC

Grouping the signs and symptoms for purposes of diagnosing, the nurse considered five diagnostic hypotheses: (1) *self-care deficit: bathing and/or hygiene* related to the impossibility of washing and drying the lower part of her body, (2) *impaired physical mobility* related to the difficulty of moving based on prosthesis precautions, (3) *risk for infection*, with the risk factors of surgical trauma and extended time in surgery, (4) *acute pain*, and (5) *impaired tissue integrity* related to surgical incision and presence of catheters (Lucena and Barros, 2006). When sitting, the hip could not be flexed beyond 90 degrees to prevent dislodging the prostheses (Almeida, Longaray, and Cezaro, 2006). *Impaired physical mobility* is frequently noted in older adults, especially those who have hip dysfunctions (Dochtermann, Titler, Wang et al., 2005; Hur, Park, Kim et al., 2005).

The nurse decided that acute pain was a related factor for the nursing diagnoses of *impaired physical mobility* and *self-care deficit: bathing and/or hygiene.* The nurse did not record the diagnosis of *impaired tissue integrity* because, with Mrs. IS being post-operative hip surgery, she would receive whatever care was needed to maintain tissue integrity. *Risk for infection* was accepted as a nursing diagnosis to guide the plan of care.

In Horta's theory, these three nursing diagnoses belong to the psychobiological needs, in the subgroups locomotion, body care, and physical security. The nurse discussed these diagnoses as the focus of care with Mrs. IS, who agreed with the plan.

NOC Outcomes

The NOC outcomes that were selected for *impaired physical mobility* were *mobility* and *ambulation*. The baseline scores were determined to be 2 (substantially compromised) and the target scores were 4 (mildly compromised).

The NOC outcome selected for *self-care deficit: bathing and/or hygiene* was *self-care: bathing*. The baseline score was determined to be 1 (severely compromised) and the target score was set as 4 (mildly compromised).

For *risk for infection*, the NOC selected was *wound healing: primary intention*. The baseline score was identified as 1 (none) and the target score was set as 4 (substantial).

NIC Interventions

The NIC interventions that were selected to achieve these outcomes and address the nursing diagnoses were *self-care assistance: bathing and/ or hygiene, positioning, teaching: prescribed activity/exercise, exercise therapy: ambulation, pain control, tube care*, and *incision site care*. On the first day after the operation Mrs. IS said, "I'd rather take a bath tomorrow" and the nurse helped her bathe in her bed. The following day Mrs. IS woke up with more energy and asked to take a shower. The nurse arranged all of the desired personal belongings and took Mrs. IS in a wheelchair to the shower, maintaining the recommended position. Mrs. IS independently washed the upper part of her body and the nurse washed her lower body.

Mrs. IS was told of the importance of keeping the abduction pillow in place to prevent joint dislocation of the prosthesis. The nurse aided the positioning of Mrs. IS to help her maintain the correct body alignment and to avoid a position that would increase the pain. The nurse also put the most used objects within Mrs. IS's reach.

After Mrs. IS rested, the nurse told her how to go through activities and the prescribed exercises, and explained the purpose and benefits they would bring to her recovery (Morgan, 2006). The nurse taught Mrs. IS how to transfer from bed to chair, avoiding over-flexing the R hip. Her husband also heard the recommendations and aided Mrs. IS to walk with crutches. Mrs. IS said, "It is not hard for me to use crutches, I used them long before the surgery."

The nurse asked Mrs. IS to communicate any pain she might feel because the physician had prescribed pain medication. Mrs. IS answered "I will let you know if I feel any pain because pain prevents me from doing my exercises. I know I must walk with crutches if I am to go home."

Ms. IS's bandage was changed after the shower and the surgical incision was healing as expected. The port-vac drain contained a very slight amount of secretions; Mrs. IS waited for the physician to remove the drain. When questioned by the nurse about how she would care for the incision when she returned home, Mrs. IS said: "I can wet it during my bath, then I can either bandage it for protection or leave it uncovered, right?" The nurse answered "yes," satisfied with Mrs. IS's interest in self care with her husband's support and assistance as needed.

Evaluation

On postoperative day five, Mrs. IS reported almost no pain and that pain was easily controlled with the prescribed pain medication. She walked with ease with Canadian crutches, and she had no edema. She walked to the bathroom to take a shower, but she needed help to wash her legs because of the positioning requirements to avoid dislodging the prosthesis.

For the NOC outcomes of *ambulation* and *mobility*, Mrs. IS reached the target goal of 4. For the *self care* outcome, Mrs. IS went from a score of 2 to 3; she still depended on another person to wash her lower body. For the outcome of *wound healing: primary intention*, Mrs. IS went from a score of 1 to 4; her surgical wound was healing satisfactorily.

References

Almeida, M.A., Longaray, V.K. Cezaro, P. (2006). Diagnósticos de enfermagem prevalentes e cuidados prescritos para pacientes ortopédicos. *Online Brasilian Journal of Nursing, 5*(3), 1–10.

Dochtermann, J., Titler, M., Wang, J.G., Reed, D., Pettit, D., Mathew-Wilson, M., Budreau, G., Bulecheck, G., Kraus, V. and Kanak, M. (2005). Describing use of nursing interventions for three groups of patients. *Journal of Nursing Scholarship, 37*(1), 57–66.

Horta, W.A. (1979) *Processo de Enfermagem*. São Paulo: EPU.

Hur, H., Park, S., Kim, S., Storey, M.J., Kim, G. (2005). Activity intolerance and impaired physical mobility in elders. *International Journal of Nursing Terminologies and Classification, 16,* 47–53.

Lucena, A.F. and Barros, A.L.B.L. (2006). Nursing diagnoses in a Brazilian intensive care unit. *International Journal of Nursing Terminologies and Classification, 17,* 139–146.

Morgan, R. (2006). Pain and reduced mobility affecting patients awaiting primary total hip replacement. *Journal of Orthopaedic Nursing, 10,* 80–85.

5.16. Using Orem's Theory for Care of a Woman with Terminal Cancer

Chie Ogasawara, RN, MEd, PhD, and Saori Yoshioka, RN, MSN

Ms. OA is a 50-year-old Japanese woman who used to work in health care. This was her fourth admission to the hospital with stage IV advanced terminal breast cancer and metastases to the liver and bone marrow. Six years ago, although she felt a lump in her right breast and swelling of the R axillary lymph nodes, she did not seek medical attention. She first went to a physician when she experienced severe pain in the upper extremity. Since then, she has been hospitalized three times for chemotherapy, radiotherapy, and a right mastectomy. This time she was admitted to the hospital on a stretcher because of severe lower back pain from a compression fracture of the thoracic spine. On admission, she was bedridden, and assessment indicated that she required total care.

Ms. OA was able to express her pains in various ways, such as "hurts like being torn by a knife," "the backbone is fragile, so I need to constantly have my back against something," and "once pain killers stop working, I tremble all over." Ms. OA was able to clearly explain the types of actions that exacerbate her pains, e.g., "In Fowler's position, the hips slide and exacerbate the pain," and "After moving around in a wheelchair three times, I felt pains around the hip bone." Ms. OA stated that "I constantly need a backrest," "If the table is set, I can eat in the semi-Fowler's position," and "When I move, I hold onto the shoulder and hip." With respect to pain management and respecting OA's wishes, pharmacological agents were prescribed, including oral morphine sulfate that provided relief. Radiotherapy to the eleventh thoracic vertebra was also effective in alleviating pain. Ms. OA performed inappropriate actions, such as crushing morphine sulfate tablets and drinking them with water.

For eating, Ms. OA required assistance to sit up in bed and adjust the food for eating. For toileting, Ms. OA wore diapers. She required assistance for all activities except grooming. Ms. OA got in and out of a wheelchair with the assistance of a PT.

With regard to social support, her key support was a colleague who is a nurse. Her colleague said that she is headstrong, stubborn, and fearful.

STOP. THINK. Which diagnoses, outcomes, and interventions would you select?

Submitter's Analysis and Use of NANDA-I, NOC, and NIC

Ms. OA's chief complaint was pain. Studies have found that chronic pain associated with distress is a frequent nursing diagnosis for patients with end-stage breast cancer (Ogasawara et. al, 2005).

For Ms. OA the nurse used the Integrated Approach to Symptom Management (IASM) (The University of California San Francisco School of Nursing Symptom Management Faculty Group, 1994), a symptom management model based on Orem's nursing theory, to assess Ms. OA's pain symptoms. Ms. OA's pain was assessed from the viewpoint of patient's perception, nurses' evaluation, and the response of pain. When applying Orem's self-care deficit theory (Orem, 2001), based on a compression fracture of the thoracic vertebra and the pain of cancer metastases to the vertebrae, Ms. OA's self-care abilities were reduced, and self-care deficits were observed. With the many cues that indicated self care deficits, the diagnoses for Ms. OA were *self care deficit: bathing/hygiene* and *self care deficit: toileting* related to acute and chronic pain.

NOC Outcomes

From the viewpoint of the IASM, the goals for Mrs. OA with the above diagnoses were based on pain, self-care ability, and quality of life. The NOC outcomes that were set for Mrs. OA were *symptom control*, *pain: psychological response*, and *pain: disruptive effects*. For *symptom control*, the overall baseline score was 2 (seldom demonstrated) and the target score was 4 (often demonstrated). For *pain: psychological response*, the overall baseline score was 1 (severe) and the target score was 4 (mild). For *pain: disruptive effects*, the overall baseline score was 1 (severe) and the target score was set as 4 (mild).

NIC Interventions

Ms. OA was forced to spend her time in bed; it was necessary to apply Orem's concept of partly compensatory nursing system (Orem, 2001). From the viewpoint of the IASM, it was important for Ms. OA to acquire the basic knowledge and skills and to make efforts to obtain support to improve her self-care ability. The nurses taught symptom management techniques to Ms. OA.

The NIC interventions used to address Ms. OA's *pain level*, as the related factor for self care deficits, were *pain management, medication management,* and *analgesic administration.* The interventions used to address her *self care deficits* were *self-care assistance: bathing/hygiene* and *self care assistance: toileting* and *self care assistance: positioning.*

The activities that were planned and administered to impart basic knowledge to OA were: (a) she was informed of her medication status and side effects, (b) she was educated about body positions to avoid exacerbating pain (sit deep into a wheelchair to reduce stress on the backbone), and (c) she was educated about narcotics, especially oral morphine.

The following basic symptom control skills were planned and taught: (a) body positions and movements to avoid exacerbating pain, (b) exercises for the legs, (c) toileting in bed while wearing diapers, (d) body position while eating, and,(e) methods for recording and notifying changes.

With respect to nursing care, when Ms. OA was first admitted, bed bath, and hand and foot baths were given due to bathing/hygiene self-care deficits. As her symptoms improved, she took showers with the help of an assistant. With respect to difficulty moving, her PT taught body positions and movements in the bed and how to transfer to and from a wheelchair. Ms. OA's support system was improved through the participation of volunteers along with her colleague.

Evaluation

The IASM and the NOC outcomes were used to evaluate the extent to which Ms. OA's symptoms, self-care ability, and quality of life were improved. Ms. OA's lower back pain was alleviated by the drugs being used. The outcomes of *symptom control* and *pain: psychological response* showed that the target scores were met. Pain, for the most part, was controlled. With respect to self-care ability, Ms. OA became able to eat meals while sitting in a wheelchair. With respect to toileting self-care, Ms. OA still wears diapers, but toileting became easier by lifting the lumbar region. With respect to bathing/hygiene self-care, Ms. OA used to take bed baths, but she became able to take showers. Her range of activity while in the wheelchair increased, and although it was once thought that Ms. OA would be confined to bed, there were plans to discharge her to home with home care services, which would improve her quality of life. Ms. OA also changed her attitude to try to do things on her own without depending as much on others.

References

Ogasawara C., Hasegawa T., Kume Y., Takahashi I., Katayama Y., Furuhashi Y., Andoh M., Yamamoto Y., Okazaki M., and Tanabe M. (2005). Nursing diagnoses and interventions of Japanese patients with end-stage breast cancer admitted for different care purposes. *International Journal of Nursing Terminologies and Classifications, 16*(3–4), 54–64.

Orem, D.E. (2001). *Nursing: Concepts of practice* (6th ed.). St. Louis: Mosby.

The University of California San Francisco School of Nursing Symptom Management Faculty Group (1994). A model for symptom management. *Journal of Nursing Scholarship, 26,* 272–226.

5.17. Cardiac Disease and Anticoagulation Therapy

Catherine Paradiso, RN, MS, APRN, BC

Mr. B is an 85-year-old Italian male with an extensive cardiac history. He had a cerebral vascular accident (CVA) 10 years ago with left hemiparesis, a myocardial infarction eight years ago, quadruple by-pass surgery with valve replacement seven years ago, hospitalization for chest pain last year resulting in cardiac arrest, and many bouts of congestive heart failure. He had been on anticoagulation therapy for seven years, since the by-pass surgery. About one year ago, he was scheduled for a cardiac catheterization for possible angioplasty, because his incidence of chest pain had increased. During the removal of a "sausage sized" thrombus in one of the coronary arteries, he experienced congestive heart failure and cardiac arrest. He was resuscitated, stabilized, and several stents were inserted in the coronary arteries. He was anticoagulated first with lovenox, and then with warfarin. He was discharged with an international normalized ratio (INR) of 2.0. His anticoagulation therapy had been managed by his private physician one time a month. His only other illness was benign prostatic hypertrophy.

This time he was admitted for gastrointestinal bleeding. He fainted while going to the bathroom and was rushed to the ED. In the ED his INR was 5.6. He was admitted to the ICU and transfused with 2 units of packed red blood cells. After his condition was stabilized, he was transferred to a medical-surgical unit of the hospital. While hospitalized, his INR was drawn twice weekly, and remained stable between 2 and 3.

Health History

Prior to his disability from cardiovascular disease, Mr. B was a restaurant supply salesman. He bragged often about the big accounts he had in Manhattan. "The 5-star restaurants were all mine ... Tavern on the Green, The Four Seasons. ... I had them all."

He lived with his wife of 60 years; they have one son who lives nearby. Their home is an apartment over a store and is up many stairs. The son reported that it is very difficult to get in and out of the apartment. Because of hemiparesis, Mr. B needs help with dressing, feeding, bathing and, sometimes, walking. His wife cares for him daily.

The son reported that over all the years since the CVA left Mr. B disabled, his parents refused to move from the apartment. Mr. B's wife is frail and has difficulty walking with severe arthritis and Paget's disease of the left leg. She reported having no energy.

The therapeutic regimen for Mr. B included 14 additional medications besides warfarin, which had to be carefully managed to prevent both the clotting and bleeding side effects of warfarin, which has many drug–drug interactions. Because of the food-drug interactions with warfarin, a diet balanced with vitamin K intake is also part of this regimen.

His son requested assistance in the home, because he thought that his parents make mistakes with the medications and diet. He also had safety concerns about their ability to climb the stairs. Mr. B is 100% service-connected through the Veterans Administration, so he has additional home care benefits, but he refused to use them, despite urging from his son.

When talking to Mr. B about his health and potential discharge, he said "They all think I am ready to drop dead. I get along just fine." He referred to his service in World War II by saying "If they didn't get me then, this sure isn't going to. It's just another bump in the road." Then he laughed.

He did not fully acknowledge disability, and reminisced about how he traveled all over the world. He had been on cruise ships to places most people only imagine, and suddenly stopped traveling when he had the CVA. The nurse saw the sense of loss in his eyes, but he bounced back by saying "When it became too hard to travel like that, I bought a country home."

He was very humorous, made jokes with the staff, and said, "You gotta kid around or you'll go nuts" and "When I don't know what to do I just kid around." When the subject of help at home was raised, he firmly said "No." When the subject was raised about having help for his wife, he said "She doesn't need it."

The nurse assessed his ability to pour and administer the complex type and amount of medications, and he insisted, "I know what I am doing." His vision was poor, yet he stated that he could "see fine." He understood why he was taking each medication in a basic way, but the nurse was unable to elicit information from him regarding details. For example, he knew that warfarin "thins" his blood, but did not know that a sub-therapeutic level can cause clotting and can result in sudden death. He did not know that an elevated INR can result in food or drug interactions with warfarin, cause bleeding, and, in turn, lead to chest pain. Considering how long he had required anticoagulation, his knowledge of food-drug interactions was limited. His wife, who cooked for him, refused to learn anything about his medications. She stated "Those drugs are all his responsibility. I do not get involved."

 STOP. THINK. Which diagnoses, outcomes, and interventions would you select?

Submitter's Analysis and Use of NANDA-I, NOC, and NIC

For many elderly people, medications are required to maintain cardiac output and extend life, especially in those with extensive cardiac histories (Katzung, 2007). All of these drugs, alone and in combinations, have risks. In this age group, it is important that the benefits of medications outweigh the risks (Cornelius, 2004). One risk is that older adults tend to dehydrate faster and experience loss of appetite. For Mr. B, the previous incidence of a large thrombus formation, insertion of cardiac stents, and extensive cardiac history placed him at high risk for cardiac complications. The bleeding side effects of warfarin are common (Brown, 2007), which is why the Joint Commission (2008) made safe anticoagulation a 2009 national patient safety goal, with all providers being liable.

The discharging nurse, in consultation with other unit nurses, chose *ineffective self health management* related to complexity of the therapeutic regimen, *deficient knowledge*, and reluctance to acknowledge the complexity and seriousness of therapeutic regimen management as the most accurate diagnoses to guide interventions. Mr. B's inability to manage his regimen was shown by this admission. Furthermore, he needed help but refused to accept the help of his son or home care services. He wanted to eat whatever he wanted, and showed no interest in understanding food and drug interactions that could be fatal.

His expressed desire to be healthy conflicted with his refusal to consider professional help in the home. He insisted that he could manage his own medications but showed no interest in knowing more about each drug. Although each medication may be required for a chronic illness, bleeding and clotting tendencies are common side effects when taken with many other medications (Wenger, Scheidt, and Weber, 2003).

A safe, anticoagulated state is achieved when the person's INR is between 2.0 and 3.0 or 2.5 and 3.5 for those with heart valve replacement (Wenger, Scheidt, and Weber, 2003). Because of the many medications Mr. B took and his refusal to integrate dietary changes aimed at balancing vitamin K intake, his INR was most likely to be variable. Another complication was that his INR was being measured monthly, instead of bi-weekly, so it was impossible to optimize his medication management. When INR was measured monthly by sending blood to a laboratory instead of doing point-of-care testing, he did not get dosing instructions until a few days after the test. The monthly testing and the time-lapse after testing allowed the INR to fluctuate to sub-therapeutic (a blood clot can form) or super-therapeutic (bleeding can occur) levels, because during this time he had eaten, drank, and taken his medications. If he had accepted a referral to the Veterans Administration Anticoagulation Home Care program, point-of-care testing would be available biweekly.

The related factors of Mr. B's *ineffective self health management*, especially *deficient knowledge*, should be addressed by the nurse, but Mr. B refused. If Mr. B was willing to learn, a NOC outcome that the discharge nurse would have chosen was *knowledge: treatment regimen*. Mr. B had been admitted for a medication side effect, which further complicated his chronic illness because the anemia associated with bleeding deprived the heart of oxygen. The other medications he was taking have side effects of orthostatic hypotension, presenting him with additional risks after discharge. Mr. B was mentally competent and able to make his own decisions, so the nurse documented the nursing diagnosis and Mr. B's decisions.

NOC Outcomes

An important outcome because Mr. B was going home to manage his own medications was *self-care: non-parenteral medication*. Mr. B's baseline score on this outcome was 2 (substantially compromised) and the goal score was 4 (mildly compromised).

The assessment data showed that all meal preparations were the responsibility of Mr. B's wife, and he managed his medications. Neither he nor his wife fully understood that food and drugs can interact in a deadly way. This admission showed that they are not able to manage the regimen independently, so the outcome selected was *discharge readiness: independent living*, with a baseline score of 3 (sometimes demonstrated) and a goal score of 5 (consistently demonstrated). The nurse thought that the outcome of *discharge readiness: supported living* was more appropriate, i.e., supported by home care services, but, again, Mr. B refused to accept help at home.

NIC Interventions

Mr. B believed he had the same capability as in earlier years. Both he and his wife were competent to make decisions, and they refused to accept help in the home.

Selecting interventions for Mr. B was difficult because he was not receptive to the nurses' interpretation of the situation. It was difficult to determine whether he fully understood, was in denial, or he did not understand. For an individual of this age, background, disability, and living situation, he may have been overwhelmed by having to integrate the regimen into his daily life. Nurses frequently encounter people with therapeutic regimens that overwhelm them, and must individualize the discharge plan to include referrals and appropriate follow-up strategies.

In this case, the complex and overwhelming nature of the regimen contributed to gastrointestinal bleeding; the bleeding complications of warfarin are preventable by effective management of diet and medications. With his refusal to allow others to help, another hospitalization was predicted for bleeding or a blood clot.

The nursing interventions that were selected to meet both outcomes were *truth telling, family involvement promotion,* and *health system guidance*. The nurse used *truth telling* by informing Mr. B, using respectful and empathic communications, that his previous self health management had been ineffective, as shown by gastrointestinal bleeding, and that the nurses thought he needed others to help him with management of this complex regimen. The discrepancy of Mr. B's desire to be well and his self health management were incompatible. Mr. B listened but did not change his mind about accepting help.

The nurse implemented the interventions of *family involvement promotion* and *health system guidance* by explaining the complexities of the therapeutic regimen to his son and providing ideas and information about possible follow-up after discharge. If Mr. B continued to refuse necessary support, the family should know how, when, and where to turn for help. Mr. B's son might later convince Mr. B to accept referral to the Veterans Administration Anticoagulation Home Care program. This would ensure that the INR would be measured bi-weekly, and point-of-care testing would be possible. This referral would make it possible for him to have a home care nurse to assess his cardiovascular status, and pour and monitor the effectiveness of medications. A dietitian could come to the home and assist his wife with food choices. It is possible that the family or other professionals would have to convince him over time.

Despite many discussions with the unit nurses and primary care physician, this couple refused a home health aid. Detailed written instructions were given them on how to access this resource if they changed their minds. They were also given written information on emergency contacts. The nurse documented all attempts at home care referrals and Mr. B's responses.

Evaluation

On discharge, Mr. B's INR was within normal limits because the warfarin dosages and diet were managed by health care providers. But the goals related to predicting optimum *self care: non-parenteral medications* and *discharge readiness: independent living* were not met. The unit nurses did what they could to convince Mr. B that he needed further assistance but the decision was Mr. B's. The nurses respected his right to make his own decisions. The nurses provided clear, written referrals and information to Mr. B and his family for follow up.

References

Brown, C. (2007). A new era of anticoagulation: Factor Xa and direct thrombin inhibitors. *U.S. Pharmacist, 32*(3), 35–47.

Cornelius, C. (2004). Drug use in the elderly: Risk or protection? *Current Opinions in Psychiatry, 17,* 443–447.

The Joint Commission. (2008). The Joint Commission announces 2009 National Patient Safety Goals for Home Care Program. Retrieved on September 13, 2008 from http://www.jointcommission.org/NewsRoom/NewsReleases/nr_09npsg_me.htm

Katzung, B. (2007). *Basic and clinical pharmacology* (10th ed.). New York: McGraw-Hill.

Wenger, N., Scheidt, S., and Weber, M. (2003). Anticoagulation at elderly age: The challenge to do better. *The American Journal of Geriatric Cardiology, 12,* 151–152.

5.18. Diabetes Self Management when Other Family Members Need Care

Coleen Kumar, RN, MS

Stella C. is an obese, 49-year-old, single, Italian-American female who has had type 2 diabetes for 10 years. Recently she experienced pain and numbness in both lower extremities, signs of diabetes complications. She made an appointment with her primary care physician, who referred her to a vascular surgeon for the painful neuropathy in her lower extremities. The surgeon ruled out peripheral vascular disease and referred Stella to the CNS diabetes educator to learn diabetes self management skills.

Stella is a college graduate who is employed as a financial controller in a small firm located close to her home. She enjoys theater, eating out, and being with family. Stella lives in an apartment with her 80-year-old widowed mother, Mary, who has mild hypertension, type 2 diabetes, and chronic rheumatoid arthritis that has limited her mobility. Stella's father passed away four years ago and she has a male sibling who is married.

Since Stella's father died, she assumed the role of head of the household. Stella's married brother tries to help with the care of their mother, but Mary puts him off, preferring to rely on Stella for all her needs. Stella maintains the house, shopping and cleaning on the weekends, although her excess weight makes heavy cleaning difficult for her. Stella said to the nurse: "I am so tired all the time. I wanted to hire someone to clean but my mother refused. She was always so good to us when we were growing up. I don't want to upset her now."

Stella spent much of her time worrying over her mother's health care, leaving little available time for caring for her own needs. She takes her medication as prescribed but has no time to think about diet management. When questioned about self monitoring of blood glucose (SMBG) she replied, "I have a monitor somewhere, but I don't really have time to use it. I try to avoid eating foods I shouldn't."

During the assessment, it became clear that Stella's knowledge about her illness was more limited than at first impression. Stella was interested in getting her diabetes under control and losing weight. "I'm not looking to be skinny, I want to feel better, have more energy," she said. Stella was five feet six inches and weighed 250 pounds. Stella said she was not as healthy as she should be and expressed concern, "My father died from complications of diabetes and my mother has diabetes. I need to do something."

As strengths, the CNS and Stella identified a close relationship with her family and having a strong sense of spirituality. Stella stated, "I get great solace from prayer and going to church."

STOP. THINK. Which diagnoses, outcomes, and interventions would you select?

Submitter's Analysis and Use of NANDA-I, NOC, and NIC

Because conceptual frameworks and models guide the plan and implementation of care in a purposeful way, Orem's self-care deficit theory was used to provide a theoretical framework to guide the CNS in helping Stella to meet self-management requirements (Orem, 2001). During the assessment and formulation of the plan of care for Stella, the CNS integrated Orem's four client-related concepts—self-care, self-care agency, therapeutic self-care demand, and self-care deficit—and two concepts that relate to nurses and their roles—nursing agency and a supportive-educative nursing system. In addition, the linking concepts called basic conditioning factors that include age, gender, developmental state, health state, socio-cultural orientation, health care system elements, family system elements, patterns of living, environmental factors, and resource availability were incorporated (Orem, 2001). With Orem's model, nursing diagnosis necessitates the investigation of the consumer's self-care agency and therapeutic self-care demand and the relationship between them. Stella and the CNS collaborated on her responses to health problems and life processes to select the most accurate nursing diagnoses.

Stella showed interest in weight loss and its relationship to her diabetes, which was a necessary condition of engagement in weight loss behavior. With the CNS, Stella determined that her sedentary lifestyle contributed to her existing poor glycemic control. Lack of physical activity and obesity could also be contributing to her feelings of fatigue (Porth, 2006). Stella's lower extremity pain could also be a barrier to action in which Stella may not increase activity in order to avoid an increase in pain.

Stella's cultural background and spiritual beliefs influenced management of her illness. She believed that most things are not in her control but are "in God's hands." In the Italian-American culture, there is an emphasis on strong religious practices (Leininger, 2005).

Stella has not asserted her power to manage her life, as indicated by not obtaining a cleaning lady because her mother said "no." This is consistent with Italian-American cultural patterns of extended and close family ties and support. This approach, however, may interfere with her self-efficacy to incorporate self management into daily routines.

Stella feels that things at home have not been the same since her father died. She has been totally responsible for the care of the household and her mother. When the demands of providing for a family member are perceived as exceeding available resources, caregivers experience stress. Stress often leads to self care deficit and feelings of burden, depression, and a sense of powerlessness (Lubkin and Larsen, 2006).

Diabetes is a self-managed illness. The specific diagnoses of *imbalanced nutrition: more than body requirements, chronic pain, powerlessness*, and *caregiver role strain* would be appropriate based on assessment data; the broad diagnosis of *ineffective self health management* related to knowledge deficits, feelings of stress, and powerlessness addresses the important issues for Stella.

NOC Outcomes

Using Orem's theory as a guide, Stella and the CNS planned for projected health outcomes. The CNS collaborated with Stella and formulated self-care requisites or health outcomes for Stella's well being and health. Self-care requisites are the expressed purposes of self-care and are attained through action (Orem, 2001). The priority outcome that was agreed upon was *diabetes self management*. It was decided that Stella's baseline score was 3 (sometimes demonstrated) but needed to be at level 5 (consistently demonstrated).

NIC Interventions

Designing effective and efficient nursing care involves selecting valid ways of assisting the people that nurses serve (Orem, 2001). The NIC interventions selected for the diagnosis of *ineffective self health management* were *assertiveness training, teaching: disease process, teaching: prescribed diet, teaching: prescribed medication,* teaching: procedure/treatment, and *family involvement promotion. Assertiveness training* was implemented so that Stella would learn how to effectively speak up for herself to her mother and brother. The rationale for the teaching interventions were related to weight loss being the single most important therapeutic objective for overweight individuals with type 2 diabetes

(American Diabetes Association [ADA], 2008). Moderate weight loss of 5 to 10% of body weight has been shown to lead to improved glycemic control (ADA, 2008). The nurse discussed with Stella the relationship between the types of food she chooses to eat and her blood sugar levels. In addition to her weight loss, success will be influenced by her diet. Adapting successfully to chronic illness includes the conviction that a meaningful quality of life is worth the struggle.

Evaluation

Stella's successful management of her illness in conjunction with increased knowledge was indicated by her self-care actions. She achieved her target scores of 5. This was indicated by Stella's behaviors. She checked her blood sugar daily and her diary indicated an average blood sugar of 140. Her food diary indicated food choices that supported good glycemic control. At the one-month follow-up visit with the CNS, Stella had lost 7.6 pounds, exceeding her short-term goal. Stella reported that the pain in her legs was improving, a result of better glycemic control. She was coping more effectively with her caregiver role by sharing some of the burden with her brother, who visited weekly. Mary agreed with Stella to hire a cleaning service. Stella was planning to attend a trip to Atlantic City with friends.

References

American Diabetes Association. (2008). Nutrition recommendations and interventions for diabetes: A position statement of the American Diabetes Association. *Diabetes Care*, *31*, S61-S78.

Leininger, M., and McFarland, M. (2005). *Culture care diversity and universality: A worldwide theory of nursing* (2nd ed.). New York: Jones and Bartlett.

Lubkin, I.M., and Larsen, P., (2006). *Chronic illness: Impact and interventions* (6th ed.). Boston, MA: Jones and Bartlett.

Orem, D. (2001). *Nursing concepts of practice* (6th ed.). St. Louis: Mosby.

Porth, C. (2006). *Pathophysiology concepts of altered health states* (6th ed.). Philadelphia: Lippincott.

5.19. Impetus of Diabetic Crisis to Improve Self Management

Emma Kontzamanis, RN, MA

CR is a 38-year-old African-American, divorced, male whose chief complaint when he was hospitalized three days ago was dry mouth, urinary frequency, polydipsia, and weight loss. Prior to that time, CR had enjoyed good health. At the time he experienced these symptoms, he was clearing asbestos from a building for his job. Because he was dressed in an air-supplied protective suit, at first, he assumed his symptoms were from dehydration and overheating. When the project ended and his symptoms persisted, he also noticed a 20-pound weight loss. He had blurred vision and mild cramping in both lower extremities. He attributed these experiences to overwork and fatigue. When he mentioned these symptoms to his sister, however, she reminded him that their grandmother developed diabetes in her 50s. His sister encouraged him to make an appointment with a primary care provider.

CR's physician referred him immediately to the ED. In the ED, his vital signs were BP 139/90, HR 90, T 99.4 °F, and oxygen saturation by pulse oximetry of 92%. His height is 5 feet 8 inches and his weight is 230 pounds, with a BMI of 35. His laboratory results were blood glucose 917 mg/dl, glycosylated hemoglobin (HbA1c) 12.5%, total cholesterol 283 mg/dl, C-reactive protein (CRP) 2.4 mg/dl, urine glucose ++++, urine protein negative, ketones trace. An IV was started and 1 liter of NS with 5 units of regular insulin was infused over one hour. CR's glucose decreased to the 300 mg/dl range, and he was admitted to a medical unit. He was diagnosed with diabetes, type 2, and diabetic ketoacidosis.

CR told the admitting nurse that he was afraid of "ending up like my grandmother." She was almost blind, had several toes amputated, received hemodialysis three times a week, and died when she was 65. The nurse asked if CR would like to discuss his condition with a nurse who specialized in the care of people with diabetes. CR said he would do anything that would keep him healthy and intact. The certified diabetic educator (CDE) visited CR that same day and discussed his usual diet and exercise pattern.

CR said he ate mostly fast foods, sometimes salads, and usually was too tired after work to do anything other than watch television and get ready for the next day. His two teenage children spent time with him every other weekend. He said they really do not like to come to his house, but it is part of his divorce agreement and he misses his children. On the alternate weekend, he spent time with friends, usually eating out and drinking several beers.

STOP. THINK. Which diagnoses, outcomes, and interventions would you select?

Submitter's Analysis and Use of NANDA-I, NOC, and NIC

CR's BMI of 35 indicates that he is obese (National Heart, Lung, and Blood Institute, n.d.). Since the mid 1970s, the prevalence of obesity has increased sharply for adults and children (Centers for Disease Control [CDC], 2008). Data from two National Health and Nutrition Examination Surveys (NHANES) show that, among adults aged 20 to 74 years, the prevalence of obesity increased from 15% (in the 1976–1980 survey) to 32.9% (in the 2003–2004 survey). The primary contributing factors are physical inactivity and unhealthy eating. People who are obese are at increased risk for several chronic diseases, including diabetes. A diabetes epidemic in the U.S. has affected 20.8 million people (CDC, 2005).

Based on CR's clinical status, the preliminary assessment of CR's diet and exercise pattern, and the current information about the causes and control of diabetes, the CDE decided the most appropriate nursing diagnosis for CR was *imbalanced nutrition: more than body requirements*. The diagnosis of *deficient knowledge* about diabetes was considered, but was not appropriate since CR realized how his lifestyle and his obesity contributed to his condition. His willingness to change his behaviors was an essential factor in identifying the nursing diagnosis. He was eager and ready to eliminate the factors that predisposed him to diabetes.

NOC Outcomes

In order to remedy CR's condition and prevent the long term effects of diabetes, the nurse and CR selected the NOC outcomes of *diabetes self management* and *blood glucose level*. Because diabetes was a new diagnosis for CR, his baseline score on *diabetes self management* was 1 (never demonstrated) and the goal score was 5 (consistently demonstrated).

His *blood glucose level* was 2 (substantial deviation from normal range) and the goal score was 5 (no deviation from normal range). His goals for the indicators were set as maintaining blood glucose levels between 60 and 110 mg/dl, adherence to a 2,000 calorie American Diabetic Association diet, and an exercise program of 20 minutes of brisk walking at least five days a week. Their discussions centered on how CR could change his eating and exercise habits to accomplish these outcomes. The possibility of eliminating insulin through these lifestyle changes was emphasized by the CDE. CR voiced his hope that this would happen and was confident that eliminating his obesity was the key to a healthy life.

NIC Interventions

The nursing interventions selected to help CR achieve his goals of weight reduction and elimination of his diabetes symptoms were *hyperglycemia management, medication administration: subcutaneous, weight reduction assistance, nutritional counseling, nutritional monitoring,* and *teaching: disease process.* For nurses to help people effectively manage their diabetes, it is important to understand behavioral change and appropriate interventions. Focusing on maintaining the quality of the person's life and working to prevent complications are important factors in teaching and coaching patients with diabetes (Seley and Weinger, 2007).

The CDE taught CR how to check his blood glucose with a glucometer and administer his insulin based on his blood glucose level. While in the hospital, his diet consisted of three balanced meals and a nighttime snack. The CDE explained how carbohydrates influenced his blood glucose and the importance of protein in eliminating the highs and lows of blood glucose. Each day, he was able to verbalize sample menus and calculate caloric intake. CR agreed to plan weekly menus for all meals and a nighttime snack before he did his weekly grocery shopping.

The importance of exercise in weight loss and its effect on blood glucose were also explained. The CDE and CR discussed how he would be able to fit 20 minutes of brisk walking into his life each day. CR decided he would leave for work 20 minutes earlier and get off the train several stops before his destination and walk to his work location. On the weekends, he planned to walk for 20 minutes in the park near his home.

Because CR lived alone, the importance of a support network to accomplish his goals was explored. The CDE asked whether his sister or a friend could serve as a support system and whether he would consider going to Overeaters Anonymous (OA). OA is a program that deals with the physical, emotional, and spiritual aspects of eating compulsively. Members share their experiences, strengths, and hopes of recovering from food addiction (Overeaters Anonymous, 2008). CR agreed to investigate an OA meeting in his local church. At the CDE's suggestion, CR also agreed to let his children know about his condition and the plan he had for eliminating his obesity and need for insulin.

Evaluation

Before discharge, CR's blood glucose was consistently between 80 and 100 mg/dl with insulin administration. He adhered to the diet provided by the CDE and used the treadmill in the Physical Therapy Department for 20 minutes a day. The NOC outcomes of *diabetes self management* and *blood glucose level* were rated as 5. The challenges of continuing this success after hospital discharge were the focus of discussions between CR and the CDE. CR agreed to weekly visits at the Diabetic Clinic where the CDE would be able to monitor and support his progress.

After three months of regular meetings with the nurse CDE, CR demonstrated success in achieving his goals of losing weight and consistently keeping his blood glucose levels within a normal range. He lost 45 pounds and, with his blood glucose consistently normal, the need for insulin injections was eliminated. His energy level increased and he was able to spend time with his children in activities such as bike riding that he was not able to do when he weighed 230 pounds.

The need for weekly visits to the CDE in the Diabetic Clinic was tapered to monthly. CR found that attending weekly OA meetings and talking to others with similar issues had helped him to stay on his diet and exercise plan. He began to enjoy life in a way that he did not think was possible when he was obese and required insulin.

References

Centers for Disease Control and Prevention. (2005). *National diabetes fact sheet: General information and national estimates on diabetes in the United States*. Retrieved July 12, 2008, from http://www.cdc.gov/diabetes/pubs/factsheet05.htm.

Centers for Disease Control and Prevention. (2008). *Physical activity and good nutrition: Essential elements to prevent chronic diseases and obesity*. Retrieved July 13, 2008, from http://www.cdc.gov/nccdphp/publications/aag/pdf/dnpa.pdf.

National Heart Lung and Blood Institute. (n.d.). Calculate your Body Mass Index. Retrieved on August 3, 2008, from http://www.nhlbisupport.com/bmi/.

Overeaters Anonymous. (2008). *A program of recovery*. Retrieved July 20, 2008, from http://www.oa.org/index.htm.

Seley, J., and Weineger, K. (2007). Executive summary: the state of the science on nursing best practices for diabetes self-management. *American Journal of Nursing. 107* (6), 6–11.

5.20. Self Management of Diabetes and Stress

MaryAnn Edelman, MS, RN

Mr. R is a 61-year-old married man who was referred by his endocrinologist to a clinical nurse specialist (CNS) because, in the last nine months, Mr. R had not kept his appointments and, at this visit, his fasting blood sugars were not as good as usual. He had a weight gain of 25 lbs and a daily fasting blood glucose level of 200 mg/dl. The current glycosylated hemoglobin level (HbA1c) was 10.8 and it should be no higher than 6. In an attempt to help Mr. R achieve the tight control he had previously demonstrated, the endocrinologist changed his oral medications and diet, and referred Mr. R to the CNS, whose expertise was helping people with diabetes self management.

The CNS used the Neuman Systems nursing model for practice (Neuman, 2002), so the assessment framework that she used was the five variables of physiologic, psychological, sociocultural, developmental, and spiritual. Mr. R had been diagnosed with type 2 diabetes six years ago. His sister had been diagnosed with type 1 diabetes at age 2 and died at age 23, following years of hemodialysis and multiple amputations from diabetic complications.

Mr. R said that his previous physical condition demonstrated good glycemic control with fasting glucose levels between 80 and 110 mg/dl, and his weight had been within the guidelines established for his height and body structure. Previously, he had kept his appointments with the endocrinologist, and there had been no evidence of complications secondary to the disease process. Both the endocrinologist and Mr. R had been confident that, if he continued on the previous path, the risk factors for complications of diabetes would be greatly reduced.

Mr. R said that during the last six years, he actively participated in self management to control symptoms and prevent complications of diabetes. After witnessing the serious complications of diabetes with

165

the untimely death of his sister, he decided that he would not want to suffer the same fate. Previously, he was meeting his personal goal of "avoiding the problems my sister had."

In discussion of coping and stress management, Mr. R indicated that nine months ago he experienced a life-changing event. He was "forced" to retire following a 40-year career in the stock exchange. "I always thought I'd stay with the company until I was ready to leave. I'm not ready yet, emotionally or financially. I've given my entire life to this company: how could they do this to me?"

When the nurse asked Mr. R what he believed to be the contributing factors to his recent weight gain and elevated glucose levels, he merely shook his head. "I couldn't say; I've been distracted since I've left my job. My routine is changed, and I guess I haven't been monitoring my weight or glucose levels during the day. When I was working, I'd check them every morning before work, in my office at lunchtime, and then as soon as I'd get home in the evening. Life is different now, and my attention seems to be more on whether or not I can pay my bills." The CNS continued discussing the situation with Mr. R to determine if he understood the relationship between the increased weight and blood glucose values. In response, he stated, "I understand how weight can affect my glucose levels, but I wasn't paying much attention to my weight. Frankly, I felt as if I'd lost control over my life since I had no input into when and how I would end my career. I was feeling anxious all the time; reaching for food seemed to calm me down enough to get through the day, so I have been overeating. I know this isn't the best thing for me to be doing, but sometimes I feel as if nothing matters. My career took a lifetime to create and its ending was out of my control, over in just minutes!"

During assessment of sociocultural status, Mr. R. described strong social supports. His wife and family incorporate the American Diabetic Association diet into their daily living routines and are supportive of all measures that facilitate an exercise program and lifestyle modifications. His wife frequently accompanied him to appointments with the physician, and together they attended informational seminars. He described strong relationships with family and friends, and enjoyed a number of recreational activities.

As part of spiritual assessment, the CNS asked Mr. R if he was aware of the feelings of powerlessness at the time they occurred. Mr. R said, "No, generally I do not think about how I feel. It doesn't seem as if my feelings count for too much of anything lately anyway! No one asked me how I'd feel about leaving my job, or if I was happy about this 'retirement.' I didn't think about how little control I had over this situation until now. I guess I have been feeling very uptight but wasn't aware of it, or that I was eating in response to these feelings."

STOP. THINK. Which diagnoses, outcomes, and interventions would you select?

Submitter's Analysis and Use of NANDA-I, NOC, and NIC

It was important that Mr. R had maintained good diabetic control until he lost his job and had to adjust to the many associated lifestyle changes. The CNS and Mr. R agreed that the stress of losing his job and the feelings of powerlessness most likely contributed to his weight gain and change in physical status. He was using food as a means of relieving the stress associated with this life-changing event. He also verbalized difficulty in maintaining management of his disease secondary to the changes in daily activities. The CNS validated with Mr. R the nursing diagnosis of *ineffective self health management* related to high stress and powerlessness.

The CNS was able to efficiently plan the appropriate interventions for Mr. R by incorporating Neuman's Model (Neuman, 2002) into his plan of care. Neuman's Model supports and enables a holistic view of people with chronic illnesses such as diabetes mellitus. Using this model, the person with diabetes is viewed as an open system in continuous interaction with the environment. The person interacts with internal and external stressors and is in a state of constant change, moving toward wellness or illness in varying degrees. The wellness of the person is uniquely defined by the person and is represented by the interrelationship of the five variables: physiologic, psychological, sociocultural, developmental, and spiritual.

A variable is an interdependent component of the person and environment and is one of the bases of holistic nursing care. The interrelationship of these variables is illustrated in Neuman's Model as functioning in harmony with environmental stressors. Tension-producing stimuli, or stressors, affect the stability of the person by invading the normal line of defense, if it is not adequately protected by the flexible line of defense. The role of a CNS includes helping people with chronic illnesses such as diabetes to adjust their flexible lines of defense to internal and external stressors and to help them optimize their normal lines of defense.

For Mr. R, assessment of the five variables demonstrated changes in the physiologic, sociocultural, and spiritual domains. His glucose levels were poorly controlled, he was experiencing personal stress in relation to his career ending abruptly, and he was not connected to, or aware of, his feelings.

The nurse collaborated with Mr. R to select the outcomes and interventions that would address these changes. This conceptualization of the person-as-partner in the health care process is supported by

Neuman's Systems Model. The relevance of consumer participation in the clinical decision-making process and the nurse working in collaboration with the consumer is essential for the nurse to customize care (Florin, Ehrenberg, and Ehnfors, 2006).

NOC Outcomes

The outcomes that the CNS and Mr. R. selected were *diabetes self-management* and *participation in health care decisions*. Mr. R's baseline score on *diabetes self management* was currently 3 (sometimes demonstrated) and the selected goal was 5 (consistently demonstrated). For *participation in health care decisions*, his baseline score was 3 and the selected goal was 5.

NIC Interventions

The focus of nursing interventions was power enhancement (Miller, 2000) and stress reduction, neither of which are listed in the NIC as nursing interventions. Stress elevates blood glucose levels (American Diabetic Association, 2008a). Two stressors that Mr. R could change were the internal stressors of perceived powerlessness and perceived financial instability. Opportunities were provided for Mr. R to explore and share his feelings about the loss of control he felt over the recent events in his life. Measures to help him to be aware of his power included having Mr. R explore those areas in his life that he was able to control. Assisting him to identify personal strengths helped Mr. R to realize he was not helpless in his current situation. Opportunities were provided for him to set realistic goals, for example, the possibility of pursuing a second career in the future. The nurse also focused on helping him adjust to new daily activities that did not center on his career. Mr. R's stress management strategies of "reaching for food" were not working to achieve his goals of weight management and glycemic control. Mr. R's stressors had invaded his normal line of defense and he had not yet adjusted his flexible line of defense to accommodate these stressors.

Nursing interventions from the NIC that were selected to achieve the outcome goals included *health education, anxiety reduction, active listening,* and *support system enhancement.* The nurse reviewed measures to help reduce Mr. R's glucose levels, which included counting the total daily intake and carbohydrates, increasing the fiber content of foods, and exercising daily as tolerated. Additional discussion centered on the importance of monitoring his glucose levels each day. *Anxiety reduction* was initiated because psychosocial well-being should be addressed in diabetes self management education (American Diabetes Association, 2008b). As part of the health education process, *anxiety reduction* was also important so that Mr. R. would hear and be able to use the information being provided. *Active listening* was needed, so that Mr. R would take the lead in deciding how he was going to "act instead of react" to the loss of his job. Reducing the anxiety level of Mr. R would additionally be supported by the nurse's active listening skills. By working in partnership with Mr. R, the CNS supported his ability to change his participation in health care decisions and improve his diabetes self management.

The CNS used the therapeutic communication techniques of open-ended questions and listening to encourage Mr. R to express and validate his feelings related to the situation. The CNS helped him to identify ways to be more aware of his feelings, to discuss them with his family and friends, and to consider joining a support group. Addressing the feelings that triggered the ineffective behavior of overeating would assist Mr. R to choose different strategies. Mr. R's wife and family supported this suggestion, and agreed to accompany him to support groups. By manipulating the environment, Mr. R began to experience a balance between his newly imposed retirement and perception of financial insecurity. He incorporated the CNS's suggestion that he "act instead of react," and he actively sought out a support group of recent retirees in the community. He met with a financial advisor and re-allocated his assets to maximize his retirement account. Mr. R mapped out a daily routine to mirror his daily activities when he was working, i.e., he began each day by monitoring his glucose, and discussed his structured daily activities with his wife. He volunteered each morning in an outreach program in his church and spent the afternoons attending a support group. The prospect of a part-time job in a realty office offered Mr. R additional encouragement.

Participating in these activities helped Mr. R to gain greater insight into his inner self. Feeling more in control, he did not experience the need to snack as frequently and, as a result, was beginning to lose some of the weight he had gained. His fasting glucose levels slowly returned to a range closer to the recommended guidelines, which served to further reinforce his self management strategies. Once Mr. R took an active role in the decision making process in his new role of retiree, his feelings of powerlessness dissipated. He became more aware of his reactions to situations and perceived greater control.

Evaluation

Within six months, Mr. R's outcome goal scores of 5 (consistent demonstration) on the outcomes of *diabetes self management* and *participation in health care decisions* were achieved. In collaboration, Mr. R and the CNS decided that his current nursing diagnosis was *effective self health management*. Mr. R knew that he could return to the CNS, if needed, for additional consultation.

References

American Diabetes Association. (2008a). Stress. Retrieved on 7/1/08 from http://www.diabetes.org/type-1diabetes/stress.jsp.

American Diabetes Association. (2008b). Standards of medical care in diabetes—2008: Position Statement. *Diabetes Care, 31,* S12-S54.

Florin J., Ehrenberg A., and Ehnfors M. (2006). Patient participation in clinical decision-making in nursing: A comparative study of nurses' and patients' perceptions. *Journal of Clinical Nursing 15,* 1498–1508.

Miller, J.F. (2000). *Coping with chronic illness: Overcoming powerlessness* (3rd ed.). Philadelphia: F.A. Davis.

Neuman, B. (2002). The Neuman systems model. In B. Neuman and J. Fawcett (eds.), *The Neuman systems model* (pp. 3–33; 351). Upper Saddle River, NJ: Prentice Hall.

5.21. Telephone Nurse Advice and an AIDS-Related Crisis

Ann M. Mayo, RN, DNSc, CNS

It was Christmas Eve and PH, a 36-year-old male with acquired immune deficiency syndrome (AIDS), telephoned the nurse advice line. He had called his primary care physician earlier in the day to report pink-tinged sputum. His physician had told him to stay home and that he did not need to be seen in the office or urgent care, but to call back if his condition changed.

At 8 pm PH called the after-hours nurse advice line. In a weakened voice, he whispered to the telephone advice nurse that he was "coughing up blood." Using a "cough" telephone protocol to direct the assessment, the nurse first determined that PH was in no respiratory distress. When asked about the color of the sputum, PH explained that he had been coughing for three days, but this evening the color of his sputum had changed from pink and now had some red streaks. When asked about his previous medical history, PH told the nurse he had human immunodeficiency virus (HIV)/AIDS and was on an up-to-date highly active antiretroviral therapy (HAART) regime.

Between protocol questions PH managed to tell the nurse he was frightened by the sight of blood. He also told the nurse that since his conversation with the physician earlier in the day, he realized it would be three more days before the clinic would be open. Because PH's earlier initial comments included "coughing up blood," the protocol disposition directed the nurse to tell PH to go to the emergency room. PH reacted negatively to this suggestion and said he was just too tired to make the trip. The nurse followed up on PH's comment with open-ended questions not included in the cough protocol. Through these questions she discovered that while PH was acutely aware of how tired he had become with his continued coughing, he also had felt weak and tired for about six weeks. In addition he said that since beginning his medications six weeks ago, he had lost his appetite.

STOP. THINK. Which diagnoses, outcomes, and interventions would you select?

Submitter's Analysis and Use of NANDA-I, NOC, and NIC

In the last two decades, telephone advice nurses have taken on important roles for consumers and the business of health care. With legal liabilities, real and perceived, protocols and guidelines for decision-making are being used in this field. Many of the protocols, however, were developed from protocols originally designed for use by physicians working in EDs (Mayo, 1998a). In a study with telephone advice nurses, the nurses verbalized that rigidly following protocols can lead to erroneous nursing diagnoses and is not always in the best interest of consumers. Nurses confident in their decision-making support the use of protocols in combination with their own "knowing" (Mayo, 1998b). These nurses believed that the best telephone nursing practice consists of taking time to connect with callers, continually expanding and applying knowledge, and using their experience to diagnose and plan care with consumers.

For PH, following the telephone advice protocol, the telephone advice nurse had a definitive plan. When the nurse discussed the plan with PH, however, and suggested that he go to the ED, he rejected this plan. Initially, the nurse considered the diagnosis of *noncompliance*, but this diagnosis was rejected because the definition of the diagnosis did not fit the situation. Once the nurse deviated from the telephone protocol questions to learn more about PH's "tiredness" and why he rejected the plan for ED disposition, the nurse realized noncompliance was not an appropriate focus for a plan of care.

Other diagnoses that were considered and rejected were *ineffective airway clearance* and *impaired gas exchange*. While PH's complaints initially prompted these diagnoses, PH's ability to easily converse over the phone and his normal mental status provided the cues to rule out these diagnoses. The diagnosis of *imbalanced nutrition: less than body requirements* would be followed up by clinic nurses at a later time. The two diagnoses appropriate for the telephone advice nurse to focus on were *fear of disease progression* and *fatigue* related to physiological status, treatments, and situational attributes.

Cues for these diagnoses were derived from a combination of PH's answers to predefined protocol questions, unsolicited comments made by him during the telephone call, and information the nurse solicited to complete the cue clusters for these diagnoses. PH's description of being frightened by the sight of blood was the major defining characteristic that supported a diagnosis of *fear of disease progression*. He articulated a feeling of emotional disruption that related to the source of blood in his sputum, and, most important, he perceived this to be a sign of worsening condition. PH identified pathological (frequent coughing, blood in sputum) and situational (no access to his MD for three days) etiologies for this fear.

Because the nurse probed as well as listened intently regarding PH's complaint of feeling tired, the story he shared provided the evidence to make a nursing diagnosis of *fatigue*. Fatigue differs from tiredness in that it is more chronic in nature, requiring adaptation on the part of the person and other people in the environment (Jenkin, Koch, and Kralik, 2006).

Based on cues provided by PH, the nurse chose to extend the assessment beyond the questions provided by the organizational protocol. The primary cues for the nurse to explore *fatigue* as a possible nursing diagnosis came from his statement that he had a diagnosis of HIV/AIDS and from his subsequent comment about being too tired to go to the emergency room. Knowledge regarding current HIV/AIDS patient symptomatology was helpful to the nurse in simultaneously expanding and refocusing an appropriate assessment beyond the limits of the telephone protocol.

Fatigue, a complex, multidimensional concept, appears to be the most frequent symptom among people with HIV/AIDS. It represents both mental and physical tiredness (Jenkin, Koch, and Kralik, 2006). People with HIV/AIDS use their feelings of fatigue to gauge the progression of the disease (Siegel, Brown-Bradley, and Lekas, 2004). PH knew that a trip to the ED would bring increased feelings of fatigue and for PH increased fatigue meant further deterioration of his already fragile health status. In this case, the nurse did not have a T-cell count, but laboratory reports such as T-cell counts are not the only cues to gauge disease progression. The person with HIV/AIDS is an additional source of information through his or her perceptions of fatigue. Therefore, realizing what significant importance "fatigue" holds for people with HIV/AIDS, patient decision-making can be understood within a different context.

NOC Outcomes

The first desired outcome for PH was *fear level*. PH's overall score was 2 (substantial) and the goal score was set as 4 (mild). If PH could manage his feelings of fear through an empathic nurse-patient relationship he could reduce his alarm about AIDS-related crisis episodes.

The second desired outcome for PH was *energy conservation*. After discussion with PH, the nurse and PH determined that his overall baseline score for energy conservation was 3 (sometimes demonstrated) and the goal score was 4 (often demonstrated).

NIC Interventions

Nursing interventions designed to control *fear* are well within the role of the telephone advice nurse and support using Olson's Theory of Empathy (Olson and Kunyk, 2004). The interventions selected were *active listening, anticipatory guidance,* and *emotional support. Active listening* on the part of the telephone advice nurse involved genuinely paying attention to PH's fears in an understanding way (Brown and Addington-Hall, 2008). This means that the nurse took time to listen to PH and not dismiss his concerns.

The nurse used *anticipatory guidance* by reassuring PH and providing information about his fears to enhance his awareness and understanding (McWilliams, Jacobson, Van Houten, Naessens, and Ytterberg, 2008). The nurse reassured PH that he was not critically ill and provided education about the symptoms that would necessitate a visit to the emergency room or a 911 call.

The nurse provided *emotional support* by discussing PH's emotions, assisting him to recognize his feelings, and being empathic in all communications. Evidence shows that emotional support is perceived by patients as important to overcoming *fear* and initiating positive action (Watt, Bobrow, and Moracco, 2008).

To help diminish PH's level of *fatigue* the nurse used the intervention of *energy management*. The nurse encouraged him to rest, prescribed naps during the day, and explained banking of energy (resting at set times to save energy). Banked energy would be needed for a trip to the ED over the weekend or a trip to the clinic next week. Until PH could be further evaluated in the clinic, he was instructed to avoid activities that involve exercise. Finlayson's (2005) pilot study indicated that energy conserving behaviors decreased fatigue severity after energy conservation was taught by teleconference.

Evaluation

Evaluating outcomes can be difficult for a telephone advice nurse because there is limited time with callers and no face-to-face contact. Evidence that PH's *fear level* was reaching the goal score of 4 included comments from him during the call that he was monitoring the intensity of his fear ("I feel less like I'm being overcome with this fear"), maintaining concentration to avoid loss of control ("I'm hearing what you are saying; I think I can do that"), and seeking information to reduce fear ("So, is coughing up blood something that I should expect?").

Evidence that PH would conserve his energy included verbalization that he would nap in the morning and afternoon over the next few days prior to his clinic appointment. The nurse evaluated that PH understood the recommendations.

References

Brown, J., and Addington-Hall, J. (2008). How people with motor neurone disease talk about living with their illness: A narrative study. *Journal of Advanced Nursing, 62*, 200–208.

Finlayson, M. (2005). A pilot study of an energy conservation project delivered by telephone conference call to people with multiple sclerosis. *Neurorehabilitation, 20*, 267–277.

Jenkin, P., Koch, T., and Kralik, D. (2006). The experience of fatigue for adults living with HIV. *Journal of Clinical Nursing, 15*, 1123–31.

Mayo, A. (1998a). The role of the telephone advice/triage nurse. *AAACN Viewpoint, 20*(6), 9–10.

Mayo, A. (1998b). *The experience of decision-making among telephone advice/triage nurses.* Hahn School of Nursing, University of San Diego, San Diego, CA. Copyright, Library of Congress (#TX4-797-530).

McWilliams, D.B., Jacobson, R.M., Van Houten, H.K., Naessens, J.M., and Ytterberg, K.L. (2008). A program of anticipatory guidance for the prevention of emergency department visits for ear pain. *Archives of Pediatrics and Adolescent Medicine, 162*, 151–156.

Olson, J.K., and Kunyk, D. (2004). Empathy. In S.J. Peterson and T.S. Bredow (eds). *Middle range theories: Application to nursing research* (pp. 151–164). Philadelphia: Lippincott Williams and Wilkins.

Siegel, K., Brown-Bradley, C.J., and Lekas, H.M. (2004). Strategies for coping with fatigue among HIV-positive individuals fifty years and older. *AIDS patient care and STDs, 18*, 275–288.

Watt, M.H., Bobrow, E.A., and Moracco, K.E. (2008). Providing support to IPV victims in the emergency department: Vignette-based interviews with IPV survivors and emergency department nurses. *Violence Against Women, 14*(6), 715–26.

5.22. Woman who Experienced a Significant Childhood Loss

Steven L. Baumann, RN, PhD, GNP-BC, PMHNP-BC

Ms. AM was an attractive 38-year-old female of Puerto-Rican descent who attended a mental health clinic in the South Bronx section of New York City (NYC) for depression, anger, and insomnia. Her providers were a psychiatric nurse practitioner and a psychiatric social worker. Recently, she entered the NYC shelter system with her two school age children to "get away" from an abusive and drug abusing husband. Ms. AM said that she was depressed, not because of her current situation, but because when she was seven years old her mother died from cancer. After her mother died, AM stayed with her father, but she described him as "not supportive," then or now. In addition, in the neighborhood where she was raised, violence, crime, and drug abuse were not only common but peer supported. It was difficult for Ms. AM to focus and not to think about how different her life would be if her mother had not died.

When she first came to the clinic, the focus of her anger was that her oldest daughter had just had a baby and had relocated to live with the family of the child's father. To make matters worse the baby's father's family was related to her husband's family and that family was putting pressure on her daughter to "not communicate" with her mother. Ms. AM had hoped that she could help her daughter with the baby and provide for them the family she did not have.

In addition to her husband being unemployed and abusing drugs, according to AM, he did not help with the children or the housework. She described him as possessive and jealous. It was common for her to receive several cell phone calls from him while she was at the mental health clinic. Ms. AM admitted that she saw other men socially, and that she had a boyfriend. It eventually became evident that her boyfriend was also possessive, jealous, and violent. Even before she left her husband, but clearly afterward, she replaced her abusive husband with someone who was strikingly similar, but younger.

Over time and with support from her health care providers, AM's relationship with her daughter improved and her daughter returned to NYC. AM was able to accomplish her goal of doing things for her daughter and grandchild.

Ms. AM recognized that her depression, anger, and insomnia, preceded her having to live in a shelter for homeless families, and even her marital and family problems. She knew it was because of the untimely death of her mother, and her inability to stop the intrusive memories that tormented her. She did not indicate an understanding that her family and personal history were affecting her current behavior.

Ms. AM asked the nurse practitioner and social worker for relief from her distressing moods and thoughts, and she hoped to provide her children and grandchildren with a better life. She was willing to do what was necessary to get a new apartment and get away from her husband. She was willing to use social services, psychotherapy, and medication as needed. She remained aggressive and impulsive, but was working to better control her behavior and moods.

STOP. THINK. Which diagnoses, outcomes, and interventions would you select?

Submitter's Analysis and Use of NANDA-I, NOC, and NIC

The trajectory of AM's life was dramatically altered by the traumatic loss of her mother at an early age. Aggravated by her current difficult choices, conflicts, and residential displacement, she suffered from severe symptoms of depression, anger, and post-traumatic stress disorder.

Stress and coping theories suggest that this family has multiple stressors and limited resources (Nichols, 2007). The trauma literature also suggests that many people who experienced traumatic events or losses at an early age often suffer prolonged symptoms of mood instability, intrusive thoughts of the trauma, and inability to focus and function (van der Kolk, Hopper, and Osterman, 2001). From previous research findings, it was expected that Ms. AM had reduced ability to cope with life's usual stressors. As in many other families with chronic coping and anxiety problems (Friedman, 2007), Ms. AM's family lacked adequate control and boundaries and there was considerable emotional reactivity to life events. The intrusiveness of traumatic thoughts and emotions from childhood and ongoing conflicts and problems are common to people who have been traumatized and there is the compulsion to repeat the trauma experience (van der Kolk et al., 2001).

Biological evidence supports that many people who have been traumatized are addicted to high levels of emotional arousal that can be created by extremely stressful lives and violent relationships (van der Kolk et al., 2001). Because such self-defeating patterns are long term, the psychiatric literature refers to people with these problems as having personality disorders (Mollar and Murphy, 2001).

In considering the nursing diagnoses for Ms. AM, *post-trauma syndrome, stress overload*, and *readiness for enhanced coping* were considered the best to guide care. If the nurse was working with Ms. AM's family while they were in the shelter, *readiness for enhanced family process* and *relocation stress syndrome* might also have been useful.

Initially, Ms. AM focused on her sleep and mood symptoms, as well as her daughter's situation and behavior. She needed a sleep aid and antidepressant, which was later augmented with a small dose of an atypical antipsychotic medication as a mood stabilizer. She needed help reducing her stressors and symptoms while increasing her resources.

There is considerable research evidence that alterations in neurological and psychosocial development occur following intense trauma, particularly when it is experienced at an early age (Malloy and Murphy, 2001; van der Kolk et al., 2001). Ms. AM's current housing, family, and relationship stressors were experienced as more stressful by her because of her inability to stop the intrusive memories of her past. *Stress overload* occurred because her perceived resources were inadequate to deal with the perceived stressors. The nursing diagnosis of *post-trauma syndrome* in this case is related to her past trauma and ongoing re-traumatizing domestic violence.

NOC Outcome

The outcomes desired for Ms. AM included reducing her most distressing symptoms and improving her coping and understanding, as well as helping her to find sufficient meaning and purpose in her life, which for her was helping her children and grandchild.

The NOC outcome that was established with Ms. AM was *coping*, with a baseline rating of 3 (sometimes demonstrated), and a goal score of 4 (often demonstrated).

NIC Interventions

The NIC interventions that were selected to help Ms. AM reach the outcome of *coping* were *coping enhancement, learning facilitation*, and *truth telling*. These interventions were part of a team approach, including the psychiatric nurse practitioner and social worker. The ability to help individuals and families explore meaning, shift patterns of relating, and see new possibilities is the essence of nursing from a human-becoming perceptive (Parse, 2007). All three approaches represent the essence of nursing, although the use of a team approach is essential.

The nurse focused on establishing a therapeutic relationship with Ms. AM and avoided preconceived notions or negative stereotypes about "such families." Ms. AM's symptoms and behaviors were strongly influenced by the traumatic loss of her mother and the need to be responsible and independent at too early an age. The nurse needed to respect Ms. AM's values, beliefs, and strengths, which in this case included her wish to make a better life for her children and her determination to do what it takes to make that a reality. Her mood and "addiction" to high levels of neurological arousal were interpreted as barriers to enhanced coping and goal attainment.

Initially, Ms. AM was encouraged to identify her strengths and abilities and increase her participation in solving her problems. She was encouraged to focus on the aspects of her situation that could be changed and begin to accept the realities of her life that could not, as all 12-step models for addictions recommend (Galanter, 2006).

In *truth telling*, at times it was useful to point out to Ms. AM when there were discrepancies between what she said she would like to obtain and her actions. These barriers were also amenable to education, therapy, and medications. With maturation of the central nervous system in mid-life, time also helped Ms. AM to deal with her early life trauma (Malloy and Murphy, 2001). The nurse working with Ms. AM realized that significant change would take time and set-backs were likely.

Ms. AM brought her children and boyfriend into therapy. Hopefully this would provide the children with positive experiences of mental health services, so they would be able to use such services in a timely fashion when needed.

Good quality nursing care provided limited assistance to Ms. AM, who had few choices but to live in homeless shelters or in neighborhoods where personal safety, family privacy, and respect was limited. The nurse, however, was an important member of the health care team. In many instances, nurses are cultural brokers and translators, both figuratively and literally, for people needing to interact with the health care system (Huggins, 2005).

Evaluation

In the course of a year, Ms. AM achieved a 4 on the outcome of *coping*. She was able to reduce the stressors in her life and family. The ability to avoid violent abusive relationships and interactions remained only partially fulfilled. She was able to use the health care and social services that were available to her and find satisfaction and purpose in caring for her family and to some degree herself. She exhibited and verbalized improved ability to establish and maintain boundaries between her and stressful others. She found an apartment for herself and the family and did not let her boyfriend live with them. It was still unclear if she was going to end her relationship with her current abusive boyfriend.

Ms. AM exhibited a greater understanding of the influence of traumatic loss in her life and somewhat better awareness of her tendency to get into stressful and violent relationships. She achieved some degree of being in control of her environment and her anger at the world. Her ability to connect her past traumas with her ongoing pattern of getting into abusive violent relationships remained only partially obtained. Knowing why she was in unhealthy relationships and other addictions was not sufficient to alter such patterns.

Ms. AM's initial symptoms and family problems did well despite her living in a shelter for homeless families for 18 months. She was able to see that her entire life was not ruined when her mother died, and that she could make progress toward reaching the goal of having a happy family.

Ms. AM demonstrated *readiness for enhanced coping* and was able to increase her sense of well being and control. The conscious decision to understand Ms. AM's behavior and mood in the context of her early life experiences enabled her to feel the support she needed to recall painful memories and seek the assistance she and her family needed.

References

Galanter, M. (2006). Spirituality in Alcoholics Anonymous: A valuable adjunct to psychiatric services. *Psychiatric Services, 57*, 307–309.

Huggins, M. (2005). Culture. In W.K. Mohr (ed.). *Psychiatric mental health nursing* (6th ed.) (pp. 79–100). Philadelphia, PA: Lippincott, Williams and Wilkins.

Mollar, M.D. and Murphy, M.F. (2001). *Becoming empowered: Symptom management for abuse and recovery from trauma*. Nine Mile Falls, WA: Psychiatric Resources Network.

Nichols, M.P. (2007). *The essentials of family therapy* (3rd. ed.). Boston: Allyn and Bacon.

Parse, R.R. (2007). The human-becoming school of thought in 2050. *Nursing Science Quarterly, 20*, 308–311.

van der Kolk, B.A., Hopper, J.W., and Osterman, J.E. (2001). Exploring the nature of traumatic memory, combining clinical knowledge with laboratory methods. *Journal of Aggression, Maltreatment and Trauma, 4*, 9–31.

5.23. Young Woman Whose Mother is Dying

Maria Müller Staub, RN, EdN, PhD

Elvira M is a 19-year "young" woman who was involved in a motor-bike accident with her mother. Her mother was driving the motorbike; Elvira was co-riding with her. The mother drove into a 79-year-old man who had tried to cross an inner city street in a pedestrian lane when the light was red. All three were brought to the ED by ambulance: mother, daughter, and the pedestrian. The mother and pedestrian were multi-trauma patients, with head injuries, and were in comas. After emergency treatments, they were transferred to the ICU in life threatening states.

Elvira had suffered only minor injuries such as bruises on her arms, but was psychologically shocked, and in a severe, unstable, emotional state, fearing what was going to happen with her mother. For Elvira, the physical and neurological exams showed no abnormalities. Elvira did not have pain, and displayed no signs of confusion. At the accident, she had only fallen from the motorbike and landed smoothly on the ground with her arms stretched out to stop the fall.

She was kept in the ED for surveillance and to be given current and careful information about the serious and deteriorating health state of her mother. Her mom was Elvira's major sorrow. Elvira was very anxious, but also aggressive and displayed helplessness and power-lessness. After getting the bad news that her mother could die of her non-operable head injuries, Elvira displayed nervous behaviors. Her father arrived about one hour after the admission of his wife and daughter, and first went to the ICU to see his wife and get information about her health state and the pedestrian who had died after suffering hemorrhages at the base of the skull. While remaining composed but understanding that his wife also was in a life threatening condition, he went to the ED to check on his daughter.

For Elvira, waiting for further information for at least one hour and not being able to be with her mother while she went through different exams and treatments at the ICU was difficult. The nurse constantly stayed with Elvira to help her bear this situation, to assess her needs, and to identify effective nursing interventions for her, while the father made telephone calls to family and friends and talked to the multi-professional care team at the ICU.

An in-depth conversation of the nurse with Elvira showed that she was in psychological treatment before the accident. Developmental problems in becoming an adult were diagnosed by a psychiatrist. Elvira said: "I don't like to leave home or go away from my mom, and I hardly went out with peers. I prefer to be with my mother."

Elvira was nervous, glimpsing unsteadily around, and walked back and forth in her small room. The physician advised her to take a tranquilizer, but she refused. She wanted constant information and to visit her mother as soon as possible, but was told this would not be possible during the next hour. "My teachers and doctors say I display disturbed social interactions," she mentioned. When the nurse asked Elvira about how she spent her free time, she said that she did not have hobbies except reading and talking with her mother. She did not engage in any sports, nor was she interested in movies or music. "Sometimes I just sit and think," she told the nurse in a voice that sounded empty, her eyes staring out through the window.

The accident worsened her unhappy situation, and the thought of losing her mother was unbearable. She said, "I can't imagine living without my mom, I'd prefer to die with her." Elvira was changing between states of nervousness and despair, frequently sobbing, and expressed lack of meaning or purpose in life and of her own acceptance. When the nurse asked her about believing in God or a higher power, she said "I'm angry toward God that he made this accident happen; he abandoned me."

The nurse selected Peplau's Model of Psychodynamic Nursing to work with Elvira (Peplau, 1952; Reynolds, 1997). Peplau describes relationship building as the key component of nursing care. The nurse thought that the most important care she could provide for Elvira was being with her, trying to build trust and starting a professional relationship during this difficult time. Peplau described four phases of the nurse-patient relationship: orientation, in which the person and the nurse mutually identify the person's problem; identification, in which the person identifies with the nurse and accepts help; exploitation, in which the person makes use of the nurse's help; and resolution, in which the person accepts new goals and frees the self from the relationship. The nurse also planned to assume one or more of the nursing roles that Peplau identified. These were the counseling role, which is working with the person on current problems; the leadership role, which is democratically working with the person; the surrogate role, which is figuratively standing in for another person in the patient's life; the stranger role, which is objectively accepting the person; the resource person, which is interpreting the medical plan to the patient; and the teaching role, which is offering information and helping the patient learn (Peplau, 1991, 1997).

After staying two hours at the ED with the nurse staying with her, the bad news came that her mother was going to die. The primary nurse accompanied Elvira and her father to say goodbye to her dying mother, who died a half hour later. When she returned to the ED, Elvira accepted a tranquilizer, cried, and was calmer.

STOP. THINK. Which diagnoses, outcomes, and interventions would you select?

Submitter's Analysis and Use of NANDA-I, NOC, and NIC

In considering the nursing diagnoses most appropriate for Elvira, diagnoses such as *delayed growth and development, social isolation, chronic sorrow, anticipatory grieving,* and *hopelessness* were disregarded. Though Elvira had previously shown deviations from age-group norms in becoming an adult, these nursing diagnoses were not the focus of nursing interventions for the nurse in the ED, and careful analysis of the nursing assessment revealed that Elvira showed *spiritual distress* related to loneliness, social alienation, and expected death of her mother. Elvira previously refused interactions with friends and peers, and had verbalized being separated from her support system if her mother would leave her. Elvira's history also revealed *ineffective coping strategies* as shown in research. Dekovic, Koning, Stams, and Buist (2008) identified pre-trauma, individual factors such as personality and coping as the most important predictors of distress related to traumatic symptoms and problem behavior.

NOC Outcomes

The NOC outcomes that the nurse and Elvira selected to address were *coping* and *personal wellbeing.* One major related factor for her *spiritual distress* was the sudden loss of her mother that was not amenable to change. The loss of her mother would influence her wellbeing during a time of grieving. The other related factors of *spiritual distress,* however, could be influenced by nursing interventions. The goals for Elvira were to feel a greater sense of control and adapt to the coming changes in her life.

The overall baseline score for coping was 3 (sometimes demonstrated) and the target score was for Elvira to maintain this level of coping during this time of grieving. The indicators to evaluate whether the target score was met or not were Elvira reporting psychological comfort, seeking information concerning treatment, and verbalizing a sense of control. The baseline score for *personal wellbeing* was 1 (not at all satisfied) and the target score for a long term goal was set as 3 (moderately satisfied). The indicators selected to evaluate were social relationships, spiritual life, ability to cope, and ability to express emotions.

NIC Interventions

The NIC interventions that the nurse implemented to support Elvira's *coping* in the ED were *anxiety reduction, calming techniques,* and *emotional support*. The physician and the nurse spoke with Elvira's psychiatrist, who supported these interventions. In studies of adolescents with traumatic grief, modified cognitive-behavioral therapy was shown to be effective in lowering depression, anxiety, and behavioral symptoms (Cohen, Mannarino, and Staron, 2006; Brown, Pearlman, and Goodman, 2004). Elvira, her father, and the psychiatrist agreed on the goal of assisting her in the coming time of grief and to use further psychological counseling to overcome her developmental problems. Before leaving the ED, appointments were made for Elvira and her father in the psychiatric outpatient clinic for the next day. The nurse assured that, after Elvira left the ED, she would receive crisis intervention and socialization enhancement. Nurses in the outpatient clinic were informed about the long term target score and the suggested indicators of *personal wellbeing* decided upon with Elvira.

Evaluation

In the evaluation phase, the nurse decided that the nursing interventions had been successful. Elvira was calmer when she left and agreed to further psychiatric sessions. By reflecting, the nurse became aware that she and Elvira had successfully participated in the first three phases of Peplau's Model, i.e., orientation, identification, and exploitation, and at least partially in the resolution phase. The nurse had acted in the counseling and teaching role, in the stranger and surrogate roles, and as a resource person for Elvira (Peplau, 1991, 1997). Despite being sad that she could not work longer with Elvira and that she would never know whether Elvira reached further improved outcomes, the nurse felt satisfied about the care given. Elvira had agreed to work with the caregivers in the outpatient clinic toward the outcome of *personal wellbeing*.

References

Brown, E.J., Pearlman, M.Y., and Goodman, R.F. (2004). Facing fears and sadness: Cognitive-behavioral therapy for childhood traumatic grief. *Harvard Review of Psychiatry, 12,* 187–198.

Cohen, J.A., Mannarino, A.P., and Staron, V.R. (2006). A pilot study of modified cognitive-behavioral therapy for childhood traumatic grief (CBT-CTG). *Journal of the American Academy of Child and Adolescent Psychiatry, 45,* 1465–73.

Dekovic, M., Koning, I.M., Stams, G.J, and Buist, K.L. (2008). Factors associated with traumatic symptoms and internalizing problems among adolescents who experienced a traumatic event. *Anxiety, Stress, and Coping, 21,* 377–386.

Peplau, H.E. (1952). *Interpersonal relations in nursing.* New York: G.P. Putnam's Sons.

Peplau, H.E. (1991). *Interpersonal relations in nursing: A conceptual framework of reference for psychodynamic nursing.* New York: Springer.

Peplau, H.E. (1997). Peplau's theory of interpersonal relations. *Nursing Science Quarterly, 10,* 162–167

Reynolds, W.J. (1997). Peplau's theory in practice. *Nursing Science Quarterly, 10,* 168–170.

5.24. Rehabilitation of a Male with a Young Family after a Stroke

Margaret J. Reilly, MS, APRN

James R is a 54-year-old white male who suffered a CVA (stroke) four weeks ago. At that time a CT scan confirmed a thrombotic CVA; a neurological evaluation concluded that the right middle cerebral artery had been affected.

He spent three weeks at a rehabilitation center (rehab) and was discharged home for skilled nursing care and additional physical (PT), occupational (OT), and speech therapies. On admission to home care services, he demonstrated right-sided paresis of his upper and lower extremities; he is right-hand dominant. He was able to ambulate with a walker and supervision, sit upright, and transfer from the bed to a wheelchair with supervision. He could feed himself if someone prepared and cut his food.

In the rehab referral, it was reported that James R had difficulty acknowledging his current physical deficits, and he often refused to participate in PT or use assistive devices. In the beginning of rehab, a one-to-one watch was ordered to limit the possibility of falls, because he impulsively tried to leave the facility to return home to care for his children. It was also noted that he expressed anger and verbal abuse toward his older brother, who along with his sister was caring for his children.

James R had expressive aphasia that initially impeded his ability to communicate. His speech had slowly improved, however, and he was now able to communicate his needs and frustrations. He struggled with the prospect of being unable to continue in his current business as owner and manager of a horse farm or fulfill his role as the primary caretaker of his children. His stroke left him unable to drive a car or ambulate without a walker. James R's only health insurance was through his estranged wife's employment.

Health History

During the admission interview, the home health care (HHC) nurse assessed that James R had been previously diagnosed with hypertension, but did not regularly take his medication. He had been 30 pounds overweight for several years, followed a diet high in fat and cholesterol, and smoked two packs of cigarettes a day for 30 years. He did not engage in a program of regular physical exercise, although as owner and manager of a horse farm he was physically active with his responsibility for the "hands-on" care of the 36 horses stabled at his farm.

He had a history of alcohol abuse, had been abstinent for 15 years, but in the last six months he began drinking again during a bitter divorce and child custody battle. His daughter told the nurse that he had "sworn" her to secrecy about his drinking, insisting that he had it "under control." She voiced regret about not contacting a family member about his drinking.

James R has been estranged from his wife of 20 years for the last eight months and the three children, ages 19, 16, and 12, currently reside with him. He lives in a rural area with limited public and private transportation.

While James R was hospitalized and in rehabilitation, his oldest brother and a sister lived at his home and cared for his children. Both must shortly return to work, however, and James R's estranged wife has shown no indication that she wants to take on the daily care of the children.

James R faced the prospect of physical and financial dependence on his siblings and children, a significant change from his role as the breadwinner and primary caretaker of his children. His social support system consisted only of his siblings and horse owners who stable their horses at his farm.

He alternated between angry outbursts at his older brother and anyone who tried to physically assist him and weeping about the future ability to care for his children and financially support them. He lamented that the stroke happened to him and not to his estranged wife. At times he was adamant that he did not need support services, and insisted that his 19-year-old daughter would take care of things. He continued to periodically refuse to participate in therapeutic exercises.

STOP. THINK. Which diagnoses, outcomes, and interventions would you select?

Submitter's Analysis and Use of NANDA-I, NOC, and NIC

On the initial home visit, the HHC nurse reviewed possible nursing diagnoses to consider for James R. These included *impaired physical mobility, impaired verbal communication, self-care deficit: bathing/hygiene, self-care deficit: dressing/grooming, risk for falls, risk for injury, impaired home maintenance, knowledge deficit: health behavior, ineffective role perfor-mance, interrupted family processes, ineffective coping*, and *powerlessness*. With further assessment, many of these diagnoses were ruled out.

The three diagnoses of *impaired physical mobility, risk for falls*, and *risk for injury* were appropriate in the immediate post-stroke period, but after three weeks at rehab, he had adapted to new ways of ambulating and transferring. He also learned adaptive methods for bathing and dressing and plans were in place for his home to be refurbished with hand-rails, ramps, grab bars, and a shower chair.

Family members assisted James R with the day-to-day running of the household until more permanent decisions could be made, so *impaired home maintenance* was ruled out. While *ineffective role perfor-mance* and *interrupted family processes* were considered, James R's core problems were more extensive than these problems.

The HHC nurse determined that the priority nursing diagnosis that addressed James R's core issues was *powerlessness*. James R was in agreement with this diagnosis. In a research study of 79 participants with end-stage renal disease, powerlessness, as conceptualized by Miller (2000), was linked to effects on quality of life and role function, both key issues for James R (Hay, 2005).

James R demonstrated the behaviors of anger over his loss of func-tional abilities, irritability regarding his dependence on others, frustra-tion and despair at his inability to fulfill his role as caretaker of his children and his business, and refusal to participate in care. Before the stroke, he had reverted back to alcohol abuse as a coping strategy, and was at risk for further use of ineffective coping strategies. Use of effec-tive coping strategies can reduce future risk of illness and promote hope and wellness (Popovich, Fox, and Bandagi, 2007).

NOC Outcomes

The NOC goals identified as appropriate for James R were *depression level, hope, coping*, and *adaptation to physical disability*. For *depression level*, at baseline his score was 2 (substantial) and the goal score was 4 (mild). For the outcomes of *hope, coping*, and *adaptation to physical disability*, the baseline scores were 2 (rarely demonstrated) and the goal scores were 4 (often demonstrated).

NIC Interventions

The nursing interventions that were selected to address the nursing diagnosis and meet the desired outcomes were *coping enhancement, counseling, decision-making support*, and *health system guidance*. The home care team enhanced James R's coping by fostering independence in daily functions and assisting him to recognize the power that he had to make decisions and arrange for positive outcomes. The nurse reviewed possible coping strategies with James R and supported strategies that they both agreed would be effective. These coping strategies included maintaining independence, having a positive attitude, and implementing new health behaviors. The nurse instructed James R on techniques to use in the home to function independently or with minimal assistance. Key people were identified to "talk through" frustrations as well as accomplishments. The nurse also provided education on lifestyle changes for health maintenance and health promotion.

The physical therapist provided exercises to build strength and the occupational therapist provided instruction on adaptive devices to allow self-sufficiency. The speech therapist supplied techniques to ensure effective communication as well as protection from aspiration. The social worker offered individual counseling as well as family counseling in adapting to new roles and lifestyles. Anti-depressant therapy was continued and group support services were identified for future use.

With the stroke diagnosis, skilled HHC nursing involved teaching self-care regimens in the home, instruction on new medications, nutrition education, and monitoring of symptoms and response to the plan of care. The HHC nurse provided decision-making support to James R by helping him to identify and select positive behaviors and actions. Family input was solicited as appropriate and new health behaviors were implemented. The nurse and social worker also provided guidance on financial resources and mechanisms for accessing the health care system.

Evaluation

After two months at home, James R benefitted from home care services. His overall target scores of 4 on the outcomes were all met.

His older brother installed hand-rails, a ramp, and grab bars in the bathroom. James R was able to manage his own hygiene and dress himself. He graduated to ambulating safely with a quad cane. Although his family was concerned that he may rely on alcohol as a coping strategy, he acknowledged that these strategies were unhealthy and agreed to regularly meet with the social worker to deter these habits. He had been started on an anti-depressant while in rehab and agreed to continue taking this medication as well as the other newly prescribed medications. He acknowledged his addictive behaviors and expressed a strong desire to "work hard to be able to take care of my children."

With the guidance of the HHC nurse, James R eventually realized he could not physically meet the needs of his 12 year-old child, and he asked his estranged wife to take responsibility for the child and she agreed. She also agreed to hold off on divorce proceedings so he could be maintained on her health insurance. At the suggestion of the home care nurse, James R met with the social worker and applied for disability to have access to health care so he would not have to rely on his estranged wife's health insurance policy.

James R's 19-year-old daughter enrolled in a local college and was his major caretaker with some help from neighbors and James R's siblings. The HHC nurse and the social worker addressed the unhealthy reliance on his 19-year-old daughter as primary caretaker. To alleviate some of the burden on her, arrangements were made for his siblings to visit weekly to assist with household maintenance and for neighbors to help with daily chores. The social worker arranged for counseling services for the daughter as well. With help from the home care nurse, James R began to consider support groups to attend after HHC services concluded. He continued to follow his medication regimen and changed his diet to limit fatty and fried foods.

Although his daughter, several neighbors, and customers assisted in maintaining the operations of the horse farm, James R realized he would not be able to supervise the necessary work that needed to be done and made a decision to sell the farm and move to a one story handicap-adapted condominium. The nurse, social worker, and family members provided support for his decision making.

References

Hay, C.G. (2005). Predictors of quality of life of elderly end-stage renal disease patients: An application of Roy's model. Doctoral dissertation, Georgia State University. Retrieved August 1, 2008, from ProQuest Nursing and Allied Health Source database. Publication No. AAT 3166438.

Miller, J.F. (2000). *Coping with chronic illness: Overcoming powerlessness* (3rd ed.). Philadelphia: F.A. Davis.

Popovich, J.M., Fox, P.G., and Bandagi, R. (2007). Coping with stroke: Psychological and social dimensions in U.S. patients. *International Journal of Psychiatric Nursing Research, 12,* 1477–1487.

5.25. Elderly Woman Who Thinks She Should Not be Discharged

Tomoko Hasegawa Katz, RN, PhD, Edmont Katz, MA, Michiyo Yagi, RN, Riyako Yoshikawa, RN, and Atsuko Higuchi, RN

Mrs. KY is a 91-year-old Japanese woman who was hospitalized for a cerebral infarction (CI) that occurred one month ago after she had fallen out of her bed. After the CI, she had a speech deficit and hemiparesis of the L arm and leg. Before the accident she lived with her daughter and son-in-law who own a small private fabric business. They work seven days a week.

Two weeks ago Mrs. KY started rehabilitation (Japanese hospitals are responsible for both short term and long term rehabilitation services) to increase independence in her activities of daily living (ADLs) but she showed no interest in being independent. She remained in her bed almost all day except when the nurse moved her to a wheelchair to go to the rehabilitation department. In spite of intensive treatment Mrs. KY still had L sided hemiparesis and she asked for help with almost all ADLs, including toileting, dressing, grooming, and hygiene.

Mrs. KY often says, "I cannot control my body, and I know that this condition will never be better." Her physician said that she would be able to regain mobility if she participated in appropriate rehabilitation and that she was in the discharge stage of hospitalization. When nurses spoke with her about rehabilitation and discharge planning, Mrs. KY expressed frustration and surprise about the need to go home so soon. She had believed that it would take a very long time to recover from a CI and that long-term intensive treatment in a hospital was the standard. She insisted on support with almost all of her ADLs.

Mrs. KY believed that her illness and physical condition were much more complex and severe than they actually were. She did not understand the need to start rehabilitation as soon as she was stabilized. She also complained about excessive physical exercise in the rehabilitation department.

STOP. THINK. Which diagnoses, outcomes, and interventions would you select?

Submitter's Analysis and Use of NANDA-I, NOC, and NIC

Mrs. KY demonstrated passivity and nonparticipation in care even though opportunities were provided. She expressed dissatisfaction over her inability to perform self-care, especially toileting, and wanted to stay in the hospital as long as possible. In addition, she did not understand the necessity and purposes of rehabilitation. The nurses decided that she was experiencing *powerlessness* related to deficient knowledge of the illness-related regimen. In a qualitative study of self determination with 17 patients in Sweden, the investigators' conclusions were that knowledge is expressed as power (Nordgren and Fridlund, 2001).

NOC Outcomes

The NOC outcome that was selected was *health beliefs: perceived ability to perform*. The baseline score was identified as 1 (very weak) and the target goal was set as 3 (moderate).

NIC Interventions

To reach the goal for *health beliefs: perceived ability to perform*, the nurses selected the NIC interventions of *teaching: individual, self-awareness enhancement*, and *mutual goal setting*. One of the nurses explained to Mrs. KY the nurses' role in helping her to improve her independence and that she would not be able to stay in the hospital much longer. When people are in arousal states, e.g., Mrs. KY receiving notice that she was being prepared to go home, they need guidance, information, and support (Woodward, 2001). When Mrs. KY understood, the nurses collaborated to teach her about her illness, treatments, and prognosis. They explained the purposes and necessity of rehabilitation.

The nurses coordinated several planning meetings with Mrs. KY's physical therapist (PT) and occupational therapist (OT) about how to interact with her. All members of the health care team worked together to establish mutual trust with her. The PT and OT spent time with Mrs. KY to discuss her perception and the reality of her physical abilities. Mrs. KY, the nurse, the PT, and the OT set a mutually agreeable goal for rehabilitation, especially for Mrs. KY to regain toileting self-care.

Mrs. KY's confidence in herself, the nurses, the PT, and the OT grew significantly as she actively interacted with them. She enjoyed interacting with her PT so much that she stayed almost all day in the rehabilitation department.

Prior to gaining an effective understanding of the rehabilitation process, Mrs. KY had experienced a feeling of neglect each time she returned to her room from rehabilitation. Before these planned interventions, she did not understand the differences in care intensity between the two settings.

From the time of initiation, two weeks of coordinated interventions resulted in Mrs. KY benefiting from an observably positive feeling about her future. As Mrs. KY's connection with the health care team steadily increased, her ability to benefit from their teaching significantly improved. She gradually came to understand the nature of the current care processes for CI. This resulted in an improved convergence of her health perceptions and realities.

Evaluation

Mrs. KY attained the outcomes that she and the nurses had set. She demonstrated that she met the target goal of 3 on *health beliefs: perceived ability to perform*. She understood that her improvement required reasonable effort in rehabilitation activities. She developed a perception that her health behavior was not too complex. She overcame *powerlessness* through increased knowledge of her health condition and treatment regimen.

References

Nordgren, S., and Fridlund, B. (2001). Patients' perceptions of self-determination as expressed in the context of care. *Journal of Advanced Nursing, 35,* 117–125.

Woodward, W. (2001). A plan for long-term care based on the nursing theory of modeling and role-modeling. In M. Lunney, *Critical thinking and nursing diagnosis: Case studies and analysis* (pp. 152–153). Philadelphia, PA: NANDA International.

5.26. Elderly Man Who is Angry

Tomoko Hasegawa Katz, RN, PhD, Edmont C. Katz, MA, Michiyo Yagi, RN, Riyako Yoshikawa, RN, and Atsuko Higuchi, RN

Mr. AM, 83 years old, was admitted to a Japanese hospital for terminal stage colon cancer with fever, pain, and high blood glucose level. For the last 10 years, he suffered from type 2 diabetes mellitus, hypertension, and rheumatoid arthritis (RA). When he was diagnosed with cancer five years ago, his cancer prognosis was poor. For two years, he has been on total parenteral nutrition (TPN).

Mr. AM lived with his wife in rural Japan. He has a son who is a priest and lives in the same city with his family. His son is out of town with his work, however, for about three weeks of every month. Whenever in town, the son and his family visit Mr. AM. He also has a daughter who lives in Tokyo, 500 miles away, with her family. According to his wife, he has devoted himself to others, and he was very respected by her, their son, and their neighbors. Mr. AM retired from his high school teaching position when he was 60. Since his retirement, he and his wife have taken care of their local temple and personal farm garden.

Soon after hospitalization, his temperature stabilized to within normal range. His critical blood values improved to glucose, 180 to 240 mg/dl; total protein, 5.4 gm/dl; and albumin, 3 gm/dl. His diet consisted of TPN and prescribed foods such as yogurt, soft rice, and soft noodles.

Mr. AM experiences back and chest pain and lower extremity weakness that make it difficult for him to independently use a commode. His wife or a nurse assist him. He has difficulty transitioning from supine to sitting positions, but is able to maintain an unassisted sitting position for a few minutes. His physician recommended lower extremity exercises to overcome toileting difficulties, but he refused. Mr. AM knew his cancer diagnosis, but did not know that he was in the terminal stage.

Since his hospitalization, Mr. AM assertively expressed his dissatis-factions. He persistently complained of body pains related to RA. When his pain became intolerable, he demanded that nurses increase his prednisone dosage. Consistently, he disregarded his care providers' instructions and frequently self-administered prednisone. His frequent expressions of frustration and anger included complaints to his family and physician as well as repeated calls to nurses with the nurse-call button. When a nurse delayed coming to him, he said, "I almost peed on the floor because you were late!" He broke his nurse-call button three times within a month. He complained, "Why has my condition gotten worse? I am in this hospital. What are the doctors and nurses doing for me?"

STOP. THINK. Which diagnoses, outcomes, and interventions would you select?

Submitter's Analysis and Use of NANDA-I, NOC, and NIC

As a teacher, a temple caretaker ("Yakuso" in Japanese), and head of a family, Mr. AM had been responsible for taking care of others and had exercised control over his life. But now his physical condition contin-ued to worsen and he felt the decline of his health to be out of control. He became frustrated over not having any control over his health status or treatments. Mr. AM said he was a very organized person, and had his own way of doing things such as personal hygiene. He was frus-trated that the nurses performed their own routines and did not ask him how he wanted things done. The nurses worked as a group to figure out the core problem and how to address it. They selected the priority diagnosis of *powerlessness* related to loss of control over dete-riorated health status and treatment. In a phenomenological study with 17 patients, Strandmark (2004) concluded that a sense of ill health is powerlessness, which occurs from a self-image of worthlessness and a sense of being imprisoned in one's life situation. Mr. AM also suffered from *acute pain* related to rheumatoid arthritis and terminal stage cancer.

NOC Outcomes

Mr. AM's nurses focused on his control over decisions and pain man-agement. The NOC outcome established for Mr. AM was *health beliefs: perceived control*. The baseline score was identified as 1 (very weak) and the target goal was set as 3 (moderate). The other selected outcome was *client satisfaction: pain management*. The baseline score for this outcome was 1 (not at all satisfied) and the target goal was set as 3 (moderately satisfied).

NIC Interventions

The NIC interventions delivered to reach the desired outcomes of *health beliefs: perceived control* and *client satisfaction: pain management* were *decision-making support* and *active listening*. Human support and intimacy with others can compensate for destructive feelings and powerlessness (Strandmark, 2004). The nurses started to display their interest in Mr. AM's complaints and frustrations rather than avoiding him. They tried to stay with and listen to him as much as time would allow. The nurses also tried to speak with Mr. AM about his pain, physical condition, and medications to determine whether there were differences between the patient's and nurses' views of his condition. They also consistently discussed with him his procedural preferences.

Mr. AM was encouraged to express his thoughts, feelings, and concerns about his health condition and future outlook. The nurses respected him and complied with his requests concerning his care, especially his personal hygiene.

Gradually, Mr. AM expressed without anger his feelings of alienation and powerlessness over his health. He said that he was frustrated because there were few opportunities for him to make decisions over his health.

Mr. AM's physical condition did not change significantly, although his pain level noticeably decreased. His expressions of dissatisfaction significantly decreased while he progressively regained his former sense of personal dignity.

Evaluation

Mr. AM achieved the outcome target of 3 on both outcomes: *health beliefs: perceived control* and *client satisfaction: pain management* after the nursing diagnosis of *powerlessness* was addressed. Mr. AM's *powerlessness* was incompletely but observably improved by *decision-making support* and *active listening* by the nurses. His acute pain was better controlled through personalized care. By working together with Mr. AM, his nurses helped him to achieve a sense of self-determination. In a qualitative study of the self-determination of 17 patients, it was concluded that feelings of self-determination could be improved by increased communication and support from nurses (Nordgren and Fridlund, 2001).

References

Nordgren, S., and Fridlund, B. (2001). Patients perceptions of self determination as expressed in the context of care. *Journal of Advanced Nursing, 35,* 117–135.

Strandmark, M. (2004). Ill health is powerlessness: A phenomenological study about worthlessness, limitation and suffering. *Scandinavian Journal of Caring Science, 18,* 135–144.

5.27. Homeless Woman's Reaction to Loss

Barbara Kraynyak Luise, RN, EdD

Maria D. is a 26-year-old mother of two children who currently resides at a shelter for homeless families with her husband, Richard, and their two children. The D. family members have been at the shelter for three weeks. They became homeless after Richard lost his job and they were unable to pay the rent for their apartment. Richard recently found a job and the family is saving for the deposit on a new apartment. Usually families are permitted to stay at the shelter for only two weeks, but an extension was approved for the D. family, since they are progressing toward their goal of a new apartment.

Richard is gone from the shelter from 8 am to 6 pm, during which time Maria is sole caregiver of the children. Maria expressed to the shelter staff that she was grateful for the home that was provided during the past three weeks but there are some aspects of shelter life that are really difficult. The days are "long" and "I miss the community where I lived. When you are in a shelter, it is very hard on you and your family. Others tell you when to get up and when to go to bed. If I want to take a shower or take a nap with my children, I have to ask permission. Some of the things I miss the most are keeping the house clean and cooking for my family. I loved our apartment and spending time there with my family. Now, I am dependent on the shelter staff."

This same day, there was a party to celebrate the birthdays of residents of the shelter whose birthdays occur during that month. The party is organized and donated each month by volunteers, including a community health nurse specialist whose research focused on helping homeless people. Each person with a birthday is recognized, honored, and presented with a small gift. Maria enjoyed the party with her children. Near the end of the party, a volunteer approached Maria to ask if she wanted to examine some clothes that had just been donated.

Maria went with the volunteer to see whether there were any clothes that she could use. While Maria was deciding on which clothes to select, the volunteers who had organized the party cleaned up the tables and discarded the cupcakes and juice boxes that Maria had saved to share that evening with her husband. When Maria returned to the party area and saw that the things she saved were not there, she became tearful, loud, and accusatory. "Someone took my plate of cupcakes and juice boxes that I was saving for my husband." When told that the volunteers had cleaned off the tables and probably threw them out, her anger increased. She pointed her finger at the volunteer, "The point is they were mine. No one had a right to touch them." She refused to be consoled by either the shelter staff or the volunteers.

 STOP. THINK. Which diagnoses, outcomes, and interventions would you select?

Submitter's Analysis and Use of NANDA, NOC, and NIC

The shelter staff members were baffled by Maria's behavior. They felt that she was overreacting to a minor incident. They might have been saying to themselves, "What is her problem? We are supporting her family until they can get money saved for a new place and this is the thanks we get." Other possible interpretations of Maria's behavior are: *self esteem disturbance, altered role performance,* and *ineffective coping.* There were some cues to support each of these diagnoses. The nurse who was working in the shelter, however, interpreted Maria's behavior as *powerlessness* related to loss of home and control of environment. Like many families who are homeless, Maria felt a lack of control over her life situation and was frustrated with her inability to act in the role of wife and mother. The dependence on others that occurred over the previous three weeks was exemplified in this incident and left her with a strong feeling of helplessness.

Even though homelessness is the lack of a home (Baumann, 1993), homeless families lose more than just their homes. With homelessness, families lose the "rootedness" that a home provides. Because of this, Maria feared that her family may begin to disintegrate because of the homeless state. To an observer, it might seem that Maria's reaction to the loss of cupcakes and juice was excessive, and indicative of serious problems. Yet, this reaction occurred in response to Maria's struggle to maintain some sense of family life.

NOC Outcome

There is no NOC outcome that has been developed for *power*, so the nurse used the outcome of *psychosocial adjustment: life change* (p. 577).

Maria was scored as a 4 (often demonstrated) with a goal score of 5 (consistently demonstrated).

NIC Interventions

The nurse acknowledged the lack of control that Maria felt at the time, which was exacerbated by this incident. The nurse suggested strategies that would enhance Maria's power (Barrett, 2000). Her statements to Maria included, "Can you forgive us for making an honest mistake? We didn't mean any harm; we were just trying to clean up after the party. You can rectify the problem by coming into the shelter pantry and picking out some goodies for your husband." Together, Maria and a volunteer were able to gather a new plate of treats that Maria would share with her husband that evening. By asking forgiveness, the nurse helped Maria to realize that she had the power to forgive. By making the suggestion that Maria select a few treats from the pantry for her and her husband, Maria knew that she had control over what was selected. In substituting for the treats that were discarded, Maria had the power to plan and carry out a special time with her husband that evening.

The nurse was aware that all possessions are meaningful to homeless people. Possessions often hold meanings for homeless people beyond their functional properties (Baumann, 1993; Drury, 2008). These tangible possessions of Maria, the cupcakes and juice, may have symbolized memories of happier times in the past. They also may have represented a way of exerting power over her situation, since she was able to obtain something special that she could share with her husband that evening. When these symbols were taken away, she exhibited the anger that is associated with *powerlessness*.

Evaluation

The nursing interventions successfully abated Maria's immediate distress. The goal score of 5 was achieved, and the nurse worked with the staff members to assist them in applying principles of supporting power for all residents of the shelter.

References

Barrett, E.A.M. (2000). The theoretical matrix for a Rogerian nursing practice. *Theoria: Journal of Nursing Theory, 9*(4), 3–7.

Baumann, S.L. (1993). The meaning of being homeless. *Scholarly Inquiry in Nursing Practice, 7*(1), 59–70.

Drury, L.J. (2008). From homeless to housed: Caring for people in transition. *Journal of Community Health Nursing, 25*(2), 91–105.

5.28. Family Stress and Alzheimer's Disease

Betty Ayotte Jensen, RN, PhD

Mrs. L, 49 years old, and Bill, her 53-year-old husband, were caring for her 71-year-old mother, Mrs. Potter, who had middle-stage dementia of the Alzheimer's type. Mr. and Mrs. L moved Mrs. Potter into their home when she was no longer able to care for herself. Both Mr. and Mrs. L work full-time outside the home; she works days and he works nights. They have two children; one is married and lives outside their home, the other lives with them and attends the local junior college.

The home health care (HHC) agency was asked to come to the home to evaluate whether the family was eligible for services that might help them with Mrs. Potter.

Mrs. L: "I don't know what I'm going to do. I feel as if my life is falling apart. I'm so tired and depressed all the time. I get up early for work but Mom is up late at night and I can't leave her alone, so I'm not getting much sleep. Mom complains constantly that she is hungry. She says no one loves her and I don't take care of her. My sister, who lives six hours away and doesn't help with Mom at all, believes what Mom tells her and calls me to complain about my care of Mom. I feel guilty that I'm gone all day but we need my paycheck to make ends meet. Mom gets a Social Security check, but I don't feel right using that. I can't take her income. She took care of me; it's my duty to take care of her. Besides, what if she gets really sick? We may need that money to pay her hospital bills.

"My husband is getting really put out about all of this. He's so impatient with her and it makes me mad. If it was his mother it would be a different story. But I still feel guilty that he has to put up with Mom's problems. We used to do lots of things together, such as long walks in the evenings. We were real close. Also, I don't think Bill finds me attractive any more. I'm afraid our marriage won't survive this.

"Sometimes I get angry at Mom when she won't bathe, or asks the same question over and over. I resent the intrusion into our lives. Then I feel so guilty. I'm a terrible daughter. My daughter and her husband have a darling baby, but I just don't have the time to spend with them. My daughter is unhappy that I'm not available to do things with her. There's so much to do taking care of Mom. My son, Jeff, is staying out late at night and complains about his grandmother. I can't ask my husband or son to help out, they have their own things, and it's my job anyway. My husband does watch Mom when I'm at work, but he also needs to be sleeping since he works at night.

"I really miss my Mom; I mean, the mother I knew. Sometimes Mom doesn't even remember who I am. She often says, 'I want to call Carla.' I have to tell her that I am Carla. That hurts. I have always enjoyed crafts. I've been a member of a handcrafts club but can rarely participate now, and I don't have time to work on crafts at home. Whenever I get my materials out, Mom tries to help, and usually makes a mess and sometimes ruins my projects. Work is now my only social life; I'd go crazy if I didn't have that.

"I expect that Mom will eventually be placed in a nursing home, but I'm afraid she won't have good care there, and won't be happy. I think I should care for her at home as long as possible, at least until she's bedbound and has to be fed."

Mr. L: "Having my mother-in-law living with us is wrecking our home. We used to be such a close family. Now my wife and I are barely speaking to each other and we are rarely intimate with each other. We used to go to the health spa twice a week and kept in good shape. I still go, but Carla has stopped, and she's gaining weight. She was always quite a looker, but she's really let herself go. Sure, I understand that we need to take care of Mom. After all, it's our duty. I wish my sister-in-law would take her for awhile, though."

"I'm really worried about my family's safety. Mom tries to help in the kitchen, but she leaves the burners on and sometimes sets dishes or even paper on them. I'm afraid she's going to burn the house down. I've got to sleep during the day, so I can't watch her every minute, but she's getting dangerous. I'm afraid to go to sleep. She lets our dog out the front door and he gets into the street. I yell at her about that, but she just does it again the next time he wants out. She also feeds him several times a day. If I hide the dog food, she opens cans of tuna for him. He's getting fat, too. One of the things that really annoys me is that we can't go anywhere. We can't leave Mom alone, so if we want to go out to eat, we have to take her with us. Her behavior can be so bizarre, it's really embarrassing. Our son won't stay alone with her and I can't blame him. He's having a real hard time with this."

Jeff: "Grandma has really messed up our lives. She says the dumbest things and she's always dirty and smelly. I know Mom tries to bathe her and wash her clothes, but Grandma puts up such a fuss that it's easier just to let her be. She wears the same things every day and won't even take them off to be washed. I used to have my friends in all the time. They thought my folks were cool. But now I stay away as much as I can. I can't bring my buddies here.

"Mom and Dad are fighting all the time now. When they start yelling I get a real bad stomach ache, so I just leave. They don't have time for me any more, either. I can't talk to either one of them; they're so busy and stressed out. I want my home and my parents back!"

STOP. THINK. Which diagnoses, outcomes, and interventions would you select?

Submitter's Analysis and Use of NANDA-I, NOC, and NIC

The diagnosis for Mrs. L was *caregiver role strain* related to care responsibilities of a family member with progressive dementia. Mrs. L expressed feelings of loss over changes in her mother, concern over her mother's future, changes in family relationships, depression, and anger. With multigenerational families, everyone in the home is affected by the presence of a family member with dementia. It is not enough to focus on only one family member without understanding the family as a group.

The diagnosis for the family as a group was *interrupted family processes* related to disruption of normal family roles and routines. This diagnosis refers to the inability of a normally functioning family to adapt in positive ways to the stressors involved. For this family, the stressors of care giving led to dysfunctional behaviors, and the emotional needs of family members were not being met.

For this intergenerational family, it was important that the nurse address issues for the primary caregiver and the family. Dementia of the Alzheimer's type is a progressive, degenerative disease that leads eventually to death (Alzheimer's Association, 2008). There is no hope for the caregivers that the situation will improve. The strain on the primary caregiver and family is great and can disrupt family function.

The nurse used the Modeling and Role-Modeling Theory (Erickson, Tomlin, and Swain, 1983) for understanding the needs of this family. Several basic needs were not being met: physiologic needs for rest, safety and security needs such as freedom from fear, need for structure and consistency, love and belonging needs, and esteem needs such as respect and importance.

NOC Outcomes

The NOC outcome selected by the nurse and the L family for *caregiver role strain* was *caregiver well-being*. The baseline score for Mrs. L was

1 (not at all satisfied) and the target score was set as 4 (very satisfied).

The NOC outcomes for *interrupted family processes* were *family coping* and *family functioning*. The baseline scores were determined to be 3 (sometimes demonstrated) and the target scores were set as 5 (consistently demonstrated).

NIC Interventions

Family care giving issues were many and complex. The nurse began by assessing the internal and external resources of individuals in the family and the family as a group. The interventions were designed to facilitate mobilization of existing resources and to identify and develop additional resources. In a qualitative study of 32 caregivers of people with Alzheimer's, additional help in care giving was a factor that improved their quality of life (Vellone, Piras, Talucci, and Cohen, 2008). The NIC interventions of *coping enhancement* and *emotional support* were foundational interventions that were used. *Coping enhancement* involved activities that facilitated the individuals in the family to adapt to the changes they were experiencing in the care recipient and in the dynamics of the family. Because Mrs. Potter's condition is chronic and deteriorating, this involved permanent changes. If coping mechanisms were not in place and in use, the physical and emotional health of Mrs. L, and indeed the entire family, was at risk. In talking with each family member, the nurse encouraged them to talk about their feelings and concerns; she also validated their feelings. Talking about feelings and fears may reduce some of the burden (Jensen, 1997). The nurse helped family members to normalize these feelings, i.e., to understand that feelings of anger, frustration, and guilt are normal responses to the stressors of care giving, related to the multiple losses they were experiencing (Erickson, 1995). As they understand that their feelings are common to caregivers, they may be able to let go of guilt and free up energy for coping.

The nurse developed and implemented a teaching plan for the family that included the disease process, the relation between loss and grief, and the relation between stress and illness. This facilitated family members' understanding of the reasons for Mrs. Potter's behaviors and their own responses, which enabled them to be more patient with her and with each other. Understanding that Mrs. L is putting her health at risk if she does not get some relief from the burden of care giving gave her the motivation to ask for help.

Using the NIC intervention of *family integrity promotion*, the nurse promoted the strengths of the family and encouraged them to identify ways they had worked together in the past to handle other crises (Erickson et al., 1983). The nurse reminded them they are a unit and needed to discuss their feelings with one another, and to work together to find solutions to some of these issues. Mr. L and son Jeff were included in problem resolution, so some of their hostility was decreasing.

The NIC interventions of *health system guidance* and *respite care* were used to meet the outcomes of *family functioning* and *family coping*. The nurse assisted the caregivers to find and use available resources. With the use of *respite care* and other resources, Mrs. L conserved energy so she could provide better care and prevent over-taxing her resources. The family was referred to community agencies for needed services. Support groups were available through the Alzheimer's Association. Respite groups offered low-cost sitters. An adult day care center near their home gave Mrs. Potter an opportunity to socialize with others and participate in enjoyable activities. The family was encouraged to hire babysitters and use day care. As they understood the health benefits to the whole family, they felt less guilty about using some of Mrs. Potter's income to pay for these services.

The NIC interventions of *family involvement promotion* and *family process maintenance* were implemented. Nursing activities were focused on supporting the unity and cohesion of the family to get the family working together to care for Mrs. Potter and to support each other and decrease the disruption of the family unit. The nurse encouraged Mr. and Mrs. L to give Jeff some of their time. Families often focus on the needs of one member to the exclusion of all others, which affects all relationships. Currently, the L family members are physically healthy, but the emotional health of all members also needs to be nurtured.

There are no easy fixes for care giving problems. The nurse built a trusting relationship with the L family, which helped them to mobilize internal and external resources for coping. Working with the family to set realistic and manageable goals nurtured the health of all family members.

Evaluation

Mrs. L's relationships with her family improved. She was more relaxed about her role as a care provider and was able to use available resources, such as respite care and day care, to give her physical and emotional relief. Mrs. L's sense of well-being was improved at the termination of nursing care of this family. Mrs. L achieved a score of 3 (satisfied), which was not at the desired level of 4 (very satisfied), but was certainly a great improvement over baseline.

The L *family functioning* markedly improved. The target score of 5 (consistently demonstrated) was met. This was a healthy family before Mrs. Potter came to live with them, so they were able to rapidly improve with nursing support.

References

Alzheimer's Association. (2008). *What is Alzheimer's?* Retrieved on August 2, 2008 from http://www.alz.org/alzheimers_disease_what_is_alzheimers. asp.

Erickson, H.C. (1995). *Modeling and role-modeling with Alzheimer's patients and their caregivers.* Research study supported by the National Institutes of Health (Grant RO1NR03032-01), the National Institute of Aging, and the National Center for Nursing Research.

Erickson, H. C, Tomlin, E. M, and Swain, M. A. P. (1983). *Modeling and role-modeling: A theory and paradigm for nursing.* Englewood Cliffs, NJ: Prentice Hall.

Jensen, B.A. (1997). Caring for caregivers. *Home Care Provider, 2,* 276–278.

Vellone, E., Piras, G., Talucci, C., and Cohen, M.Z. (2008). Quality of life for caregivers of people with Alzheimer's Disease. *Journal of Advanced Nursing, 61,* 222–231.

5.29. Family Struggling with Ostomy Care at Home

Arlene Farren, RN, PhD, AOCN and Gail Champagne, RN, BSN

Mr. R is a 65-year-old male with prostatic cancer who recently experienced tumor compression of the sigmoid colon, requiring a sigmoid colostomy. Following postoperative recovery in the hospital, he was admitted to a home care service. The initial report from the hospital-based nurse included information about the family unit (wife, adult daughter, and his sister) and Mr. R's difficulty learning ostomy care and irrigation of the stoma. During the hospital stay, Mrs. R did colostomy care once and performed several irrigations. The plan of the HHC nurse was to continue teaching Mr. R and his wife the colostomy care that was begun in the hospital, including teaching daily irrigations of the colon.

At home, Mr. R expressed difficulty in learning self care of the colostomy. For example, he told the HHC nurse, "I can't really see the thing (stoma). I'm having a really hard time with all of this (irrigating equipment). Why do I have to learn this (ostomy care)? Can my wife do it like she did in the hospital?" Mr. R's physician said the option of omitting daily irrigations was not possible.

Mrs. R is employed full time and seemed overwhelmed with the procedures. She expressed feelings of anxiety, frustration, and fear of damaging the stoma. When Mrs. R. provided stoma care and irrigation before going to work, she was often one to one and a half hours late for work, which was an additional stressor for her.

The HHC nurse approached other family members to enlist their assistance with the ostomy care and support for Mr. and Mrs. R. The daughter stated, "I can't even look at that thing," and refused. His sister refused without comment. Whenever the HHC nurse discussed the treatment or procedure, the daughter and sister exited the room.

Over several weeks, attempts at teaching Mr. R self care continued to be generally unsuccessful. He was able to change the wafer after more than expected instruction and supervision by the nurse. The nurse tried several strategies to assist Mr. R. For example, a large magnifying mirror and increased lighting but Mr. R continued to state that he could not see the stoma well enough to do the procedure.

STOP. THINK. Which diagnoses, outcomes, and interventions would you select?

Submitter's Analysis and Use of NANDA-I, NOC, and NIC

After having little success with previous approaches, the HHC nurse used Rogers' (1970, 1992) Science of Unitary Human Beings (SUHB) to analyze and plan for helping the R family. Roger's four key postulates and three principles were then used as the basis for nursing care (Rogers, 1970, 1992). The nurse accepted that Mr. R and his family are open energy fields that have a distinguishing characteristic of the field called pattern. Pandimensionality is defined as a nonlinear domain without spatial and temporal attributes (Rogers, 1992). Pandimensionality gives rise to the relative present in which past, present, and future are experienced as one.

Rogers' (1992) principles of homeodynamics describe continuous change of field. There are three principles—helicy, resonancy, and integrality. Helicy describes change as innovative or a new way of doing things that emerges from creativity (Butcher, 2008). Resonancy describes the wave frequency of change as low-high frequency pattern. Integrality is defined as the continuous mutual human-environmental field process. Rogers (1990) stated that the SUHB is equally applicable to groups. In this case, the group energy field was the family; it was irreducible and integral with its own environmental field.

Using this perspective, the HHC nurse saw it was best to engage with the group or family field. It is the family that needed support and help. The R family is unitary, more than a collection of members, and more than Mr. R's ostomy or prostate cancer complications. The family journey toward well-being required appreciating a pattern beyond Mr. R's and family members seeming unwillingness to learn. The nurse understood that the group field, as with other fields, "have an awareness of their wholeness and of their integrality with the environment where both change together in a dynamic way (Phillips, 1997, p. 22)." This was crucial for the care of the R family.

Based on the postulates and homeodynamic principles, family field change was manifested as an innovative, growing diversity of field pattern in which people knowingly participate. It is the patterning process that gives rise to unitary well-being. Family assessment, an awareness of field manifestations, enabled the nurse to appreciate the family pattern in mutual process. The mutual process of nurse-family provided opportunities to participate through patterning-healing modalities that pattern the environment for well-being.

Manifestations of the R family suggested that distress was present in the field and included family statements and behaviors. For example, Mr. R expressed his difficulties in statements to the HHC nurse. Mrs. R was overwhelmed. The nurse heard expressions of anxiety and fear. Mrs. R had experienced a changed pattern of lateness at work, which increased her stress. The R family daughter and Mr. R's sister refused to engage in Mr. R's physical care. The refusal of assistance with care was upsetting to each individual and the family as a whole. The behaviors of leaving the room were manifestations of distress.

The integral nature of the family pattern was clearly evident. There was a consistent story that unfolded with themes such as "I can't deal with this," "I can't do it," "I'm afraid," "I need help." The nurses' teaching was not accomplishing its goal, which supported an ongoing pattern disruption in the R family field.

A priority diagnosis was *disturbed family energy field* related to family crisis. Other diagnoses that were considered but did not fit with Roger's SUHB were *disturbed body image, ineffective self health management,* and *compromised family coping.* In relation to the diagnostic statement, although a causative relationship is incongruent with Rogers' science, it simply stated that the "related to" factor of family crisis means that the group field is experiencing disruption.

NOC Outcomes: Manifestations of Family Well-being

Using Roger's SUHB, the NOC outcomes were viewed as manifestations of family field patterning that would be observed for change. Several outcomes in the class of family well-being were considered appropriate. The HHC nurse and the family agreed that a change in *family functioning* was desired. The baseline outcome rating was 2 (rarely demonstrated) and the family said that 4 (often demonstrated) was the best target rating they could hope to achieve. During this discussion, the family revealed concerns and grief for a perceived loss of family functioning associated with Mr. R's illness and fear of his poor prognosis.

Family coping was another priority outcome. The overall rating was determined to be a 2 (rarely demonstrated) and the family identified a realistic target rating of 4 (often demonstrated). Examples of indicators included expressing feelings and emotions openly among members and using family-centered stress reduction strategies.

NIC Interventions: Patterning of the Family-Environmental Field for Change

The HHC nurse, in mutual process with the family, engaged opportunities to pattern the field for well-being and created opportunities for change. To make progress toward enhanced *family functioning* and *family coping*, the nurse used the NIC interventions of *anxiety reduction, caregiver support, case management, family involvement promotion, presence,* and *teaching: psychomotor skill.*

The nurse used "centering" to prepare to experience the integrality of field and intention for well-being and used a quiet presence with the family. *Anxiety reduction* activities were implemented, such as a calm, reassuring approach, seeking to understand the family's perspective of the situation, supporting the use of appropriate defense mechanisms, and instructing the family on stress and anxiety reduction.

Using *caregiver support*, the HHC nurse accepted expressions of negative emotions from the family and acknowledged the difficulties they were experiencing. In all interactions, the nurse used therapeutic verbal and non-verbal communication approaches. The nurse encouraged all to accept the interdependency that was occurring and encouraged attendance at support groups within the community for families dealing with similar issues. The nurse facilitated a discussion that tried to establish realistic expectations of the family. The nurse used activities of the case management intervention, including referrals to a family therapist and community groups for support and resources such as a referral to ostomy-mate for a family visit. Telephone follow-up (more frequent at first, becoming less frequent as comfort increased) was used between visits. The nurse prepared the R family for termination of the relationship from the first visit while reassuring the family of the full course of home care services.

For the R family, it was essential to promote family involvement to pattern the environment for well-being. The HHC nurse realized that it was essential to identify the family's capability for and preference for involvement. As trust and the desire for involvement grew, the nurse encouraged the family to expand involvement in developing the plan of care. The nurse assisted the family to identify other situational stressors such as work and anticipatory grieving and worked with the family from a strength- and potential-based perspective, focusing on how they could participate and maintain an ongoing discussion of options. Contracting with the family was considered but not used at this time.

During the course of home care, the HHC nurse used *teaching: psychomotor skill* (ostomy care and irrigation). The nurse provided expert demonstration and explanation of the procedures. Some of the activities included implementing an individualized procedure for changing and irrigating that included: (a) using therapeutic touch prior to the procedure; (b) patterning the environment before the procedure with relaxing music that was quiet with gentle tones and an aroma that was a clean, gentle fragrance such as lavender or chamomile; (c) describing the "tools" or equipment in terms of pleasing sensory details; (d) gently touching the skin and describing in a positive and descriptive manner what was being done each time; (e) when complete, using a positive affirmation that reflected imaging wholeness and wellness; and (f) allowing time for questions and comments.

The nurse first asked the family to participate by providing space for the equipment, the procedure, and so forth. The nurse made the necessary initial ordering and assured timely delivery of the items, gently increasing the family participation based on their cues. Additional activities regarding the actual procedure and care included the use of imagery—imaging and visioning the process during the bag change and procedure; monitoring for pain, discomfort, and other concerns on each visit; and when appropriate or acceptable, using photography to gently introduce the physical manifestations, equipment, procedure, and completion, as well as integrated pictures of the family as a whole.

Evaluation: Ongoing Pattern Appreciation

After three weeks of home care services, the family and nurse agreed upon an overall rating for *family functioning* as 3 (sometimes demonstrated), improved although less improved than desired. Family *coping* was rated as a 3 with improvement on all applicable indicators. At this point, the frequency of in-home visits decreased and the home care nurse increased the frequency of telephone follow-up. Because the target outcome was not yet met, ongoing monitoring was needed to identify the need for increased intensity of nursing services.

References

Butcher, H.K. (2008). Innovations column. *Visions, 15,* 29.

Phillips, J.R. (1997). Evolution of the science of unitary human beings. In M. Madrid (ed.). *Patterns of Rogerian knowing* (pp. 11–27). New York: National League for Nursing Press.

Rogers, M.E. (1970). *An introduction to the theoretical basis of nursing.* Philadelphia: F.A. Davis Company.

Rogers, M.E. (1990). Nursing: Science of unitary irreducible human beings: Update 1990. In E.A.M. Barrett (ed.). *Visions of Rogers' science-based nursing* (pp. 5–11). New York: National League for Nursing.

Rogers, M.E. (1992). Nursing science and the space age. *Nursing Science Quarterly, 5,* 27–34.

5.30. Nonparticipation in Rehabilitation with a Colostomy

Maria Müller Staub, RN, EdN, PhD

Peter B is a 52-year-old male with multiple health problems who was diagnosed with colon cancer. He was admitted to a rehabilitation center (rehab) after hospitalization for surgery. Tumor surgery was successful but he needed a stoma.

Three years ago he suffered an MI and had two subsequent bypass surgeries. He has had chronic bronchitis and smoked three packages of cigarettes a day. In the hospital, he coughed for about an hour each morning. Peter B said that he drinks "about one bottle of wine a day."

As a freelance journalist, he usually worked at home. He had a sedentary lifestyle and did not like to walk. He said he only went out to a nearby restaurant.

Peter B lived with his 86-year-old mother who has dementia in a three-bedroom apartment on the third floor. His mother has suffered from arthritis for 20 years, with severely impaired mobility. She can only move with a walker and is not able to care for herself. Her physician requested a visiting nurse every day, but she only allowed the nurse to come one time a week.

The caregivers reported that the apartment was in a deteriorated state, and that Peter B and his mother did not eat well because Mrs. B was no longer able to cook. Mrs. B was convinced, however, that she cooked perfect meals twice a day.

When the nurse asked Peter B how he felt about this situation, he said: "The household is her job, I never used to do it and as long as she is in charge, it is her will to do it as she likes."

Peter B is 5 feet, 8 inches tall and weighs 187 lbs, with a BMI of 27. He had thin legs and arms with little muscle strength; his waist diameter, however, was above normal with ascites. When asked about his life and work style, he said "it's OK, we will go on and manage things," then he changed the topic by telling a joke.

The first four days of rehab, Peter B displayed normal postoperative recovery, using little pain medication, but he had a self-care deficit in bathing/hygiene and in dressing, because he felt too weak to do it. When asked if he slept well and if he felt rested in the morning, he said: "Good question, this depends on how I dream—usually I have no dreams—and how do you sleep?" The nurse said: "Fine, but I'm asking YOU, because you feel tired. Sleeping well during recovery is important. So, how was your sleep?" Peter B said, "It depends and it is the same as home, this is not of importance." During the daytime and until after 10 pm he was out of his room visiting the hospital restaurant and came only to his room for stoma care and meals. The nurses on duty reported he smelled from alcohol and cigarettes when coming back.

During dressing changes, he never looked at the stoma, but he told stories or made jokes. He refused to engage in learning to take responsibility for stoma care. On the fifth day, he stayed in bed, telling the nurse he felt tired. In the evening, he had pain in the bowel and his body temperature was 102 °F. A urinary tract infection and pneumonia were diagnosed the next day, and he was put on IV antibiotics.

When the nurse asked Peter B how he felt about his situation, he said he viewed himself as an optimist, taking things in life as they come, and always being ready for a joke. "I have nothing to say anyway. It's the same everywhere in the world, woman have the say, be it here or at home." When his infections were diagnosed, he asked to be allowed to smoke in his room or go to the restaurant with a friend. When the nurse reminded him that smoking was not permitted in the hospital and smoking was the worst he could do for his pneumonia, he became angry and said "Then I will go home tomorrow; it makes no sense that I'm here anyway." When asked how the treatment would be organized and what he thought about his self-care, he said: "I'll be OK. I don't need help, bad guys always stay alive." As during the previous days, he did not engage in discussing his health problems, his self-care deficits, or taking care of the stoma.

STOP. THINK. Which diagnoses, outcomes, and interventions would you select?

Submitter's Analysis and Use of NANDA-I, NOC, and NIC

The rehab nurses discussed how to plan care with Peter B, since no nurse seemed to be able to work collaboratively toward commonly agreed outcomes. In considering the nursing diagnoses most appropriate for Peter B, they discussed *delayed surgical recovery, ineffective airway clearance, self-care deficit, hyperthermia, imbalanced nutrition: less than body requirements, ineffective self health management, insomnia, ineffective coping, chronic low self-esteem, disturbed body image* related to the stoma, and sedentary lifestyle. One nurse said: "Yes, he has most of these problems, but in my view, the main problem is that we can't connect with him to talk about all that. I feel that he is denying what is going on. When I asked him about his cancer, he said "First: bad boys don't die, and second: This was only a minor thing, I'm OK. By the way, did you see the football game last night?" Without him being able to discuss his health patterns and behavior, we will not be able to help him."

The nurses chose the diagnosis of *defensive coping* related to inadequate level of social support created by the characteristic of relationships (his mother was the one having a say, but suffered dementia) and *situational crisis* related to the occurrence of cancer, complications, and uncertainty. Peter B's behaviors met the definition and defining characteristics of this diagnosis. He clearly showed the defining characteristics of *defensive coping* such as denial of obvious problems, projections of responsibility related to self-care and stoma care, rationalization, difficulties establishing relationships with caregivers, and sometimes ridiculous behaviors.

NOC Outcomes

The NOC outcomes chosen were *acceptance of health status* and *self-esteem*. The goal was for Peter B to accept having had cancer leading to a stoma, and to accept responsibility for stoma care. His baseline score on this outcome was 2 (rarely demonstrated) and his target score was 4 (often demonstrated). The outcome of *self esteem* was chosen because he had mentioned several times "I have nothing to say, women have the say" and "I'm a bad guy." The nurses assumed that he was coping by drinking more than one bottle of alcohol at home and that he was also drinking with visitors in the hospital restaurant. Addictive behaviors, e.g., Peter B's drinking and smoking, are related to ineffective coping and low self-esteem. Studies have shown that self-efficacy strongly predicted adherence behavior, and drinking relapse episodes were predicted by low self-efficacy (Tracey, 2007; Schweitzer, Head, and Dwyer, 2007; Cooney, Litt, Cooney, Pilkey, Steinberg, and Oncken, 2007). His baseline score on *self esteem* was 3 (sometimes positive) and the target score was 4 (often positive).

NIC Interventions

To reach the outcomes chosen, the nurses decided to choose one nurse, Carla V, to work with Peter B. Carla V chose the nursing interventions of *self esteem enhancement, emotional support, presence, active listening, cognitive restructuring, truth telling*, and *body image enhancement*. Carla V was convinced that Peter B would be able to better grasp his situation and feel more control, and that his optimistic tendency would help him to reach the selected outcomes. However, she suspected that she would not be able to openly discuss these desired outcomes with him.

When she entered Peter B's room the next day, he looked at her and said, "It's nice that you are working today." Carla V responded, "Yes, I'm glad to be here. How do you feel this morning?" And, with one eye winking, she continued, "How were your dreams last night"? He said, "Wonderful, I dreamt being at the beach, without this sac on my belly." The nurse said, "This is truly a dream, I mean this is what you really dream of, being able to live without this sac!?" He responded, "I know I never will." This conversation was the start of many conversations that Carla V and Peter B had during the following days. Carla and the care team learned to know Peter B from another side, when he told her that he had been in a clinic to recover from alcoholism last year but did not manage to "stay dry" for long. He even exposed his perception that "the problems with my mother, my job, and my health are so overwhelming, I think I just try to swallow it all down with alcohol."

Carla V used the intervention of *self-esteem enhancement* and learned that *truth telling* was not necessary since Peter B went on to openly talk about his health and behavior problems, but *truth reassuring* (Hancock et al., 2007) and *cognitive restructuring* were the appropriate interventions (Pender, Murdaugh, and Parsons, 2006). Ten days later, he mentioned: "If I have a chance to go on with my own life, I'll go to AA." Carla responded, "Going to Alcoholics Anonymous (AA) could be your only chance to go on." "Then please show me how to change the sac on my belly, and bring these brochures that you previously mentioned about nutrition for people with stomas!" he said.

Evaluation

In 16 days, Peter B left rehab. His target scores for both outcomes were met. He had contacted AA and agreed to start the program. The nursing diagnoses *delayed surgical recovery, ineffective airway clearance, hyperthermia*, and *insomnia* had subsided, and he had recovered from pneumonia and the urinary tract infection. He had ordered a visiting nurse daily and required home maintenance service to take responsibility despite knowing his mother could oppose. "I'll let her believe SHE is cooking twice a day, but now I'm the one to make sure WE BOTH eat twice a day," he said.

References

Cooney, N.L., Litt, M.D., Cooney, J.L., Pilkey, D.T., Steinberg, H.R., and Oncken, C.A. (2007). Alcohol and tobacco cessation in alcohol-dependent smokers: analysis of real-time reports. *Psychology of Addictive Behaviors*, 21, 277–286.

Hancock, K., Clayton, J., Parker, S., Wal der, S., Butow, P., Carrick, S., et al. (2007). Truth-telling in discussing prognosis in advanced life-limiting illnesses: A systematic review. *Palliative Medicine, 21,* 507–517.

Pender, N.J., Murdaugh, C.L., and Parsons, M.A. (2006). *Health promotion in nursing practice* (5th ed.). Upper Saddle River, NJ: Pearson Prentice Hall.

Schweitzer, R.D., Head, K., and Dwyer, J.W. (2007). Psychological factors and treatment adherence behavior in patients with chronic heart failure. *Journal of Cardiovascular Nursing, 22,* 76–83.

Tracey, J. (2007). The mind of the alcoholic. *Journal of the American College of Dentists, 74*(4), 18–23.

5.31. Man with Urinary Incontinence After Prostate Surgery

Annemarie Dowling-Castronovo, RN, MA, GNP

BV is a 65-year-old Caucasian male who had a radical prostatectomy for prostate cancer two months ago. His past medical history is unremarkable with the exception of an elevated prostate specific antigen (PSA) six months ago and a subsequent diagnostic evaluation that resulted in the diagnosis of prostate cancer. He came to the urologist's office for follow-up. During routine screening by the urological nurse, BV was visibly anxious as he described his experiences with "leaking" urine. He stated, "I am thankful that the doc got all the cancer, but this leaking is really getting to me. I did all those Kegels, but they just are not working."

During further assessment, the nurse learned that BV was experiencing urinary leakage when he laughed or turned in various positions, especially bending. He denied the experience of uncontrollable urges to urinate. He had no complaints of incomplete bladder emptying, urinary dribbling, hesitancy, or frequency. There was no record of a completed bladder diary. Although he had begun taking evening walks with his wife, he was reluctant to play golf because of his fear of leakage. He had a difficult time identifying dietary and fluid intake that may be contributing to the leakage. He demonstrated relief when he replied that he had no "bed-wetting." BV described his wife as supportive: "She is the one who helped me figure out what pad [incontinence pad] to use."

BV expressed frustration because he thought that he was doing "what the doctor ordered" and was not "totally dry." Despite this frustration he was enormously grateful that he was "cancer free." He is a retired businessman who continues to do consultant work. BV worried about returning to this work because of "the annoying leakage."

BV asked the nurse how to best manage the urinary leakage, "Is this leakage normal?" He also described his lack of confidence with performing the Kegels.

STOP. THINK. Which diagnoses, outcomes, and interventions would you select?

Submitter's Analysis of Data and Use of NANDA-I, NOC, and NIC

Considering the nursing diagnoses most appropriate for BV, diagnoses such as *self care deficit, urinary incontinence: functional/urge* or *urinary retention* were immediately disregarded. BV did not exhibit functional impairments and his symptoms were not consistent with urge incontinence or overflow urinary incontinence. His symptoms, e.g., urinary leakage with increased abdominal pressure such as sneezing, were consistent with the diagnosis of *stress urinary incontinence* (Abrams et al., 2003). Assessment, diagnosis, and treatment of urinary incontinence should be highly individualized. Therefore, the nurse and BV mutually discussed and agreed on this diagnosis and the treatment plan. While BV expressed the desire to be completely dry, the nurse realized that a more objective, detailed account of his urinary leakage was needed as a baseline for setting future goals. In addition, it was unclear whether BV was appropriately performing his Kegels (Kegel, 1956). The nurse further assessed and noted that there were no perianal skin alterations and no complaints of constipation or fecal incontinence. The diagnosis of *stress urinary incontinence* was validated when urinary incontinence was reproduced when the nurse asked BV to cough.

The diagnosis of *ineffective self health management* was also considered but since BV may not have had sufficient instruction and support prior to this encounter, it was ethically important not to blame him for the problem by saying his actions were "ineffective" (Redman, 2005). In addition, it was likely that he was more concerned with the cancer removal, and now that he knew he was "cancer free" he was trying to deal with the urinary leakage. Based on these data, *readiness for enhanced self health management* was also selected as a nursing diagnosis.

NOC Outcomes

The NOC outcome that was selected for the diagnosis of *stress urinary incontinence* was *urinary continence*. His baseline score was 3 (sometimes demonstrated) and the goal score was 5 (consistently demonstrated).

The NOC outcome that was selected for *readiness for enhanced self health management* was *treatment behavior: illness or injury*. The baseline score was determined to be 3 (sometimes demonstrated) and the target score was 5 (consistently demonstrated).

NIC Interventions

The nursing interventions selected to help BV achieve urinary continence were *pelvic muscle exercise, urinary incontinence care*, and *biofeedback* (Gray, 2008). The nurse spoke to BV about doing a detailed and
complete three-day bladder diary (International Consultation on
Incontinence, 2000; Jeyaseelan, Roe, and Oldham, 2000). The nurse
assessed BV's current understanding of a bladder diary and provided
needed information, verbally and written, so that the bladder diary
would be completed as accurately as possible. Medications were
reviewed and none were noted to have adverse urological activity,
which could have contributed to his urinary incontinence.

The nurse planned with BV to complete a *biofeedback* session to
assess pelvic floor muscle activity. The biofeedback session with surface
electrodes identified that BV needed instruction in how to isolate his
pelvic muscles without contracting either his abdominal or gluteal
muscles. A post-prostatectomy support group was explored with BV,
but he declined participation.

The above interventions also helped BV with his *treatment behavior:
incontinence*. Another NIC intervention that the nurse used to treat
this diagnosis was *mutual goal setting*. Based on the data from the
bladder diary and the biofeedback session, an individualized plan of
care was devised with BV. The nurse met with him for three visits
over a six-week period. As time went on, BV expressed less frustration with urinary leakage. His bladder diary initially identified three
to six small urinary leaks per day, defined as the need to change an
incontinence pad. BV expressed that completion of the diary enabled
him to have an increased awareness of when he leaked urine. With
biofeedback therapy BV was able to reach the goal to perform 10 pelvic
floor muscle exercises three times a day (total = 30). The nurse assessed
that BV was ready to learn the "knack" (Miller, Ashton-Miller, and
DeLancey, 1998), a pelvic floor muscle contraction prior to an activity
that results in urine leakage and in a female sample has resulted in
control of urine leakage (Miller et al., 1998). BV verbalized that he
would practice the knack with his swing of a golf club in his
backyard.

Evaluation

In the six-week period, the score on the NOC outcome of *urinary continence* improved to 4, not as good as hoped for but much better than
it had been. The score on *treatment behavior: illness or injury* was 5. BV
verbalized that he was achieving his personal goals. He reported occasional urinary leaks, about once a day. He still wore pads during the
day, but did not wear them at night; his confidence had increased that
he would not "start wetting the bed." He continued to perform pelvic
floor muscle exercises and the knack helped to give him the confidence

to play a short course of golf with his wife. In addition to being pleased with his increased control of urinary elimination, he was pleased that he did not have erectile dysfunction.

References

Abrams, P., Cardozo, L., Fall, M., Griffiths, D., Rosier, P., Ulmsten, U., van Kerrebroeck, P., Victor, A., and Wein, A. (2003). The standardisation of terminology of lower urinary tract function: Report from the standardization sub-committee of the International Continence Society. *Urology, 61,* 37–49.

Gray, M. (2008). Stress urinary incontinence. In B. Ackley and G. Ladwig, *Nursing diagnosis handbook: An evidence-based guide to planning care* (8th ed., pp. 462–468). St. Louis, MO: Mosby/Elsevier.

International Consultation on Incontinence (2000). Assessment and treatment of urinary incontinence. *Lancet, 355,* 2153–2158.

Jeyaseelan, S.M., Roe, B.H., and Oldham, J.A. (2000). The use of frequency/volume charts to assess urinary incontinence. *Physical Therapy Reviews, 5,* 141–146.

Kegel, A.H. (1956). Stress incontinence of urine in women: Physiologic treatment. *International College of Surgeons, 25,* 487–499.

Miller, J.M., Ashton-Miller, J.A., and DeLancey, J.O. (1998). A pelvic muscle precontraction can reduce cough-related urine loss in selected women with mild SUI. *Journal of the American Geriatrics Society, 46,* 870–874.

Redman, B.K. (2005). The ethics of self-management preparation for chronic illness. *Nursing Ethics, 12,* 360–369.

5.32. Palliative Care and the Outcome of Comfort

Maria Aurora Fernandez–Roibas, RN and
Carme Espinosa–Fresnedo, RN, MS

Manuel was an 83-year-old man who was hospitalized in the palliative care unit for about one month before he died because he could no longer live on his own. Manuel had been a widow for the last five years. He had two daughters and one son. When he was home, his older daughter visited him every day and supervised his nutrition, hygiene, and home maintenance. Manuel's son visited him from time to time, but his relationship with his son and with his younger daughter had not been very close. Up until hospitalization, he lived on his own in a rural area in Lugo, Northwest Spain. He was autonomous in activities of daily living and every day he took long walks. His neighbors helped him as needed.

About one year ago, he began to experience loss of voice, but he thought the difficulties were associated with a cough. When the cough did not improve, he decided to visit his family physician, and afterwards a specialist in otolaryngology. Neither physician identified any pathology in the vowel strings that could contribute to a loss of voice. About one month later, Manuel found a tumor in the clavicle region and the loss of voice was still there. He did not want to speak to the neighbors because they detected his difficulties in speaking, and then questioned him about the reason. He began to feel neck pain and tiredness. Again he visited the specialist and a CAT scan was performed. After that he was sent to surgery for a biopsy of the supraclavicular tumor.

Manuel was very worried about being in the hospital, because he had never before been hospitalized. He did not like the hospital schedule, the need of being without his own clothes, and the whole day doing nothing. He said, "If I have to live like this I would rather die, unless the doctors can find something to make me feel better."

After the biopsy, the physician informed Manuel's daughter that there is nothing that could be done except palliative care. The cancer was too large and inoperable. Manuel returned home, but he was tired and experienced diarrhea. He did not want anyone to visit, only his daughter and his sister who lived quite close to him.

A few weeks after the biopsy, at 3 am he suffered severe dyspnea. When he tried to get up from bed, he was not able to, so he was taken to the palliative care unit of the hospital.

Nursing Assessment on the Palliative Care Unit

When Manuel arrived on the unit he was conscious, oriented, and cooperative. He could not walk or stand. The surgical wound from the biopsy was painful and the pain radiated to his head. He said he had pain in his legs and he was very tired. He had no appetite and swallowing pills was painful. He choked on liquids such as soup. With the loss of voice, he did not want to speak or be spoken to.

His skin was intact, but, using the Braden scale, he presented with a moderate risk for impaired tissue integrity with a score of 14 (Prevention Plus, 2001). Manuel had an intravenous catheter in his right hand, and soft tissue edema was beginning in both hands.

Manuel did not have teeth in the inferior maxillary region, so he ate a soft diet, such as soups, yogurt, and milk. His usual frequency of defecation was one stool a day, but after suffering diarrhea at home, he had not defecated for the last two days. Using the Barthel scale (Grixti, 2005), he was dependant for all activities of daily living. Manuel's vital signs were: BP 120/60, heart rate 80; temperature, 98.2 °F; and oxygen saturation, 94% on natural air. His diagnosis was thyroid adenocarcinoma, stage IV, with metastasis to the liver.

As the principal caregiver, Manuel's older daughter said that the family decided not to tell Manuel his diagnosis. They did not want him to be afraid; they wanted him to enjoy what was left of his life.

Manuel's daughter participated in his care, but she thought that he was angry. He kept his eyes closed and did not want to talk. She thought that he was angry with her.

STOP. THINK. Which diagnoses, outcomes, and interventions would you select?

Submitter's Analysis and Use of NANDA-I, NOC, and NIC

In considering Manuel's situation, the nurses considered the diagnoses of *chronic pain, fatigue, impaired bed mobility, risk for impaired tissue integ-*

rity, bathing/hygiene self care deficit, toileting self care deficit, feeding self care deficit, dressing/grooming self care deficit, risk for falls, risk for aspiration, and *hopelessness.*

To prioritize nursing diagnoses, a reasoning web, following Pesut and Herman's (1999) Outcome Present-State Test (OPT), model was used. The case was framed as a palliative care situation, in the context of Manuel's cultural patterns. In the Northwest part of Spain it is quite common for the family to be told bad news, but not the patient. Often, this is because the family wants to protect the person from being upset about the diagnosis.

A nursing plan of care was devised for Manuel's inability to provide self care and the existing problems and risk states; these diagnoses and the plans of care were routinely managed in the palliative care unit. In addition, the nurses were concerned about Manuel's and his daughter's emotional state. Using the web format of the OPT model, the nurse clustered the cues and decided that the most important diagnosis to address for Manuel was *hopelessness*. Hope is important for human life, even in palliative care. Even if Manuel's daughter did not want to tell her father about his poor prognosis, Manuel probably knew he was dying. His verbal expressions, his reluctance to speak and eat, and keeping his eyes closed may have been manifestations of his knowing about the real situation. Taking into account the situation in the cultural context, Manuel may have been trying to protect his daughter from the pain of knowing he was dying.

The nurse also considered the importance of working with Manuel's family to help them maintain their relationship in this phase of Manuel's life. In this sense, a nursing diagnosis of *risk for compromised family coping* was identified as needing further assessment to validate the existence of risk factors. This diagnosis exists in NANDA-I as an actual nursing diagnosis, but not as a risk diagnosis. Obviously, if nurses are able to treat the actual nursing diagnosis, they must also be able to identify the existence of risk factors and prevent the diagnosis.

Manuel's chronic pain was diagnosed and treated by the nurses and physicians. The nurses thought that the diagnosis of *discomfort* should be available on the NANDA list. This is a "discomfort" situation: *pain, self care deficit in all the activities of daily living, hopelessness, grieving,* and probably other responses. The nurses decided on the diagnosis of *hopelessness* because the defining characteristics matched the evidence in this case.

NOC Outcomes

Manuel needed to be in a state of comfort and needed relief from discomfort (Kolkaba and Kolkaba, 1991; Moneymaker, 2005), so the outcome selected for Manuel was *comfort status.* The definition and indicators of this outcome were a good fit with Manuel's situation. The overall baseline score was identified as 1 (severely compromised) and the target score was identified as 4 (mildly compromised).

NIC Interventions

For the diagnoses of *chronic pain* and *self care deficit*, the NIC interventions of *pain management* and *self care assistance* were implemented. Pain control was achieved through analgesia administration. Self care assistance was useful to assist Manuel in achieving physical well-being and safety.

To address Manuel's *comfort status*, the nurse chose *counseling*. *Counseling* is a broad intervention in which the nurse uses an interactive helping process that focuses on the needs, problems, and feelings of patients and significant others to enhance or support coping, problem solving, and interpersonal relationships. In this case, the nurse focused on Manuel's needs; once the physical needs were addressed through administration of the appropriate analgesia, Manuel could explain what else was worrying him. The nurse helped Manuel to express his feelings about dying or being dependant upon others, and she also helped Manuel to express his feelings related to his daughter and other family members. Use of this intervention included other interventions such as *presence* and *active listening* with both Manuel and his family.

Evaluation

Manuel died as expected. He and his family never talked openly about the dying process, but a feeling of comprehensiveness was present in their relationship. He did not feel pain and he expressed achievement of the target goal of 4 on the *comfort status* outcome. At the end, a comfortable death was achieved.

In the case of Manuel, the use of NANDA-I, NOC, and NIC enabled the nurse to identify a flaw in the NANDA-I language: the broad diagnosis of *discomfort* needs to be developed to improve the nursing discipline and nursing care. Some nurses think that the use of standardized nursing languages leads to standardization of the care of individual patients. However, when standardized nursing languages are used correctly, the care of people is not standardized. These languages enable the individualization of care plans, taking into account the actual needs of each patient.

References

Grixti, R. (2005). Evaluation of the Barthel ADL Index Scale Year 2004. Retrieved on August 18, 2008, from www.sahha.gov.mt/showdoc.aspx?id=195andfile source=4andfile=Pbarthel04.pdf.

Kolkaba, K.Y., and Kolkaba, R.J. (1991). An analysis of the concept of comfort. *Journal of Advanced Nursing 16*, 1301–1316.

Moneymaker K. (2005). Comfort measures only. *Journal of Palliative Medicine, 8*, 688.

Pesut, D.J., and Herman, J. (1999). *Clinical reasoning: The art and science of critical and creative thinking*. Boston: Delmar.

Prevention Plus. (2001). *Braden Scale*. Retrieved on August 20, 2008, from www.bradenscale.com/braden.pdf.

5.33. Hospice and Palliative Care

Roseann Nahmod, RN, MS, BC-NE

Abraham is a 78-year-old Jewish male who is 5 feet, 4 inches and used to weigh 150 pounds. Six months ago, Abraham presented at his primary physician's office with complaints of coughing up blood-tinged sputum and feeling fatigued.

Until Abraham got sick, he worked part time as a building maintenance employee in a health care facility. He lives with his wife Sarah and they have two grown children and three grandchildren. His usual weekly activities included attending various health lectures at the senior center, evening prayers at the synagogue, and weekly bus trips to gambling casinos in Atlantic City. The family maintains a kosher diet, primarily vegetables and grains. Abraham has had type 2 diabetes for 20 years and has smoked two packs of cigarettes a day for 42 years.

Following a series of blood work, chest X-rays, and computed axial tomography (CT) scans, Abraham's results were hemoglobin (HGB) 14.5 grams per deciliter (gm/dl) and hematocrit (HCT) 43.6%. His CT scan detailed the following: 2.2 × 2.8 cm speculated mass within left lower lung lobe. An additional 3.5 × 2.7 spiculated hilar mass was observed in the left upper lobe with narrowing of the left upper lobe bronchus. Central lobular emphysematous changes were noted; his medical diagnosis was stage IV lung cancer.

During the months that followed, Abraham experienced a regimen of chemotherapy and radiation, with two series of six-week treatments. Chemotherapy-induced nausea contributed to a weight drop to 141 pounds, HGB drop to 8 gm/dl, and HCT drop to 24%. Periodic injections of procrit (40,000 units) were given to increase his red blood cell production.

As the disease quickly progressed, Abraham struggled to maintain his weight. His wife tried diligently to coax him to eat and drink any tolerable foods and to meet his physical and emotional needs. Though

225

reluctant at first to have strangers in her home, Sarah finally accepted that help was needed with Abraham's care and agreed to contact hospice care services.

The hospice nurse and other team members were slowly welcomed by the family. During the first few visits, the hospice team gathered data about Abraham and his family's cultural beliefs, customs, and communication style. Effective communication within a cultural context was needed to ensure that Abraham's needs were being met and to prevent misinterpretation or misunderstanding.

A nebulizer and portable oxygen tanks were provided to be used as needed for his bouts of shortness of breath. The cancer had spread to his spine, and pain, at times, was described as unbearable. While at rest, Abraham reported his pain as a 4 on the pain scale but changes in position or attempts to ambulate increased his pain level to 8, 9, or 10. When this happened, his response to encouragement and support from family was "I can't take the pain. My life is over. I want to die." To the hospice nurse, he stated that he was fearful of pain and requested that the hospice team not let him suffer.

Sarah, age 82, was trying to do everything for him, including turning and positioning in bed every two hours. She expressed concern for his suffering and asked many questions that indicated a preoccupation with care giving routines. When asked about her own health status, she said she was not sleeping at night and felt nervous about the many care giving activities.

STOP. THINK. Which diagnoses, outcomes, and interventions would you select?

Submitter's Analysis and Use of NANDA-I, NOC, and NIC

Hospice and palliative care is comprehensive, interdisciplinary care for people with advanced, progressive, life-threatening illness and their families (Morrison et al., 2007). The purpose of hospice care is to help people with life-threatening illnesses and their families to achieve the best possible quality of life throughout the course of the illness by preventing and relieving suffering, controlling symptoms, providing psychosocial support, and preserving opportunities for personal and family development.

From his physical examination, health history, and family assessment, two nursing diagnoses that the hospice nurse ruled out were *self care deficit* and *activity intolerance*. This was because Abraham's condition was recognized as terminal, and diagnoses such as these would not be addressed because improvements were not expected. *Imbalanced nutrition* was considered important but only to maintain the best possible nutrition in this circumstance. Other nursing diagnoses that hospice nurses generally address at various times in the dying process are *fear, death anxiety, hopelessness, grieving*, and *readiness for enhanced family processes*.

The high priority diagnoses at this time, however, were *acute pain* for Abraham and *risk of caregiver role strain* for Sarah. Aggressive management of acute cancer pain was necessary to relieve Abraham's suffering. For Sarah, it was important to prevent *caregiver role strain*, so that her own health would be maintained throughout the process of providing care for Abraham. The supports that were available from hospice services and other family members would make this possible.

NOC Outcomes

The priority outcome for Abraham was *pain level* with a baseline score of 1 (severe) and a goal score of 4 (mild). The priority outcome for Sarah was *caregiver role endurance*. The baseline score was determined as 3 (moderately adequate) and the goal score was set as 5 (totally adequate).

NIC Interventions

Watson's 10 caritas processes were used by the hospice nurses to help Abraham and his family (Watson, 2006, 2007). Within the philosophy and science of caring, Watson defines nursing as establishing a transpersonal caring relationship that supports quality of life, including a peaceful death. This is considered as a moral commitment of the nurse. This caring approach is humanistic and altruistic, consisting of the instillation of faith and hope, formation of helping and trusting human care relationships, and formation of supportive, protective, and/or corrective mental, physical, societal, and spiritual environment.

The NIC nursing intervention for Abraham's pain was *pain management*, using a multidisciplinary approach. After consultation with the hospice nurse, Abraham's daughter set up a tape player with Hebrew and Arabic music to encourage relaxation and pain relief. Extra pillows and other physical support measures were used to improve overall comfort. Abraham continued to use the pain scale and was successful in selecting pain relief modalities such as prayer. The hospice nurse was notified if current pain relief measures were unsuccessful or current complaints were a significant change from Abraham's past experience of pain. When these activities were no longer effective in controlling pain, the nurse communicated the physician's prescription for liquid roxonol and morphine to be introduced as part of the therapeutic regimen. The nurse taught Abraham's son how to pre-fill syringes of roxanol with the correct dose, so the medication could be given to him before bedtime and in the middle of the night. The pain was being managed, but he slept more and more hours and resisted the family's attempts for him to be out of bed. This was expected and supported. By administering the pain medications at bedtime, Abraham and the family were able to obtain a few hours of continuous sleep.

The primary NIC intervention used for Sarah was *caregiver support*. Since their marriage 66 years ago, Sarah had provided homemaker tasks. For her to relinquish tasks such as preparing meals or managing the many facets of the home was extremely difficult. The hospice team encouraged Sarah to manage her stress and to use health maintenance strategies, including accepting meals from others, to sustain her own physical and mental health. The children took turns spending the night to provide respite care for Sarah. Additional hospice resources were used as needed and respite care was offered.

Evaluation

Abraham's breathing became shallow most of the time, though he was not in distress, and his face was pale and sunken. Significant changes in his weight were obvious by his thin, cachexic frame. He was kept warm and comfortable, surrounded by his family. He died quietly, calmly, with his family by his side. The hospice care services enabled him to die in familiar surroundings.

Abraham and his family said they benefited from the hospice care he received. He was kept pain free and the family welcomed the hospice team's support and guidance as affairs were put in order and dialogue was encouraged. They said that the hospice team demonstrated knowledge and compassion during the time of death and immediately thereafter. At a bereavement visit several weeks after Abraham's death, the family told the nurse that the hospice team's encouragement to say goodbye was an extremely beneficial aspect of hospice care services.

References

Morrison, L.J., Scott, O.J., Block, S.D., and American Board of Hospice and Palliative Medicine Competencies Work Group. (2007). Developing initial competency-based outcomes for the hospice and palliative medicine subspecialist: Phase I of the hospice and palliative medicine competencies project. *Journal of Palliative Medicine, 10,* 313–330.

Watson, J. (2006). Part one: Jean Watson's theory of human caring. In M.E. Parker (ed.), *Nursing theories and nursing practice* (2nd ed., pp. 295–302). Philadelphia: F.A. Davis.

Watson, J. (2007). Theoretical questions and concerns: Response from a caring science framework. *Nursing Science Quarterly, 20*(1), 13–15.

5.34. Two-Year-Old Bess's Response to Parents' Divorce

Susan Mee, RN, MS, and Sandra Frick-Helms, PhD, RN, RPT-S

Two-year-old Bess was brought to the nurse therapist's office by her father. Bess's parents had been separated for 11 months. She did not see her mother for the first six months of the separation and contact after that was sporadic and infrequent. Her father met and became engaged to a woman affectionately referred to as "Mama Sally." Two months ago, Bess's biological mother moved back to the vicinity and filed for legal custody of Bess. Bess now spends one evening per week and every other weekend with her biological mother. Her father stated that Bess's behavior has dramatically changed. He said she gets frustrated frequently and easily, and has begun to "act out" by displaying the violently oppositional behavior of tantrums, crying, hitting, kicking, throwing things, and screaming, "NO!" This behavior was especially evident after visits with her mother. After an episode of violent behavior, Bess was lethargic and despondent. When her father or Mama Sally said "I love you," Bess frequently got upset and yelled, "No, only Mommy loves me."

Child-centered therapeutic play (TP) sessions were begun with Bess as a diagnostic modality. Two of the behavior categories that emerged in the TP sessions were (a) Bess named a doll "Mommy" (biological mother) and alternated "making Mommy go potty" or making her take a bath because "Mommy all dirty," and (b) Bess played with a small horse that she slapped on the nose while sternly repeating, "spit it out," and "NO, horsey, NO!" Bess nurtured the doll she named Mommy by crooning to her and having her go "nite nite." She also buried Mommy's face in the sand and "locked her in the garage."

The father reported that Bess's mother was pregnant and Bess had said that "only Mommy was her 'real mother' because Bess 'grew in Mommy's tummy.'" Bess started lashing out at Mama Sally, saying, "You not my real mommy; real Mommy have Bess in her tummy." Bess began to act insecure and displayed fear when leaving for visits with her mommy. Bess also began to retain feces. The nurse therapist educated the father and his fiancée to conduct TP sessions with Bess. In these sessions, Bess tested them by ostentatiously sucking on a baby bottle (she had been weaned from a bottle six months previously) and involving them, particularly her father, in play that involved the "real Mommy."

 STOP. THINK. Which diagnoses, outcomes, and interventions would you select?

Submitter's Analysis and Use of NANDA-I, NOC, and NIC

One of the difficulties in the interpretation of affective states in small children is their inability to express complex feelings because of their lack of verbal skills and life experiences (Camastral, 2008; Del Po and Frick, 1988; Rye, 2008). After working with Bess, the nurse therapist believed that Bess was experiencing moderate to severe *powerlessness*, but the nurse therapist could not rely on verbal expressions of having no control as a critical cue for the diagnosis. Because Bess was only 2 years old, it was necessary to infer a feeling of lack of control by examining the behaviors described by her father and feelings she expressed through play. For children, play takes the place of verbal skills seen in adults (Del Po and Frick, 1988; Camastral, 2008; Rye, 2008). Therapeutic play (TP) uses toys to help children communicate their perceptions. In non-directive TP, the child controls the process and content of play; the therapist empathically responds, enabling the child's free expression.

The first cue to *powerlessness* was dramatically altered behavior, signaling a general negative affective state. When Bess's oppositional behavior and frequent loud "NOs" were viewed in a developmental context, they were interpreted as an attempt to gain control or mastery of a situation or event. Children in this developmental stage are struggling to attain a sense of autonomy or independence (Erikson, 1963). Autonomy is gained through mastery of situations, events, and feelings. One of the frequent ways that striving for autonomy is manifested in toddlers is through oppositional behavior.

Cues provided by Bess's play served to reinforce the impression that she perceived herself as struggling to attain and maintain control. She showed a desire to control when she made Mommy go potty and take a bath, buried Mommy's face in the sand, and locked her in the garage. Potty training is often considered the major struggle of toddlers striving for autonomy. Bess never made the Daddy or Mama Sally dolls go potty. Instead, she played out these normally occurring events with the Mommy doll, in essence, controlling Mommy.

Other defining characteristics of *powerlessness* displayed by Bess were lethargy and despondence, the expressions of frustration, the doubt she expressed about her relationship with Daddy and Mama Sally, the fear that she displayed prior to visiting Mommy, her fear of alienation, and the strong feelings displayed in oppositional behaviors. A two-year-old is just beginning to learn behaviors necessary for satisfactory role performance. This learning usually occurs because of consistent positive responses from caretakers. In Bess's first year of life, she was rewarded for positive responses from caretakers by receiving positive, nurturing responses in return. Bess then learned that behaving positively toward her mother did not result in consistent nurturing from her mother; rather, her mother kept "abandoning" her. Since she did not know how to behave, there were dramatic alterations in her behavior.

While Bess was with her mother, she was dependent on her for care and emotional safety, yet Bess had learned that she could not rely on her mother. Bess responded to this unrewarded dependence by showing irritability, resentment, anger, and guilt after visits with her mother. Anger and resentment toward her mother could be seen in her play, including the tone of voice used to remonstrate the toy horse. Children who have had consistently positive experiences with nurturance tend to play out more nurturant roles in pretend play. Children who have had negative nurturing experiences tend to play either the aggressor or victim; Bess consistently played the aggressor.

NOC Outcomes

Two NOC outcomes were selected to address powerlessness: *coping* and *psychosocial adjustment: life change*. On *coping*, Bess's baseline score was determined to be 2 (rarely demonstrated) and the target score was set as 4 (often demonstrated). On *psychosocial adjustment*, Bess's baseline score was determined to be 3 (sometimes demonstrated) and the target score was set as 4 (often demonstrated).

NIC Interventions

The NIC interventions of *therapeutic play, active listening, developmental enhancement, constipation/impaction management, coping enhancement,* and *security enhancement* were selected. The nurse continued to monitor Bess's state of *powerlessness* and to support and enhance coping processes. Therapeutic play gave Bess the opportunity to practice with past and present concerns (Frick-Helms, 1994; 1997). In addition, the nurse therapist helped her father devise rituals that would convincingly demonstrate to Bess that she would be returning home to Daddy and Mama Sally. Because choices regarding visitation could not be made by Bess, each of these rituals was designed to be under Bess's control. After several repetitions of these rituals, Bess began to initiate them whenever going to visit Mommy and her fear behaviors significantly decreased.

As the nurse therapist worked with Bess, additional cues to the diagnosis of *powerlessness* occurred. Bess was clearly reluctant to express her feelings. Whenever her anger was reflected to her in TP sessions with statements such as, "Bess is mad; Bess is really mad at Mommy," Bess vehemently denied such feelings. In the U.S. culture, children are typically taught at an early age that anger and aggression are unacceptable behaviors and feelings (Golden, 2003). Another cue was that Bess had been retaining feces for three weeks when she came to a play session visibly "out-of-sorts." Retention of feces is a sign of serious emotional difficulty in a child and is thought to be an attempt at controlling. She slammed objects down forcefully, threw toys, and defiantly broke previously set limits. The nurse therapist reflected this anger repeatedly. Suddenly Bess stopped and, looking straight at the nurse therapist, yelled, "I'M MAD!" For the rest of the session she expressed her anger repeatedly and even whispered, "I'm afraid." After this session, she had a massive bowel movement and she no longer retained feces.

Therapeutic play provided Bess with the opportunity to feel safe enough to express her negative feelings; it enhanced her feelings of power. The test of whether interventions have been successful in alleviating a response is to determine that the defining characteristics have disappeared or decreased in intensity or frequency (Frick-Helms, 1994b).

Evaluation

In two months, the target scores were met for the two outcomes and the play therapy sessions were completed. In six months, a follow up telephone call was made; the father said that there was no return of the defining characteristics of *powerlessness*. This case study is a description of an actual situation in which a diagnosis was made and successfully treated, which validated the accuracy of the diagnosis.

References

Camastral, S. (2008). No small change: Process oriented play therapy for children of separating parents. *Australian and New Zealand Journal of Family Therapy, 29*, 100–106.

DelPo, E., and Frick, S. (1988). Directed and nondirected play as therapeutic modalities. *Children's Health Care, 16*, 261–267.

Erikson, E. (1963). *Childhood and society*. New York: Norton.

Frick-Helms, S. (1994). Promoting healthy play. In C. Betz, M. Hunsberger, and S., Wright (eds.). *Family centered nursing care of children* (pp. 601–626). Philadelphia: Saunders.

Frick-Helms, S. (1997). Boys cry better than girls: Play therapy behaviors of children residing in a shelter for battered women. *Journal of Play Therapy, 6*(1), 73–91.

Golden, H. (2003). *Healthy anger: How to help children and teens manage their anger.* NY: Oxford University Press.

Rye, N. (2008). Understanding therapies: Play therapy as a mental health intervention for children and adolescents. *Journal of Family Health Care, 18*(1), 17–29.

5.35. Challenges in Helping a Person to Accept Long-Term Care

Arlene A. Kasten, MSN, RN, GNP, BC

With his gruff demands, frequent snarls, and impatient responses, Henry's behaviors were considered "frustrating" by nurses on the unit. Providing holistic nursing care for Henry was difficult; many of the nurses complained that they did not know how to please him. At 78, Henry required continuous oxygen for his chronic obstructive lung disease, he had urinary incontinence, and he needed several creams and ointments for his leathery, edematous lower legs. Although he had independently managed his colostomy care for years, he now demanded staff to "do something with this!" He resisted any encouragement to remain independent in meeting hygiene needs. He was unsteady and unable to ambulate safely without assistance. When asked how he would be able to live by himself, his response was, "I was doing just fine." His children expressed concern, however, for his failing health and inability to manage personal hygiene, health problems, and home.

His children brought him to a large hospital in the city from a rural area about 300 miles to the north. The children all lived in or within an hour's drive of the city. Even if he accepted their help, it would be a hardship for his children to frequently drive the distance to his home to provide the help that he needed. His children arranged for Henry to be admitted to a nursing home after hospitalization.

Efforts to help Henry accept nursing home placement were met with anger toward his children and the staff. When nurses tried to explore the reality of the situation, it only served to solidify his anger and resistance. He insisted that no one could talk with him about going to a nursing home. His telephone conversations with his children were as gruff as his dialogue with the hospital staff. He was overheard speaking more gently, however, to a grandchild.

On one occasion, Henry had just spoken with his daughter-in-law about the planned move to the nursing home. The nurse worked with

Henry to help him process his conversation and his situation; the nurse asked questions and encouraged him to talk about the situation. He suddenly broke into tears. "Mary! Mary did not call me. Does she know where I am? Is she all right? Oh how I miss my Mary," he cried. He explained through his tears that Mary was a lady friend who lived near his home. He took her to the physician and to do her shopping. "Who will do those things for her if I am not there?"

STOP. THINK. Which diagnoses, outcomes, and interventions would you select?

Submitter's Analysis and Use of NANDA-I, NOC, and NIC

The nurses' difficulty in providing holistic nursing care to Henry led to a team discussion of what they could do to resolve this dilemma. Analysis of his behaviors generated many possible diagnoses such as *anger, ineffective coping, low self esteem*, and others. These were each rejected as not helpful enough to guide a plan of care. A care plan to set limits was discussed that included identification of unacceptable behavior and statements of consequences for those behaviors. The nursing staff did not feel comfortable with this solution, however, and continued to analyze the situation. The nursing staff was challenged to accurately describe Henry's responses to his situation so they could help him with his psychological and emotional concerns as well as meet his needs for management of complex chronic therapeutic regimens.

Further analysis of Henry's harsh words and gruffness, his present situation, and his background led to a diagnosis of *powerlessness* related to deficient knowledge about his health status, decisional conflict, and loss of independence secondary to physical inabilities. The symptoms that Henry exhibited were anger, acting out, inappropriate dependence, and anxiety. A phenomenological study of the experience of powerlessness of 40 people with chronic conditions, found that subjects experienced feelings of insecurity and threat to personal and social identity (Aujoulat, Luminet, and Decacche, 2007).

Considering Henry's background and current experiences, he was a prime candidate for the experience of *powerlessness*. Before he retired, he was a supervisor. He had also held several supervisory positions during his career, one of which was maintenance supervisor in the nursing home he was scheduled to enter. He had his own perceptions of what life would be like as a patient in a nursing home. There were numerous changes and losses in his life. He was losing his independence, his home, his health, and his Mary. In a qualitative study of 16 men with depression, the findings were similar to previous studies that showed men may need to emphasize control, strength, and responsibility for others (Emslie, Ridge, Ziebland, and Hunt, 2006). A study of 25 people with ill health found that the essence of ill health is powerlessness (Strandmark, 2004).

NOC Outcomes

Two NOC outcomes were selected for Henry: *personal autonomy* and *acceptance: health status*. For *personal autonomy*, the baseline score was 2 (substantially compromised) and the target score was 5 (not compromised). For *acceptance: health status*, the baseline score was 2 (rarely demonstrated) and the target score was 4 (often demonstrated).

NIC Interventions

When addressing a complex nursing diagnosis such as *powerlessness* as it relates to chronic illnesses, nurses should consider many possible interventions (Miller, 2000). The NIC interventions that were selected for Henry were *decision-making support, presence, anticipatory guidance, self awareness enhancement,* and *coping enhancement*. Providing information to Henry about his children and the staff's concerns about his acceptance of his current health status was considered foundational, but this intervention was not implemented until the nurse helped Henry with *decision making support*.

The nursing intervention of *decision making support* was applied by taking the time to explore possible options with Henry that might be more acceptable. It was discussed that he could go to a nursing home near his northern community for a while until he regained some strength. Mary could visit. ... "No, Mary is not well enough to visit me." The tears continued to flow. The nurse offered to place a telephone call to Mary after which Henry's eyes brightened and the tears ceased. His tears resumed, however, when he spoke with Mary, telling her that he missed her and loved her. Eventually, he told her of his dilemma. They talked for a while longer. Henry motioned to the nurse that he was finished with his conversation. The nurse took him back to his room and waited for Henry to compose himself. With calm resolve, Henry reported that Mary told him to stay in the city, near his children. She was scheduled for hip surgery and would be living with her daughter. Henry was calmer and expressed acceptance that Mary would not need him. His anger seemed to dissolve, at least temporarily, after his loss of control of helping Mary was resolved. The simple task of dialing the telephone to call Mary contributed to improved self determination and control.

After this, other interventions that were used before Henry left the hospital were *environmental restructuring* and *reminiscence therapy*. He was most responsive to *reminiscence therapy*, which enabled him to resolve his relationship with Mary, thus facilitating acceptance of nursing home placement. Henry and his family were encouraged to participate in team discussions so that they could work together to facilitate an acceptable resolution of Henry's concerns. Addressing the etiologies of his *powerlessness* through the interventions of *decision making support, presence*, and *providing information* reduced Henry's feelings of powerlessness. The nurse assisted Henry in resolving the problem, supported his self-esteem, and upheld his dignity. Additionally, the nurse shared the assessment, diagnosis, and interventions with other nurses, social service professionals, physicians, nurse practitioners, and other members of the health care team.

Evaluation

One week later, when Henry was being discharged to a long-term care setting, the outcomes were evaluated. On the outcome of *personal autonomy*, Henry achieved a score of 5. On the outcome of *acceptance: health status*, Henry achieved the goal score of 4. Henry's mood was improved and he said that he knew that he must go to a long-term care setting and he would make the best of it.

References

Aujoulat, I., Luminet, O., and Decacche, A. (2007). The perspective of patients on their experience of powerlessness. *Qualitative Health Research, 17*, 772–785.

Emslie, C., Ridge, D., Ziebland, S., and Hunt, K. (2006). Men's accounts of depression: Reconstructing or resisting hegemonic masculinity? *Social Science and Medicine, 62*, 2246–2257.

Miller, J.F. (2000). *Coping with chronic illness: Overcoming powerlessness* (3rd ed.). Philadelphia: F.A. Davis.

Strandmark, M.K. (2004). Ill health is powerlessness: A phenomenological study about worthlessness, limitations and suffering. *Scandinavian Journal of Caring Science, 18*, 135–144.

5.36. Woman with a History of Being Battered

Judy Carlson, EdD, RN, CS, FNP

Mary, 34, was a battered woman who recently moved into a new apartment with her 11-year-old daughter. It had been six weeks since Mary left a shelter for abused women. Mary was married twice to men who were batterers, the first time for 12 years and the second for two years. Being abused by men was a way of life for Mary, starting when she was very young.

In her teenage years her father shot her mother and subsequently killed himself. Mary received counseling after this tragedy to help her understand that she had a right not to be abused and did not deserve abuse. Recently at the women's shelter after receiving two months of counseling, Mary realized that in both her marriages she had chosen men who represented father figures to her. Perhaps, she realized, this was related to "my search for the love my father did not give me." The last battering that Mary received at the hands of her second husband was so severe it almost killed her.

Mary experienced various health problems from years of battering, including chronic back pain, sleeplessness, and fatigue. Recently, she had a poor appetite from abscesses of three of her teeth. With much prompting by the nurse and the social worker, she called the clinic to make an appointment to be seen by the dentist. When Mary was told they could only see her if it was an emergency, she did not make the appointment.

Mary indicated that for the first time she felt safe from her husband because he did not know where she was and it had been some time since she had contact with him. Her statements indicated her continued resolve to remain free from abuse. She expressed a desire to complete her high school diploma and get a job but did not think it was likely because she was always told she was "dumb." Although she was aware of the importance of exercise to her rehabilitation, she stopped her walking routine because "it did not really help anyway." There were several women Mary met at the shelter whom she could contact, but Mary voiced that "the time is not right" and "friendships never really work out anyway." Mary had not been to a support group since she left the shelter because "I have so much to do."

Mary was happy to have an apartment of her own and felt it would never have been possible without the help of the counselor from the shelter. Although the nurse thought Mary's three-room apartment was attractive and comfortable, Mary frequently cleaned and rearranged the furniture to get it "to her liking" but never quite succeeded in this effort.

STOP. THINK. Which diagnoses, outcomes, and interventions would you select?

Submitter's Analysis and Use of NANDA-I, NOC, and NIC

For Mary, several human responses on the NANDA-I list were considered to be relatively accurate: *impaired social interaction, social isolation, situational low self esteem, chronic low self esteem,* and *powerlessness.* These NANDA-I diagnoses, however, reflect only some of the cues in this case, while a concept that is not yet on the NANDA-I approved list, learned helplessness, offers a better explanation for Mary's behavior. Although the concept of helplessness was accepted as a NANDA label in 1994 with the group of diagnoses submitted by the Psychiatric Mental Health Group of the American Nurses Association, a definition for the label was not included and it was not approved for the NANDA-I list.

Learned helplessness was defined as perceived inability to influence or control outcomes, which is learned through environmental circumstances and leads to suppression of subsequent behaviors that affect outcomes (Abramson, Seligman, and Teasdale, 1978). The theory of learned helplessness includes the concept of attribution, which refers to the beliefs that people have about the reasons that events occur. The dimensions of attribution are blame placement (internal or external), duration (short- or long-term), and occurrence (all situations or only some situations). The causation that people attribute to uncontrollable events determines the nature and chronicity of learned helplessness (Clements and Sawhney, 2000). People with internal blame placement and long-standing experiences of helplessness in many situations have a more severe form of learned helplessness than people who have external blame placement and short-term or few experiences of helplessness. Mary was experiencing chronic helplessness that she generalized to many aspects of her life. Learned helplessness was used as a framework for Walker's (1984) studies of battered women and in research studies was linked to the experiences of battered women (Bergai, Gershon, and Shalev, 2007; Bhandari, Levitch, Ball, Everett, Geden, and Bullock, 2008).

Differences between learned helplessness and *powerlessness* are related to the way people process events in attempts to control outcomes (McDermott, 1995). With *powerlessness*, the self is not involved and does not change in response to power struggles. When desired outcomes are not accomplished, rage is experienced and *powerlessness* occurs. With learned helplessness, there is high involvement of the self when desired outcomes are not achieved. When events cannot be controlled, the self is at great risk and becomes diminished. With each exposure and thwarted attempt at controlling outcomes, greater degrees of helplessness are experienced (Bergai, Gershon, and Shalev, 2007).

The defining characteristics that the nurse used to make this diagnosis for Mary were numerous expressions of being inadequate, consistent avoidance of seeking information for self care, verbalizations of inability to perform self care, inadequate follow up on self care activities, verbalized negative self concept, loneliness, and social withdrawal (Nehls and Sallman, 2008) and the uneasiness and dissatisfaction Mary felt toward everything she did.

NOC Outcomes

The NOC outcome that the nurse selected for learned helplessness was *personal resiliency*. The baseline score was determined to be 1 (never demonstrated), even though she had improved some aspects of her life, such as feeling safe. The target score was 3 (sometimes demonstrated). The assumption is that the more personal resiliency Mary would demonstrate, the less helpless she would feel.

NIC Interventions

The NIC interventions that the nurse selected to work with Mary were *self efficacy enhancement, self awareness enhancement, self-responsibility facilitation, cognitive restructuring, self esteem enhancement, support system enhancement, socialization enhancement,* and *behavior modification* related to social skills. First, the nurse helped Mary to become aware that her responses were learned and, therefore, could be changed. A battered woman such as Mary must recognize the possibility that she can maintain a protected lifestyle (i.e., a life free of battering).

If the most accurate diagnosis of Mary's response was determined to be *powerlessness*, the nursing interventions would differ. The emphasis for *powerlessness* would have been on *communication enhancement, assertiveness training,* and *learning facilitation* (Miller, 2000; Fallot and Harris, 2002). The fact that the choice of nursing interventions listed in

NIC is different for each concept supports acceptance of learned help-lessness as a new diagnosis—one that differs from *powerlessness.*

The nurse emphasized *self efficacy enhancement* to strengthen Mary's confidence in her ability to perform a health behavior. The nurse explored with Mary her perception to perform desired behaviors such as making friends with other women, the benefits of executing the desired behaviors, her perception of risks of not executing these behaviors, and her perception of barriers to changing her behaviors. The nurse provided information about these behaviors, assisted Mary in committing to a plan of action, and reinforced her confidence in making behavior changes and taking action. The nurse provided a supportive environment and modeled desired behaviors. The nurse used role playing to help Mary gain experience in responding differently, after which the nurse provided positive reinforcement. Role playing also provided an opportunity for mastery of new behaviors. The nurse used positive persuasive statements such as, "I feel a growing sense of confidence in you."

The nurse encouraged Mary to interact with others and held a networking lunch for Mary. Through role playing and desensitization relaxation methods, the nurse helped prepare Mary for future experiences.

Evaluation

After working with Mary for three months, the nurse and Mary determined that Mary met the target outcome of 3, which was a 30% improvement. Mary had developed additional coping strategies and was able at times to exhibit a positive mood. At times, she expressed self efficacy, sought emotional support, used more strategies to avoid violent situations, and weighed alternatives to problem solving. She began to adapt to adversities as challenges and kept herself from returning to abusive relationships. She also participated in social activities.

References

Abramson, I. Seligman, M., and Teasdale, J. (1978). Learned helplessness in humans: Critique and reformulation. *Journal of Abnormal Psychology, 87,* 49–75.

Bergai, N., Gershon, B., and Shalev, A. (2007). Posttraumatic stress disorder and depression in battered women: The mediating role of learned helplessness. *Journal of Family Violence, 232,* 267–275.

Bhandari, S., Levitch, A., Ball, K., Everett, K., Geden, E., and Bullock, L. (2008). Comparative analyses of stressors experienced by rural low-income pregnant women experiencing intimate partner violence and those who are not. *Journal of Obstetric, Gynecologic and Neonatal Nursing, 37,* 492–501.

Clements, C., and Sawhney, D. (2000). Coping with domestic violence: Control attributions, dysphoria, and hopelessness. *Journal of Traumatic Stress, 13,* 219–240.

Fallot, R., and Harris, M. (2002). The Trauma Recovery and Empowerment Model (TREM): Conceptual and practical issues in a group intervention for women. *Community Mental Health Journal, 6,* 475–485.

McDermott, M.A. (1995). Learned helplessness: A more discriminating nursing diagnosis. In M. Rantz and P. LeMone (eds). *Classification of nursing diagnoses: Proceedings of the eleventh national conference* (pp. 212–213). Glendale, CA: CINAHL Information Systems.

Miller, J.F. (2000). *Coping with chronic illness: Overcoming powerlessness* (3rd ed.). Philadelphia: F.A. Davis.

Nehls, N., and Sallman, J. (2008). Women living with a history of physical and/ or sexual abuse, substance use, and mental health problems. *Qualitative Health Research, 15,* 365–381.

Walker, L. (1984). *The battered women syndrome.* New York: Springer.

5.37. Woman in Labor with Complications

Danna L. Sims, RN, MS

Mrs. SG is a 34-year-old female who has had no significant health problems other than unexplained infertility. *In vitro* fertilization resulted in a confirmed pregnancy and, at 37 weeks gestation, SG presented in labor with abdominal contractions, rupture of the amniotic membranes, 4 cm dilatation, 80% effacement, at −1 station. Labor started about three hours prior to arrival to the labor and delivery (L and D) unit of the hospital. Mrs. SG stated that her membranes ruptured approximately one hour prior to arrival. Mrs. SG said that she was "nervous" and she attempted controlled breathing techniques with her husband as her support person and labor coach.

After five hours of pitocin-enhanced labor with epidural pain management, SG delivered a 7 pound, 2 ounce viable female infant with Apgar scores of 9 at one minute and five minutes. The infant was transported to the regular newborn nursery. During the recovery period in L and D, Mrs. SG experienced excessive vaginal bleeding with a boggy fundus and expression of multiple large clots. Significant free flow was noted on fundal palpation, and vigorous fundal massage was given. Postpartum hemorrhaging was continuous, so her physician performed two vaginal explorations. A vaginal hematoma was noted on examination and her physician was able to express multiple large clots containing placental tissue. Vaginal bleeding was persistent and active, even after vaginal exploration. Pitocin, methergine, and hemobate were given without success and the vaginal bleeding persisted as heavy and continuous. The physician prescribed packed red blood cells to be given immediately and Mrs. SG was taken to the operating room for a dilatation and curettage (D and C). Informed consent was obtained for any procedures forthcoming. The D and C procedure was unsuccessful to stop the bleeding, so the physician performed a vaginal hysterectomy with additional transfusions of packed red blood cells.

Mrs. SG believed that she was in good health regardless of her past history of unexplained infertility. Aside from this gynecological history, her first menstrual onset was at 13 years of age, with irregular cycles fluctuating from intervals of every 28 days to every 32 days, lasting five or six days, with moderate flow. Sexual activity started at 18 years of age and birth control methods consisted of barrier precautions and a three-year history of birth control pills.

Infertility testing included sperm count, blood tests, ovulatory testing, diagnostic sonogram, hysteroscopy, hysterosalpingogram, laparoscopy, and pharmacological agents. Infertility findings concluded with a diagnosis of decreased ovulation. Mrs. SG stated, "Aside from my infertility, I was never seriously ill and never had any major surgeries other than the ones I had during my infertility problems."

Despite nausea and vomiting during the first trimester, and some complaints of constipation toward the end of the third trimester, Mrs. SG maintained good nutritional intake throughout the pregnancy. Weight gain was steady, resulting in an overall gain of 29 pounds. Prenatal vitamins were taken throughout the pregnancy; a multivitamin with folic acid supplement was started two years prior to the pregnancy.

Mrs. SG reported no significant limitations to her activities. She continued to work as a medical secretary for a private physician's office until one week prior to delivery. Prior to the pregnancy, Mrs. SG walked 30 minutes three times a week and continued walking exercises until the beginning of the third trimester. Her physician did not limit her activities once she became pregnant, and suggested activity as tolerated. Her normal sleep pattern each night ranged from six to seven hours. She had increased complaints of fatigue for the last month and experienced some overall discomfort during the last month of pregnancy, alleviated by rest and side-lying position.

Mrs. SG had been married for six years. Her husband remained supportive and comforting and took the role of support person through the labor and delivery process. Mrs. SG was alert and oriented and all five senses were intact. She and her husband understood the severity and implications of her postpartum bleeding going into the surgery, with the possibility of a vaginal hysterectomy and permanent infertility. Mrs. SG stated, "We tried so long to get pregnant and now with these problems I will never have another child again." She expressed concern over how much "effort it took to get pregnant" and the realization that "now I permanently can never have another baby ever again. I disappointed my husband." Saddened about the inability to conceive more children and disappointed about the delivery outcome, she asked if her mother could stay overnight with her because her husband needed to go home and get some sleep for work in the morning. On a positive note, Mrs. SG stated, "I should be grateful to have a healthy child."

STOP. THINK. Which diagnoses, outcomes, and interventions would you select?

Submitter's Analysis and Use of NANDA-I, NOC, and NIC

When considering the most appropriate nursing diagnosis for Mrs. SG, the nurses clustered the cues of an unexpected hysterectomy of a 34 year-old-woman who had planned to have additional children, the unexpected loss of a body part (her uterus), expressed sadness, statements of inability to conceive again after the hysterectomy surgery, and statements about disappointing her husband. Mrs. SG exhibited the phenomena of *grieving* related to significant losses, which was the nurses' diagnosis. The nurses also recorded the diagnosis of *readiness for enhanced role performance*. This diagnosis was identified and treated for many new mothers such as Mrs. SG. The outcome and interventions for the first diagnosis are presented here because the diagnosis of *grieving* is not routine in L and D units.

NOC Outcome

The NOC outcome that was selected with Mrs. SG was *coping*. Based on the experience of grief and loss, Mrs. SG rated herself as 3 (sometimes demonstrated) and thought that her goal at this point in time was only to maintain an overall score of 3. She knew that it would take time to resolve her grief over these unexpected losses. Mrs. SG's ability to state, "I should be grateful to have a healthy child," indicated that, in time, she would be able to move forward in the maternal role.

NIC Interventions

The NIC interventions for Mrs. SG included *teaching: individual, presence* and *emotional support*. Teaching consisted of instructing Mrs. SG and her family about the phases of the grieving process. Part of grieving is to set up new roles and behaviors because grieving is a pervasive experience that affects every aspect of a person's life (Reed, 2003). When family and friends visited Mrs. SG, the nurse described the grief process and encouraged them to be supportive. This was important so that the grief process could be better understood and accepted by people in her environment.

Teaching also included identification of community resources for bereavement support (Florczak, 2008). This would help to prevent complicated or prolonged grieving. Some bereaved people develop severe, long-term reactions to their loss. This kind of reaction may later be associated with adverse health outcomes (Hawton, 2007). Mrs. SG would be going home very soon and would probably need further support.

Presence by the nurse consisted of being there to listen to Mrs. SG and her family express their feelings and concerns. Significant others were encouraged to participate, especially with a situation of a young woman not being able to have more children. This can affect the entire family, especially the husband (Reed, 2003). By encouraging expression of these feelings, coping and healing can begin. The grief response in some women may be so great that their relationships become strained.

Emotional support incorporated making empathetic statements about the grief, supporting her progression through personal grieving stages, and assisting Mrs. SG in identifying personal coping strategies that she had used in the past and that could be used for this crisis. Emotional support was also implemented by discussing any cultural, religious, and social customs that she associated with loss. The nurse told Mrs. SG that dealing with psychological and emotional states such as anxiety, fear, and depression would be crucial for her and her husband. Previous conflicts may need to be resolved at this time, such as the infertility, inability to conceive, and how that affected this permanent infertility issue. Throughout the nurse's provision of emotional support, reinforcement of progress was verbalized.

Evaluation

The target score on *coping* was met. Mrs. SG expressed her feelings on her perceived body image and inability to be able to conceive more children. She recognized that even though it was a major and extreme disappointment to have such finiteness in her reproductive life, she was grateful to have become pregnant with all of her years of trying to conceive. She expressed thankfulness for now having a healthy newborn. Mrs. SG acknowledged the steps in the grieving process (denial, anger, bargaining, depression, and acceptance). She acknowledged the community resources that were available to her and her family. She was able to conclude that her inability to become pregnant was part of her grief.

References

Florczak, K. (2008). The persistent yet ever-changing nature of grieving a loss. *Nursing Science Quarterly, 21,* 7–11.

Hawton, K. (2007). Complicated grief after bereavement. *British Medical Journal, 334,* 962–963.

Reed, K. (2003). Grief is more than tears. *Nursing Science Quarterly, 16,* 77–81.

5.38. Integration of Neuman's Systems Model in Postpartum Nursing

Eileen Gigliotti, RN, PhD

Cheryl, a 29-year-old married primapara, vaginally delivered a healthy, full term eight pound boy yesterday afternoon. On admission she stated that she planned to breastfeed but had bottle fed during the evening and night shifts related to "difficulty in getting him to latch on." That morning, at feeding time, the nurse asked if she would like help and Cheryl agreed hesitantly to try again. The nurse showed Cheryl how to position him and guide the areola to his mouth. He latched on initially but lost his grasp when Cheryl pulled back. With the next attempt, he latched on and Cheryl jerked abruptly exclaiming, "Ouch, that hurts." In response to her movement, he lost his grasp. After several more unsuccessful attempts to latch on, the baby began crying and then fell asleep.

The nurse noted that Cheryl had made extensive preparations to breastfeed, including nursing gowns and bras, as well as having several breastfeeding books on her bedside table. Cheryl did not appear to be in any discomfort physically, and her nipples were erect with no signs of inversion. Finally, the baby had been alert, rooted, and sucked well, and the record showed that he had taken two ounces of formula at the last two feedings.

A co-worker called and inquired about her breastfeeding experiences and seemed to be giving much advice. When Cheryl's husband and mother arrived together, her husband became anxious about the baby's lack of breastfeeding and said, "Did he eat anything?" Cheryl responded, "I'm trying my best! You saw him last night, he takes the bottle so well but he just does not like the breast. Maybe I can pump the milk and give it to him; he sucks so well from a bottle." Cheryl's mother said, "Maybe he's not getting anything. That happened to me, so I bottle fed. That way you're sure the baby is getting enough." Cheryl glanced at her silent but distressed husband and said to the nurse, "Could you get me a bottle? I gave him one last night and he went right to sleep, I'll try again this afternoon."

STOP. THINK. Which diagnoses, outcomes, and interventions would you select?

Submitter's Analysis and Use of NANDA-I, NOC, and NIC

When considering competing diagnoses, the nurse considered the accuracy of both the response and the etiology. The nurse, whose practice was guided by the Neuman systems model (NSM) (Neuman, 2002), knew that though the NSM terminology is complex, it is the essence of the model that guides practice (Gigliotti, 2008). That is, when people are exposed to environmental stressors, their coping mechanisms (both short [flexible line of defense] as well as long term [lines of resistance]) keep them in a state of dynamic equilibrium (their usual health state). Thus, nursing is concerned with assessing the person or family's perceptions of the health problem or life process, which is considered as the stressor, as well as their coping resources, and then assisting them in coping with this stressor.

This involves asking ourselves and the person or family the NSM assessment questions (Neuman, 2002) that focus on both the nurse's and consumer's perceptions of the health problem, lifestyle changes, coping resources, and needs from the nurse and others. The key is that the nurse assesses what the person or family sees as the major problem and works with the person or family to use their resources to solve their own problem. This is in contrast to the nurse deciding what the problem is and then doing for the person or family to solve the problem. In fact, as Gigliotti (2008) notes, "not only is it impossible to solve someone else's problem but, unless we ask, we don't even know what the problem is" (p. 44).

Accordingly, the nurse first assessed her own perception of the problem. From her initial assessment, she perceived that Cheryl had intellectual knowledge of breastfeeding but lacked experience with the process and was anxious about the baby getting enough milk. The nurse also perceived that Cheryl had breastfeeding support from co-workers and her husband but her mother preferred bottle feeding; thus she was getting conflicting advice. The nurse realized, however, that she had no knowledge of how breastfeeding would fit with Cheryl's lifestyle or what she needed from others in this situation.

Ineffective breastfeeding related to maternal/infant physiological etiology can be ruled out given the data (infant's strong suck and retention of two ounces of formula, mother's good nipple structure). *Knowledge deficit* related to lack of exposure is a possibility but Cheryl has asked no questions concerning the baby's infant feeding pattern so it is unlikely as the main problem. Finally, *ineffective individual coping* related to situational crisis would be a premature diagnosis because Cheryl has not demonstrated an inability to solve problems. Thus, the nurse tentatively formed the diagnosis: *anxiety* related to situational crisis (initiation of breastfeeding). This diagnosis assumed that Cheryl desired to breastfeed but was anxious and needed reassurance and assistance.

The nurse then asked Cheryl what she saw as the major problem, how this situation would affect her lifestyle, what she could do to help herself, and what she needed from others, including the nurse. During their conversation, Cheryl said that she knew that breast-feeding was best and her husband and co-workers assumed she would breastfeed. She said she never felt comfortable with that choice and did not foresee enjoying it but did not see how she could not breastfeed, knowing all the benefits. Cheryl said she real-ized she had been blaming the baby for not latching on when it was really she who was reluctant. She thought that a compromise might be to express the milk and bottle feed. She said that her husband would most likely support her decision and what she needed from the nurse was information about pumping breast milk, honest information about formula, and support for her ultimate decision.

After gaining insight into Cheryl's perceptions, the nurse realized that her initial perceptions and Cheryl's were incongruent. She shared with Cheryl that she saw her as a well educated woman who was in a supportive relationship and had a healthy baby; thus, her resources were high. She asked if it was correct that Cheryl was experiencing *decisional conflict* related to the benefits and problems of infant feeding choice. That is, she saw breastfeeding as best but was not enthusiastic about breastfeeding; likewise, she liked the idea of bottle feeding but saw formula as a poor nutritional choice. Cheryl agreed that the nurse's perceptions were correct.

NOC Outcome

The NOC outcome that was selected with Cheryl was *decision making*, with a baseline score of 3 (moderately compromised) and a goal score of 5 (not compromised). The selected indicators and Cheryl's baseline and goal scores were as follows: (a) identified relevant information regarding breast milk, pumping breast milk, and formula with a baseline score of 3 and a goal score of 5; (b) acknowledged social context of the situation with a baseline score of 4 and a goal score of 5; and (c) selected among alternatives with a baseline score of 2 and a goal score of 5.

NIC Interventions

The NIC interventions that the nurse selected to help Cheryl were *decision making support* and *values clarification. Decision making support* activities emphasized the need, as described above, to determine whether there are differences between Cheryl's and the nurse's perceptions of the situation. These intervention descriptions also emphasize collaborative decision making, providing information as needed, and supporting the person or family in their decision. These activities are congruent with Nelson's (2006) nursing practice theory of breastfeeding, which proposes a non-paternalistic process that respects the rights of the mother to make the decision. Nelson notes that the salutary experience (which may include not breastfeeding) is one that is beneficial to both mother and baby. In addition, this theory includes need for support and recognition of each mother and infant dyad's uniqueness.

Furthermore, in a qualitative study of breastfeeding practices, Arthur, Godfrey, and Renfrew (2007) called attention to women's feelings that it is a moral imperative to breastfeed to be a "good mother." That is, in the effort to encourage breastfeeding, the message is sent that to not breastfeed is not to be "a good mother." Thus, Cheryl needed information about alternatives as well as help with clarifying her values concerning breastfeeding and mothering to make a decision.

As before, to help Cheryl with values clarification, the nurse's values on this topic also needed to be clear. Toward this end, Gigliotti (1995) created a breastfeeding values clarification exercise. The nurse knew that if Cheryl was to openly discuss the decision to breast or bottle feed, an attitude of acceptance of both choices must be communicated. The nurse informed Cheryl that formula feeding was a viable option and encouraged her to discuss the pros and cons of breast and formula feeding as well as pumping breast milk and bottle feeding. The nurse assured Cheryl that she would be able to meet her child's complex needs by choosing the method that was right for her. Accordingly, formula information was provided and the breast pumping option was thoroughly explored. Finally, the social consequences of both breast and formula feeding were discussed along with anticipation of possible feelings of guilt.

Evaluation

With encouragement, Cheryl talked openly about how breastfeeding fit with her lifestyle, the feasibility of pumping breast milk for bottle feeding, and her husband's feelings about breastfeeding. Cheryl said that her husband liked the idea of the health benefits of breast milk but she knew he would support breast or bottle feeding. After careful consideration, Cheryl made a decision between the two choices, thus achieving an overall score of 5 (not compromised) on each of the above decision making indicators and the overall outcome rating. She decided that she would be happier with formula and bottle feeding. Though she did not look forward to telling her co-worker, she laughed and said, "Hey it's my decision, and I can handle that."

With careful assessment and mutual goal setting, the nurse assisted Cheryl in making an informed decision, while respecting her individual needs. Without using a nursing model of practice, the nurse might have formulated the diagnosis without Cheryl's input and treated the wrong problem. Furthermore, Cheryl would likely have switched to formula feeding anyway but experienced lifelong guilt and feelings of being a bad mother.

References

Gigliotti, E. (1995). When women decide *not* to breast-feed. *MCN: The American Journal of Maternal Child Nursing. 20,* 315–321.

Gigliotti, E. (2008). The value of nursing models in practice. *Dokuz Eylul University School of Nursing Electronic Journal, 1* (1), 42–50. Http://www.deuhyoedergi.org/index.php?option=com_contentandtask=viewandid=22 andItemid=35.

Marshall, J.L., Godfrey, M., Renfrew, M.J. (2007). Being a good mother; Managing breast feeding and merging identities. *Social Science and Medicine. 55* (10), 2147–2159.

Nelson, A.M. (2006). Toward a situation-specific theory of breast feeding. *Research and Theory for Nursing Practice. 20* (1), 9–27.

Neuman, B. (2002). The Neuman systems model. In B. Neuman and J. Fawcett (eds.), *The Neuman systems model* (pp. 3–33; p.351). Upper Saddle River, NJ: Prentice Hall.

5.39. Business Woman with Stress in Her Personal Life

Maria Müller Staub, RN, EdN, PhD

Eliza S is a 48-year-old woman who was born in Switzerland and now has an executive position in New York, USA for an international pharmaceutical firm. In New York, she went to a Swiss psychotherapist for extreme fatigue and many personal problems that were upsetting her. During the last year, Eliza S had worked more than 60 hours a week in her job and was very successful, but suffered sleep deprivation. After discussing these and other issues, the psychotherapist advised her to go to a psychiatric clinic in Switzerland for one month so she could rest and resolve some of her personal problems. She took a one-month leave from work and went to Switzerland for treatment.

Eliza S had been living separately from her third husband, Greg, who lived in their Swiss home. Three years ago, he had become the CEO of a Swiss firm, but he lost this position and has been jobless for the past year.

Shortly after entering the clinic, she started to manage her stay in the clinic similarly to managing her job by asking for specific therapies and developing an organized plan for her treatment, including jogging, music therapy, psychological counseling sessions, and only short times to rest between appointments. In counseling sessions, she was restless, expressed feelings of emptiness, acted tired, and complained of endless, pondering thoughts.

When the nurse asked Eliza S about her past life, she said that she was born into a wealthy Swiss family and went to a kibbutz in Israel when she was 18, where she fell in love with an Israeli. They married one year later and moved to the USA and had a daughter, Simona. At that time, Eliza S studied psychology and worked part-time in an insurance company. Problems in raising and educating their daughter rose early in the marriage and Eliza's husband had difficulty adjusting to the US lifestyle, including the studies and work of his wife. When

Simona was four years old, the couple decided to divorce. The husband chose to go back to Israel and took his daughter with him, while Eliza stayed in New York. Eliza visited Simona and her ex-husband several times a year, but lost track of Simona after age 16, when Simona refused the visits of her mother.

Soon after finishing her master's degrees in psychology, Eliza S obtained an executive position in a pharmaceutical company and she subsequently chose to study pharmacology. After completing her pharmacology degree, she changed jobs, becoming a top executive of a firm where she was responsible for successful mergers. Eliza S always liked her jobs and was an active woman, enjoying music, theater, and sports activities.

Three years after the divorce from her first husband, she married again, but was divorced from her second husband after four years of marriage. In counseling, her feelings about relationships were explored. "Being refused by Simona makes me sad, maybe I should try again to contact her," she said. "Maybe my main problem is that I'm not able to bond with others; after I was living with Greg for two years, he obtained his Swiss position and we decided to 'live separate-together,' but now this relationship is also deteriorating." "I fear I will lose my position if I stay away longer. The costs of my house are so high that I am considering selling it, and I am also thinking of separating from Greg. I'm so, so extremely tired, but I need to make decisions quickly, otherwise even more things will go astray," Eliza S said.

Eliza S struggled to resolve her problems of fatigue, her husband's loss of a job, their deteriorating relationship, and financial problems related to the expenses of two houses, high travel costs, and one income. Eliza S sometimes opened up, showed her feelings, and wept. Most of the time, however, she was controlled and restless.

STOP. THINK. Which diagnoses, outcomes, and interventions would you select?

Submitter's Analysis and Use of NANDA-I, NOC, and NIC

In reviewing the many issues of concern, the nurse and Eliza identified the possible diagnoses of *sleep deprivation, fatigue, impaired social interactions, impaired parenting,* and *decisional conflict* as the bases for a plan of care. Eliza S clearly suffered from *sleep deprivation*, with the defining characteristics of decreased ability to function, tiredness, inability to concentrate, and restlessness. She also exhibited the related factors of *sustained inadequate sleep hygiene* from working too many hours and prolonged psychological discomfort. The *sleep deprivation*, the many hours of work in a responsible position, and *decisional conflict* contributed to the experience of *fatigue*. There were insufficient data to support the diagnoses of *impaired social interactions* and *impaired parenting* and it seemed that intervening for these diagnoses would not make a significant difference in Eliza's present well being.

The nurse and Eliza S chose the diagnosis of *decisional conflict* regarding possible sale of her house, separation from her husband, and resignation from her job. Eliza S was under great pressure to make decisions that would have significant effects on her lifestyle and personal well being. *Decisional conflict* was identified as a contributing factor to inadequate sleep patterns and feelings of fatigue. Another reason that this diagnosis was considered as the most important to address was that most of the time Eliza S was controlled and restless; organizing things provided the best relief for her.

NOC Outcomes

Eliza S and her primary nurse chose the outcome of *decision making*, with Eliza specifying it as "selling or not selling the house," "deciding about keeping my position," and "resolving my relationship problems." The baseline score was set as 2 (substantially compromised) and the target score was set as 4 (mildly compromised).

NIC Interventions

The NIC interventions that Eliza S and her nurse selected were *decision making support, emotional support* and *guided imagery*. According to Eliza S's priorities, the nurse supported her in identifying the benefits of selling her house and the benefits of trying to keep it. The nurse also asked her to explain possibilities when predicting the changes that would occur with selling versus not selling the house.

In *guided imagery* sessions Eliza was supported in opening up and envisioning new ways of living after having made a decision. The literature supports using *guided imagery* to regain general mental and physical well being and to relieve stress. Studies explained the mechanism through which relaxation by means of guided imagery is effective in reducing stress (Watanabe, Fukuda, and Shirakawa, 2005; Watanabe, Fukuda, Hara, Maeda, Ohira and Shirakawa, 2006; Kwekkeboom, Hau, Wanta, and Bumpus, 2008). The possibility of giving up the job, house, and lifestyle in New York was compared to staying with her husband in Switzerland. Eliza was precise in her thinking, even though these conflicts remained for about two weeks. The nurse, working with the interdisciplinary team, also addressed her fatigue and insisted on a more relaxed schedule of Eliza's therapeutic activities. After several days of a more relaxed schedule, Eliza started to sleep better and felt less tired. She participated in psychological group counseling sessions, went to music therapy, and joined a jogging group. Coming back, she said "I always jogged alone but it is much easier with others—I like to run in a group!"

In the second week, Eliza S started consults with a lawyer to discuss possibilities about selling the house. At that point, she left the clinic, flew to New York, and placed the house for sale. At the same time, she decided to keep her job. She returned to the clinic after her trip to New York.

Evaluation

After 20 days, Eliza S insisted on leaving the clinic. She and the nurse decided that she still had *decisional conflict* regarding her relationship with her husband, so they rated her outcome as 3 (moderately compromised), instead of the desired 4.

Eliza S felt calm, slept better, and reported being less tired. She expressed relief about having organized the selling of her house. "I'm so glad I was able to come to a decision. I am ready now for the decisions to follow. First I need to go back to work. I know other things remain open, such as my relationship with my husband," she said. The nurses and the psychotherapist would have liked to continue working with Eliza about the possible roots of her problems in maintaining relationships and in having a better work-life balance, but they had to accept her will to leave the clinic. When evaluating the care given, Eliza S had improved in *decision making*, even though not to the extent she had planned with the nurse.

References

Kwekkebom, K.L., Hau, H., Wanta, B., and Bumpus, M. (2008). Patients' perceptions of the effectiveness of guided imagery and progressive muscle relaxation interventions used for cancer pain. *Complementary Therapies in Clinical Practice, 14*, 185–194.

Watanabe, E., Fukuda, S., and Shirakawa, T. (2005). Effects among healthy subjects of the duration of regularly practicing a guided imagery program. *BMC Complementary and Alternative Medicine, 20*(5), 21.

Watanabe, E., Fukuda, S., Hara, H., Maeda, Y., Ohira, H., and Shirakawa, T. (2006). Differences in relaxation by means of guided imagery in a healthy community sample. *Alternative Therapies in Health and Medicine, 12*, 60–66.

Case Studies with a Primary Focus on Risk Diagnoses and Associated Outcomes and Interventions

6

6.1. Role of Nurses in the Protection of Children

Andrea Karolys, RN, BSN

Ramon is a one-year-old infant who was referred to public health field nursing after being returned to his home with his mother from the children's home of the county. Ramon, his three-year-old sister Maria, and 13-year-old sister Teresa, had been removed from their home by the juvenile court while their mother Guadalupe completed a drug rehabilitation program. Guadalupe is presently unemployed and is supported by a federal and state funded agency. Her family support consisted of her mother who has a history of alcoholism. Guadalupe has a ninth grade education.

The public health nurse (PHN) was referred to the home to check on Ramon's growth and development and to connect Guadalupe and the family to community resources. Upon arrival to the apartment complex, the PHN walked through a broken gated area by a pool to access the staircase leading to the family's second story apartment. A three-year-old was riding a tricycle unattended at the top of the stairs on a second story walkway. The PHN noted that the glass picture window had been duct taped along broken edges and the door had two large holes. After knocking on the door three times, the door opened slowly, and a woman who said she was Guadalupe peered through the security chain, and eventually opened the door for the PHN to enter the apartment. Her breath reeked of alcohol. The room was dark and sparsely furnished. Mosquitoes circled the cans of food that were open on a kitchen table cluttered with half eaten bowls of cereal. The room smelled of natural gas and foul food. Roaches were noted on the walls.

Before beginning the visit routines, the PHN asked Guadalupe to call Maria into the house from the second story walkway. Ramon was crying in a playpen, surrounded by soiled blankets, a bottle of red punch, and small toy Legos. The PHN noted an unfilled antibiotic prescription for Teresa dated one week before the home visit. When asked about this, Guadalupe said she did not fill the prescription because she could not locate the children's Medi Cal cards (California Medicaid). Teresa complained of a chronic cough and had stayed home from school with a fever.

Further assessment revealed that Guadalupe was aware that Teresa needed the medication but her boyfriend had spent the money to buy beer for a party. She and the boyfriend had fought about this issue, which was how the front door glass was broken. Guadalupe explained that her boyfriend had been recently released from jail for cocaine possession. She also shared with the PHN that she has a hard time taking care of the kids when Teresa goes to school so she likes having her home.

STOP. THINK. Which diagnoses, outcomes, and interventions would you select?

Submitter's Analysis and Use of NANDA-I, NOC, and NIC

Positive coping strategies were not demonstrated within this family and the needs of various family members were not being met. Despite having been through drug and alcohol rehabilitation and having been the recipient of extensive social service interventions, Guadalupe had not been able to convert this help into positive family processes. Nursing assessment of family processes revealed that Guadalupe demonstrated a dysfunctional pattern of substance abuse as indicated by repeated adverse consequences and failure to fulfill important obligations at home. Although the PHN considered the nursing diagnoses of *ineffective family management of therapeutic regimen, noncompliance, ineffective individual coping*, and at *risk for violence*, the children's *risk for injury* and *need for positive parenting* were considered more important at this time.

The most important diagnosis that the PHN selected was *risk for injury*. This diagnosis was supported by observation of safety hazards at the entrance of the apartment complex, lack of gating around the pool, and broken windows and doors. The three-year-old child who was riding a tricycle in a dangerous area on the balcony was at risk for injury. All three children were at risk for injury in the cluttered, unsafe apartment, including an appliance that leaked gas. The presence of rotten food and possibility of malnutrition was also a risk factor. The children were at risk for injury from the lack of attention to these hazards by their mother. The one-year-old infant, with small toys in the crib, was at risk for choking.

A second priority diagnosis for this visit was *impaired parenting* related to deficient knowledge, lack of support, and ineffective coping strategies. The family processes did not support positive parenting roles and was an etiology of the two diagnoses. The mother had not created an environment to promote the well being of her children. Some of the cues that were characteristic of the diagnosis were: blatant inattention to the developmental, safety, and emotional needs of the children; lack of attention to the health care needs of Teresa; neglect of Teresa's schooling; putting Teresa in the inappropriate role of care-giver/parent; and verbalization of inability to care for her children. Additional risk factors of this diagnosis included lack of support from significant others, a violent relationship with her boyfriend, and finan-cial stressors. This mother's history of drug abuse, evidence of current alcohol abuse, and lack of knowledge and motivation to care for her children made this situation a high priority concern of the PHN.

NOC Outcomes

The NOC outcomes that were selected for this family based on these two diagnoses were *risk control* and *parenting performance*. The baseline score on *risk control* was 2 (rarely demonstrated) and the target score was 4 (often demonstrated). The baseline score on *parenting performance* was 2 (rarely demonstrated) and the target score was 4 (often demonstrated).

NIC Interventions

For both outcomes the PHN used the NIC interventions of *risk identi-fication, parent education: infant, parent education: childbearing family*, and *parent education: adolescent*. The nurse discussed environmental and child safety issues with Guadalupe, including caring for her children under the influence of alcohol and other chemical substances. The PHN told Guadalupe that she would report this information to social ser-vices. During this visit, the mother was taught to remove all small objects from the infant's crib (American Academy of Pediatrics [AAP], 2006). Other topics that were taught were risks related to the nutrition of the one-, three-, and 13-year-old children, including risks to the infant of dental caries and malnutrition (AAP, 2004).

Teaching about safety included never leaving the three-year old and one-year old unattended and the dangers of falls when a child rides a tricycle on a second story balcony near a staircase (AAP, 2001). The laws related to child abuse were explained so that Guadalupe would understand the seriousness of the situation.

Additional NIC interventions that were used were *referral* and *case management*. The nurse referred the mother to social services and con-nected the 13-year old with counseling resources. Additionally, the mother was referred to Aid to Families with Dependent Children (AFDC), as well as medical and food resources. The mother was given a referral for the three-year-old for a Head Start preschool program near the home. The PHN encouraged Guadalupe to re-enter the county's alcohol and drug rehabilitation program with her children, where she would receive parenting and home skills classes and counseling to address parenting skills and domestic violence.

The challenges presented by cases such as Guadalupe and her children can be met by experienced PHNs because of their knowledge and skills related to history taking; physical examination; communication; family assessment and intervention; collaborative processes with families, communities, and other providers; and use of community and social service resources. The findings of family assessments are considered in the context of the community, environment, and acculturated practices. Public health nursing is multifaceted to include health education, counseling, culture brokerage, and referral to other providers. The goal is to help families surmount the complex barriers to health care such as poverty, prejudice, and lack of resources.

Public health nurses are challenged to participate in private and public partnerships to provide education and resources in the community. Opportunities are available in the community, e.g., health fairs to explain health promotion, health protection, and community resources for the achievement of optimum family health. In order to achieve the complex goals of this public health agency, the public health field nurses renovated the nursing documentation system to include NANDA-I, NOC, and NIC. Use of these standardized nursing vocabularies has clarified the work of PHNs for communication to others. For example, reports to referral sources to demonstrate the health outcomes of consumers are clearer since implementation.

Evaluation

The target scores on the two NOC outcomes were not met but the children were protected by removing them from the mother. Despite extensive teaching and biweekly joint home visitation with social services, the family exhausted all PHN resources. Guadalupe continued to abuse alcohol, despite extensive nursing and social service interventions. The risk for injury to the children and the parenting skills did not improve. Subsequently, the three children were placed in long term foster care. The mother became pregnant again and was treated in the county methadone program for pregnant addicted mothers.

References

American Academy of Pediatrics, Committee on Injury and Poison Prevention. (2001). Falls from heights: Windows, roofs, balconies. Retrieved on September 18, 2008, from http://aappolicy.aappublications.org/.

American Academy of Pediatrics, Committee on Injury and Poison Prevention. (2006). *Choking prevention and first aid for infants and children*. Retrieved on

September 16, 2008, from http://aap.org/parenting corner_Q_and_A:Choking prevention.

American Academy of Pediatrics, Committee on Nutrition. (2004). *Pediatric nutrition handbook* (5th ed.). Elk Grove Village, IL: Author.

6.2. Responses to Mechanical Ventilation

Leo M. Lunney, RN

Mr. S is a 71-year-old male. He came to the ED by ambulance in respiratory distress with oxygen delivered at 30% by a venti-mask. The physical examination revealed: HR 120, sinus tachycardia; BP, 170/91; RR, 40; and SaO_2 65%. An ABG was immediately obtained. Ausculation revealed severely decreased breath sounds in all lung fields and bilateral apical wheezing. The chest X-ray showed chronic changes consistent with chronic obstructive pulmonary disease (COPD).

Considering Mr. S's serious condition, the nurse briefly interviewed him; he said that he had been treated for COPD for 10 years and had been smoking three packs of cigarettes a day. Usually Mr. S used home oxygen for ambulation only, but for the past 10 days had continuously used oxygen. He also stated that he usually does not use oxygen more than 2 liters/m by nasal cannula and it was necessary to use 4 l/m to partially relieve distress.

The ED physician ordered xopenex (1.25 mg) by nebulizer and solu-cortef (125 mg) IV to be given immediately. The ABG results showed PH, 7.20; PO_2, 48; PCO_2, 68; HCO_3, 20; SaO_2, 68%. The respiratory care practitioner (RCP) recommended a course of bi-level positive airway pressure (BIPAP) non-invasive ventilation prior to intubation. Respiratory distress persisted and the SaO_2 continued in the 78 to 80% range. The next ABG results indicated that mechanical ventilation was necessary, so the RCP started to intubate Mr. S with a dual lumen 7.5 endotracheal tube (ETT). The ETT mistakenly entered the esophageal cavity, however, so it was discarded and a new dual lumen ETT was used with success. This procedure follows the guidelines for prevention of hospital-associated pneumonias (Centers for Disease Prevention and Control [CDC], 2004). The dual lumen ETT was used to prevent pooling of secretions on the top of the ETT balloon. A chest X-ray confirmed proper placement of the ETT and the device was secured. Mr.

S was admitted to the medical intensive care unit (MICU) with a medical diagnosis of exacerbation COPD.

STOP. THINK. Which diagnoses, outcomes, and interventions would you select?

Submitter's Analysis and Use of NANDA, NOC, and NIC

With the information provided about Mr. S by the ED staff members, the MICU nurses immediately diagnosed *impaired gas exchange*, *risk for infection*, and *risk for compromised human dignity*. The diagnosis of *impaired gas exchange* was already being treated by mechanical ventilation. Mechanical ventilation supported respiration while the inflammatory and obstructive processes at the alveolar capillary level were being treated.

With this necessary invasion of Mr. S's respiratory tract, the *risk for infection* was high, so daily assessments were performed to establish the continued necessity for mechanical ventilator support (CDC, 2004; Sinuff, Muscedere, Cook, Dodek, Heyland, and Canadian Critical Care Trials Group, 2008). Prior to the implementation of evidenced-based guidelines for prevention of ventilator associated pneumonia (VAP), the CDC (1997) reported that there were 4.2 to 16.3 cases of VAP per 1,000 ventilator days. At that time, VAP was the leading cause of mortality and morbidity in ICU settings and mortality rates of people diagnosed with VAP was 20 to 50%. The critical nature of this hospital-acquired infection led to the development of evidence-based practice (EBP) guidelines (CDC, 2004). In a review of studies since 2004, Gastmeier and Geffers (2007) concluded that multi-module programs based on EBP resulted in reduction of VAP from 31 to 57%.

Mr. S was at *risk for compromised human dignity* because mechanical ventilation and his physical status placed him in a vulnerable situation in which he no longer could make decisions for himself. He was unable to effectively communicate and had lost control of bodily functions (Schou and Egerod, 2008).

Use of NOC Outcomes

Based on the standardized routines in the MICU, the nurses immediately knew that their outcomes selection would include *mechanical ventilation response*, *infection severity*, and *coping*. On *mechanical ventilation response* and *infection severity*, Mr. S's baseline scores were 5 (no deviation from normal range) and the target scores were to remain at 5. On *coping*, his baseline score was 5 (consistently demonstrated) and the goal was to remain at 5.

Use of NIC Interventions

On arrival to the MICU, the nurses immediately implemented the mechanical ventilation protocol that was established through an extensive literature review of research findings related to VAP and the CDC guidelines for prevention of hospital-based pneumonias. An evidenced-based practice project revealed that simple procedures could reduce the incidence of infection (Pfeifer, Orser, Gefen, McGuiness, and Hannon, 2001). The emphasis on reducing VAP is multinational, e.g., in the United Kingdom it was established as a national initiative (Pellowe, 2007). In the MICU where Mr. S was admitted, there have been no incidences of VAP for two years since implementing this EVP protocol. To implement the protocol, the nurse manager educated all MICU personnel on the specifics of the protocol and accountability procedures were set up to enforce compliance as described by Larson, Quiros, and Lin (2007). The NIC interventions that were part of this protocol were *positioning, airway management, airway suctioning, mechanical ventilation (vent) management: invasive oxygen therapy, infection protection, and coping enhancement.*

The head of the bed was placed at 45 degrees (CDC, 2004) to decrease the risk of aspiration of stomach contents. In previous research, the supine position was shown to increase the risk for aspiration (Hess, 2005).

For airway management and airway suctioning, the second ETT lumen was connected to intermittent suction. The in-line suction catheter was placed between the ventilator circuit and the mechanical ventilator. The consulting physician pulmonology specialist activated the vent management protocol, which included sedation to reduce discomfort and pain (Jacob, Lubszky, Friolet, Rothen, Kolarova, and Takala, 2007).

The immediate focus when people are mechanically ventilated is extubation (CDC, 2004). This is because the ETT acts as a portal into the lungs; the goal is to limit intubation time to prevent the seeding of bacteria into the lungs. Each morning, in collaboration, the nurse and RCP performed an assessment of possible vent discontinuation. This activity was coordinated with a daily sedation interruption to enable assessment of other responses, such as neurological, of Mr. S. As with other ventilated patients, Mr. S was scored on multiple parameters and it was determined that he would tolerate a spontaneous breathing trial, which is an effective indicator for the probability of extubation success (Ely, 2001). At 60 minutes of the breathing trail Mr. S exhibited respiratory changes. His RR increased to 36 and he desaturated to 85%. The breathing trial was discontinued and he was returned to his original ventilator settings and sedation regimen.

The nurses provided oral care hourly to limit bacterial growth within the naso-oral cavity (CDC, 2004). The integrity of a closed system was maintained, e.g., the ventilator circuits and in-line suction catheters were changed when soiled or every seven days. A disposable endotracheal tube (ETT) cuff manometer was used every two hours to detect balloon air leaks. A seal between the balloon and the trachea wall was necessary to prevent infiltration of contaminated oral secretions into the lungs.

Vigorous hand washing standards were maintained. Implementation of the CDC hand hygiene guidelines was a collaborative effort of hospital administration, nurse managers, and clinical staff (Haas and Larson, 2008).

To minimize the risk of compromised human dignity and promote optimum coping with these procedures, the nurses implemented the NIC interventions of *environmental management: comfort* and *coping enhancement*. They ensured that the lighting, noises, and room temperature were as comfortable as possible. While at the bedside, they spoke to Mr. S with dignity and respect and explained to him their immediate and long-term goals. Because the MICU was air conditioned, they provided blankets to avoid undue exposure to drafts and chilling.

Evaluation

On day three, the vent discontinuation assessment supported the advancement to a spontaneous breathing trail. At 120 minutes there were no abnormal respiratory and hemodynamic responses to the trial and ABGs were drawn. With the results of the ABGs and clinical observations of the nurse and RCP, the pulmonologist decided to extubate Mr. S, which was successful.

Mr. S did not remember the vent experience because the sedation drug, diprivan, had an amnesiac effect. Between the time of extubation and discharge, the nurses taught Mr. S how to avoid COPD exacerbation when he returned home, including the antigen role of cigarette smoke. Mr. S's wife acknowledged the MICU nurses' diligence and care of Mr. S. In five days, Mr. S was discharged from the hospital.

References

Centers for Disease Control. (1997). *Guideline for Prevention of Nosocomial Infection*. Morbidity and Mortality Weekly Report, 46, (No. RR-1).

Centers for Disease Control. (2004). Guidelines for preventing health care associated pneumonia, 2003. *Morbidity and Mortality Weekly Report, 53*, RR-3. Retrieved on September 29, 2008, from http://www.cdc.gov/mmwr/PDF/rr/rr5303.pdf.

Ely, W., Meade, M., Haponick, E. (2001). Mechanical ventilator weaning protocols driven by nonphysician health-care professional: Evidence-based clinical practice guideline. *Chest, 120*, 454S-463S.

Gastmeier, P., and Geffers, C. (2007). Prevention of ventilator-associated pneumonia: Analysis of studies published since 2004. *Journal of Hospital Infection, 67*, 1–8.

Haas, J.P., and Larson, E.L. (2008). Compliance with hand hygiene guidelines: Where are we in 2008? *American Journal of Nursing, 108*(8), 40–45.

Hess, D.R. (2005). Patient positioning and ventilator-associated pneumonia. *Respiratory Care, 50*, 892–898.

Jacob, S., Lubszky, S., Friolt, R., Rothen, H., Kolarova, A., and Takala, J. (2007). Sedation and weaning from mechanical ventilation: Effects of process optimization outside a clinical trial. *Journal of Critical Care, 22*, 219–228.

Larson, E.L., Quiros, D., and Lin, S.X. (2007). Dissemination of the CDC's hand hygiene guidelines and impact of infection rates. *American Journal of Infection Control, 35*, 666–675.

Pellowe, C. (2007). Managing and leading the infection prevention initiative. *Journal of Nursing Management, 15*, 567–573.

Pfeifer, L.T., Orser, L., Gefen, C., McGuinness, R., and Hannon, C.V. (2001). Preventing ventilator associated pneumonia: What all nurses should know. *American Journal of Nursing, 101*(8), 24AA–24GG.

Schou, L., and Egerod, I. (2008). A qualitative study into the lived experience of post-CABG patients during mechanical ventilator weaning. *Intensive and Critical Care Nursing, 24*, 171–179.

Sinuff, T., Muscedere, J., Cook, D., Dodek, P., Heyland, D., and Canadian Critical Care Trials Group. (2008). Ventilator-associated pneumonia: Improving outcomes through guidelines implementation. *Journal of Critical Care, 23*, 18–125.

6.3. Family Caregiving at End of Life

Paul Germano, RN, BS and Margaret M. Terjesen, RN, MS

ES is a 75-year-old female who has had recent surgery for a malignant neoplasm of her bronchus and lungs. Her cancer has metastasized to the lymph nodes and her long term prognosis is poor. Nonetheless, ES was receiving treatment for her cancer.

The chemotherapy treatment for the illness contributed to anemia and muscle weakness. ES was also suffering from depression, which she attributed to her current condition. The disease and treatment had left her so physically and mentally debilitated that she had no energy or desire to get out of bed. This immobility created an additional problem of a stage 2 decubitus on her R hip. ES preferred to lie on her R side while in bed. Physical therapy (PT) had been prescribed for ES but she was often too tired and unmotivated to participate in this regimen. Based on ES's current condition, she was eligible for Medicare, a home health care (HHC) nurse, and PT services.

Prior to this, ES was independent and provided for her family. Now her condition required the continued assistance of her 76-year-old husband and 42-year-old daughter. Both assisted ES with her activities of daily living which included personal hygiene, toileting, changing the decubitus ulcer dressing, preparing meals, administering her medications, and transporting her for chemotherapy treatments and other medical appointments.

To the HHC nurse, the care required for ES seemed like a huge burden for her family, but the family was willing to provide whatever personal care and other services ES required. The HHC nurse evaluated the care provided by the family and judged it to be competent. While fully capable of managing these duties, however, the family reported being overwhelmed and frustrated at times. ES's daughter stated, "I feel bad whenever I change my mother's dressing because she screams in pain." ES's husband joked that now he has to do all the cooking, and if her disease does not kill her, his cooking will. ES's family was stoic in the face of the challenge presented to them. It was apparent, however, that they needed assistance in managing ES's condition and the family dynamic that the illness created.

Although this family was financially solvent, paying for an around-the-clock HHC aid would create a financial burden. ES was not eligible for the Medicaid program, which might supply an around-the-clock aid, because the family's finances were above the allowable limit. Her family had accepted the responsibility of ES's care and had displayed tremendous resolve and adeptness in attending to her needs. They knew her condition was terminal. ES's daughter desired to effectively change the dressings without causing unnecessary pain. ES's husband wanted to know how to make his wife feel more at ease.

 STOP. THINK. Which diagnoses, outcomes, and interventions would you select?

Submitter's Analysis and Use of NANDA-I, NOC, and NIC

When considering appropriate nursing diagnoses for ES and her family, the nurse clustered the data of: the family understood that her condition was terminal, family accepted her impending death, family desired to make her last days as fulfilling as possible. Their coping skills were sufficient and they demonstrated great determination to make ES's last days as comfortable as possible. ES's family had shouldered the tremendous burden of managing and sustaining her health. The family had shown that they were extremely involved and capable to achieve that end. They also were aware that they wanted additional knowledge for future care, and had expressed a willingness to learn from the HHC nurse.

Three nursing diagnoses were identified to assist this family care for ES: *risk for infection, acute pain,* and *readiness for enhanced family therapeutic regimen management. Risk for infection* was secondary to a compromised immune system and limited mobility. This diagnosis took on a high priority because ES was high risk with her condition and treatment, and her family was lacking knowledge regarding this risk. While ES's daughter was adept at changing her mother's bandages, the nurse noted that she did not use aseptic technique. Additionally, ES's bedroom was crowded with many objects that could be a breeding place for microorganisms.

The *acute pain* was secondary to the disease process as evidenced by ES's complaints and her expressions when her family offered care. ES's pain was long standing and often severe. ES and her family were in need of effectively managing her opioid analgesic regimen to better allay her discomfort and enable the family to attend to her needs.

The *readiness for enhanced family therapeutic regimen management* diagnosis strongly related to the complexity of ES's illness and the family dynamic. In a systematic review of research related to informal caregiver's needs in end of life care, the results showed that caregivers need additional practical information on how to help people who are dying (Bee, Barnes, and Luker, 2008). ES's condition brought with it a host of issues and demands on her caretakers. Her family had managed them satisfactorily but her increasingly debilitated state presented a continuing challenge to her family and they were ambivalent about better management. While displaying adeptness in handling this crisis, the family's competence in managing ES's health could be augmented by the HHC nurse.

NOC Outcomes

In conjunction with the family, the following outcomes were selected to guide nursing care: *infection severity, pain level,* and *treatment behavior: illness or injury*. The baseline score for *infection severity* was 5 (none) and the target score was to remain at 5. The baseline score for *pain level* was 2 (substantial) and the goal score was 4 (mild). The baseline score for *treatment behavior: illness or injury* was 4 (often demonstrated) and the target score was 5 (consistently demonstrated).

NIC Interventions

The nursing interventions selected to address the outcome of *infection severity* were *infection protection, home maintenance assistance,* and *positioning*. The nurse taught ES's family aseptic technique for performing dressing changes and tactfully suggested the removal of non-essential objects from her room. The nurse encouraged regular turning and positioning while in bed and increased mobility as tolerated to prevent infection and additional skin breakdown and to promote healing. Additionally, the nurse furnished information on how to maintain a safe and clean environment to prevent injury and retard the growth of microorganisms.

The NIC intervention of *pain management* was provided to help the family to relieve the distress created by ES's disease process. Teaching the family the principles of pain management, such as the administration of the analgesic prior to dressing changes or PT exercises, enabled ES to better tolerate treatment. Teaching ES nonpharmacological methods of pain relief also augmented the analgesic regimen. Techniques such as relaxation, guided imagery, distraction, biofeedback, and hot or cold compresses were discussed with the family as possibilities.

The NIC interventions for the diagnosis of *readiness for enhanced family therapeutic regimen* were *teaching: disease process, teaching: prescribed activity and exercise,* and *teaching: prescribed medication.* Identifying the changes in ES's physical condition from both the disease process and the medication regimen gave the family the ability to anticipate ES's needs and modify their care-giving tactics. The progression of ES's illness required the family to make continued adjustments to her activities, nutrition, and pain management. ES did not feel the same every day, so having this knowledge helped the family to better cope with new or different problems created by the illness or medication regimen as they arose. This was especially true for physical activity.

Instructing the patient, and her family, on the purpose for and benefits of prescribed physical activity and the means to conserve energy while attempting these activities provided the additional motivation needed to get ES out of bed. In addition, ES and her family were informed about the importance of turning and positioning ES every two hours when she was in bed. The goal of adherence to a physical activity regimen and turning and positioning in bed was to prevent further skin breakdown. Additionally, instructing ES and her family on the benefits, side effects, and correct administration of the medication regimen helped to regulate the sequelae of ES's illness and better manage her activities. For example, administering her pain medication 30 minutes before dressing changes contributed to less distress and her daughter did not feel guilty about causing pain. Knowing the side effects also allowed ES and her family to plan, or not plan, other activities.

Support system enhancement was provided to help the family cope with the stress of managing her care. While ES had Medicare and was not eligible for a full time HHC aid, finding other community resources diminished some of the family's burden. ES was eligible for programs such as Meals on Wheels to spare her husband from having to prepare the meals. She and her family admitted that they were too proud to look for help and were not aware of the available programs. A list of the social services available in the area was provided to ES and her family. The use of these services made a difference in managing ES's health and maintaining her family's health.

Evaluation

The outcomes as planned were met. ES remained free of infection and her pain level was maintained at mild most of the time. ES and her family described extensive knowledge of the effects of the disease, signs and symptoms of complications, and the expected course of the disease. They described how to balance rest and activity, factors that decreased the ability to perform activity, the purpose of activity, and its expected effects. Their knowledge of the medication regimen was also substantial—as they were able to describe the action, administration, and the benefits and side effects of the medication regimen. ES and her family still expressed a reluctance to use community services. Continued encouragement and guidance was required to achieve this goal.

Nurses' Reflection

Working with ES and her family was an enlightening experience. Faced with tremendous adversity, and imminent death, ES and her family retained their resolve and were determined to make her remaining days as fulfilling as possible. They were a resilient family, determined to manage this crisis on their own. They determined, however, that should the situation become overwhelming, they would seek additional help. Knowing that they can and will do everything possible to alleviate ES's condition, and remain as a cohesive group, was an inspiration. It was a privilege and our utmost fortunate pleasure to have made the acquaintance of this extraordinary family.

Reference

Bee, P.E., Barnes, P., and Luker, K.A. (2008). A systematic review of informal caregiver's needs to providing home-based end-of-life care to people with cancer. *Journal of Clinical Nursing*, July 1, epub, ahead of print.

6.4. Man with Renal Calculi and Stent Placement

Mary G. McCaffery-Tesoro, MS, RN, C, OCN

JR, a 61-year-old white male with a diagnosis of renal calculi who was admitted to the hospital on the morning of surgery for cystoscopy, lithotripsy, and stent placement, was admitted to the medical-surgical unit following the procedure for observation. He was scheduled for discharge the next day.

The admitting data showed that he was alert and oriented with complaints of left flank pain that he rated as 7 on a 10-point scale. There was an intravenous (IV) D5 ½ NS infusing at 80 ml/hr to the left hand. His vital signs were within normal range. The physical examination was unremarkable with the exception of left costrovetebral tenderness, the use of oxygen (O_2) 2 liters a minute by nasal cannula, and a BMI of 32.

His significant past health history included a history of renal calculi one year ago, hypertension (HTN), and sleep apnea. JR stopped smoking 10 years prior. At home, he takes inderal 10 mg twice per day for the HTN and uses a bi-level positive airway pressure (BIPAP) machine for sleep apnea. He has no known allergies.

When discussing his actual and anticipated needs, JR asked for pain medication and asked to keep his BIPAP machine at the bedside for sleep. When discussing his acceptable pain threshold he stated, "0, no pain." JR stated that the physician had not obtained a sample of his "stone" and he did not know what type they were. He stated that he was satisfied with his home life and that he and his wife have a very good relationship. JR is a retired diamond cutter and he was very proud of the level of professionalism he incorporated into his work. He said that he expected the same professionalism from health care providers.

JR was asked to void in a urinal so his urine could be assessed for color and amount and strained for the possible passage of calculi or gravel. His urine was amber in color and the output was approximately 70 ml/hr without evidence of calculi. JR's blood urea nitrogen and creatinine were 10 and 0.8, respectively. His intake of oral fluids was adequate, supplemented by IV fluids. His input was congruent with his output. JR complained of left flank pain 9/10 only when voiding and was medicated with two percocet without relief of this episodic pain. He verbalized acceptance of this episodic pain because it only occurred during voiding and he was concerned that an increase of analgesia may compromise his respiratory function.

JR maintained a saturated oxygen concentration (SaO$_2$) of 92 to 94% receiving oxygen (2 to 4 liters). The BIPAP machine was at the bedside to be used at bedtime. Pulse oximetry was continuously monitored, with the alarm set to ring when the level dropped below 90%. When JR fell asleep in the chair, his SaO$_2$ dropped to 85% and when he awakened the level returned to 92%. The respiratory therapist and pulmonary physician attended and it was discussed with JR that nurses would make frequent rounds (q 15 to 30 minutes).

JR's vital signs remained stable with a maximum T 99 °F. He verbalized the need to measure and strain urine to capture any sand or stone for analysis and to measure output. He also was able to verbalize the manifestations of urinary tract infection. JR verbalized approval of the BIPAP machine used in the hospital and demonstrated use. When his sleep apnea was discussed he shared that he is on a weight reduction regimen, which he hoped would positively impact his breathing status. JR was able to verbalize a low calorie, high fiber diet that he had been managing at home. His BMI is currently 32 and JR states that he has lost 10 pounds in the last three months by following a low calorie, high fiber diet. Unfortunately, JR continues to experience pain in the left flank area upon micturation and there is a plan to incorporate new pain management measures that do not cause him to become sleepy.

STOP. THINK. Which diagnoses, outcomes, and interventions would you select?

Submitter's Analysis and Use of NANDA-I, NOC, and NIC

The nursing diagnoses of *acute pain* and *risk for ineffective breathing pattern* were identified. Management of pain and routine responsibilities associated with care of people with urinary calculi were basic standards of care on the unit and those problems were being effectively managed.

While JR's admitting complaint focused on renal calculi and the associated pain, it was his *risk for ineffective breathing pattern* related to history of sleep apnea that was a high priority for the nurse because it posed the greatest risk to an uncomplicated hospitalization. In a literature review of obstructive sleep apnea, Lamm, Poeschel, and Smith (2008) concluded that this problem can lead to serious complications and needs to be addressed by nurses.

Obstructive sleep apnea occurs when there is a complete or partial obstruction of the upper airway during sleep (Tomlinson, 2007). Complications of this disorder include loud snoring, elevated blood pressure, decreased oxygen saturation, and frequent arousals during sleep. It is most common in those over 65 years of age and among obese adults. The nurse's assessment of this risk was based on JR's admitting history and the nurse's observation of diminished oxygen saturation, from 94% to 85%, when JR fell asleep.

NOC Outcomes

The nurse collaborated with JR, the physician, and the respiratory therapist to determine appropriate and acceptable outcome goals and interventions. The NOC outcomes of *respiratory status: airway patency*, *respiratory status: gas exchange*, and *respiratory status: ventilation* were selected to monitor this risk. His baseline score was rated as 5 (no deviation from normal range) when awake and the goal was to maintain a rating of 5, even when asleep. Airway patency and respiratory ventilation were measured by assessment of ease, rate, depth, and rhythm of breathing as well as assessment of breath sounds. Gas exchange was measured by assessment of cognitive status, skin color, and oxygen saturation measurement. JR's input related to the comfort and ease of breathing was solicited throughout the process.

NIC Interventions

The NIC interventions that were selected to meet these outcomes were *airway management, positioning, respiratory monitoring, ventilation assistance*, and *teaching: disease process*. The nurse scheduled frequent assessments of JR's respiratory and cognitive status, used continuous pulse oximetry, and monitored oxygen administration by nasal cannula from 2 to 4 liters a minute to maintain a pulse oximetry reading from 92 to 94%.

The nurse assigned JR to a room in close proximity to the nurses' station, assisted his positioning in a chair during the day and elevated the head of the bed to 45 degrees when he was resting in bed and sleeping at night, and encouraged his use of the BIPAP machine when sleeping.

In teaching about the disease process, the nurse reviewed what JR already knew and clarified anything that he questioned. They discussed the relation of excess weight to sleep apnea. JR agreed to a nutrition consultation for exploration of his eating patterns and ways that he could improve them for weight loss.

Evaluation

JR maintained a *respiratory status* outcome rating of 4 to 5 (slight deviation from normal to normal) during his hospital stay. While asleep and using the BIPAP machine, he maintained an oxygen saturation level of 92% or greater. When he fell asleep during the day without the BIPAP machine his saturation dropped to 88%, which triggered the pulse oximeter alarm and alerted both JR and the nurse to the drop in oxygenation. Once JR woke up and adjusted his positioning to maintain his airway, his oxygen level again reached 92%.

Prior to discharge, JR was able to verbalize the indications and instructions for his discharge medications of ampicillin and inderal as well as his next physician appointment. He had social support from his wife and children at home. He planned to return in two weeks to undergo subsequent cystoscopy with lithotripsy to remove the remaining calculi. JR was discharged with an appropriate diet plan for him and his wife. He planned to continue the use of the BIPAP machine and oxygen therapy at home and to consult with his private pulmonologist after discharge to discuss continuation and an exercise program.

References

Lamm, J., Poeschcel, J., and Smith, S. (2008). Obtaining a thorough health history and routinely screening for obstructive sleep apnea. *Journal of the American Academy of Nurse Practitioners, 20*, 225–229.

Tomlinson, M. (2007). Obstructive sleep apnea syndrome: Diagnosis and management. *Nursing Standard, 21*(48), 49–56, 58, 60.

6.5. Helping a Man with Low Literacy

Cynthia E. Degazon, PhD, RN and Bobbie Jean Perdue, PhD, RN

Mr. Jones is a 73-year-old African American male, retired bus driver who never married, had no children, lived alone, and was currently receiving Medicaid. Born in the rural south, Mr. Jones migrated to the north when he was 25 years of age. As a child in Mississippi, where his family still resides, Mr. Jones attended elementary school for only four years. Mr. Jones spoke with a very heavy accent and certain monosyllabic words were difficult to discern. In his writing he used printed letters spaced far apart.

One week ago, Mr. Jones was discharged from the hospital with medical diagnoses of peripheral vascular disease, hypertension, type 2 diabetes mellitus, and hyperlipidemia. He was given prescriptions for six medications, to be taken at varying times during the day. In addition, Mr. Jones was placed on a low sodium, low cholesterol diabetic diet and instructed to take a 20-minute walk at least three times per week. While in the hospital, Mr. Jones received verbal and written discharge instructions about how to carry out a treatment protocol to manage his chronic illnesses. A referral was also made to a home health care (HHC) agency for a HHC nurse to monitor his clinical status, assist him with implementation of the therapeutic regimen, and provide nutritional and exercise education. Because Mr. Jones was learning how to manage newly diagnosed illnesses, the HHC agency assigned a nurse case manager to help him with his chronic illness management education. An HHC aid was assigned to assist him with personal care, food shopping, and food preparation three days a week.

A senior baccalaureate nursing student who was precepted by the nurse case manager was assigned to visit Mr. Jones for weekly follow-up care. In the initial visit, the student nurse (SN) performed a head-to-toe physical assessment, a family assessment, and a functional health history focusing on self care activities with emphasis on medication administration, diet management, and exercise. In reviewing the purpose of each medication with Mr. Jones, the SN counted the number of pills in each of the six bottles and inferred that Mr. Jones had not been taking his medications as prescribed.

As part of the nutritional history, the SN asked about foods that Mr. Jones had eaten in the previous 24 hours. Mr. Jones responded that for breakfast he usually had toast with butter and jam and coffee; for lunch he had a cold cut sandwich such as bologna, ham, or cheese, and for dinner he ate mashed potatoes, green beans, and fried or baked chicken. Further questions were asked to explore how Mr. Jones communicated his food preferences to the HHC aid who prepared the meals. Mr. Jones stated that the HHC aid prepared his meals as he liked them: the potatoes with a generous amount of butter to make them creamy. She did not remove the skin from the chicken before baking or frying.

The SN also assessed Mr. Jones's knowledge about his medication regimen. Mr. Jones was not able to accurately describe the frequency, the dosage or the purpose of any of the medications. He also expressed the belief that by taking one of each pill daily, instead of the two pills prescribed for his blood pressure, he would have met the requirements for adequate medication management. Mr. Jones acknowledged that while he did not walk the three times per week as suggested, he walked to the store once per week and planned to increase his frequency when the weather became warmer. As the SN concluded the visit, Mr. Jones said that he wanted the pain in his legs to go away and to sleep though the night without having to go to the bathroom two to three times, and that he was committed to do what was necessary to take care of himself.

The SN recognized that the HHC aid was an essential member of the interdisciplinary team caring for Mr. Jones and discussed with her the care she provided to Mr. Jones. The HHC aid said, "I am aware that Mr. Jones is on a low sodium and low cholesterol diet, but I made fried chicken for him because he likes it and I wanted to please him." The SN recognized that the HHC aid had not been present for previous teaching, and that additional classes would be needed. The SN worked with the aid to develop a self-management education plan that the HHC aid could use with Mr. Jones.

STOP. THINK. Which diagnoses, outcomes, and interventions would you select?

Submitter's Analysis and Use of NANDA-I, NOC, and NIC

When the SN presented Mr. Jones's case to classmates in post conference, they weighed the evidence before identifying a nursing diagnosis that would be discussed and validated with Mr. Jones to adequately address his health challenges. The students were challenged by the professor to discuss discrepancies between Mr. Jones's behavior and his discharge instructions.

After analyzing the presenting data, it was hypothesized that Mr. Jones had low literacy skills as evidenced by his report of four years of elementary school, his writing style, and his inability to follow the written discharge instructions, even though they were visible on the table. When queried, Mr. Jones could not recall the purpose and frequency of his medications. He was also unable to select appropriate substitutes from the exchange list for meal planning; he reported that the dietitian spoke too quickly and used words that he did not understand. Research findings have shown that limited health literacy is independently associated with health status, higher use of health services, and worse health outcomes (U.S. Department of Health and Human Services, 2000; White, Chen, and Atchison, 2008). The discharge instructions in the form of a written teaching plan were judged inadequate to help Mr. Jones with the problem solving and self efficacy skills needed to manage his chronic conditions. The students concluded that the nurse who planned Mr. Jones's discharge did not accurately assess his clinical comprehension, his understanding of how to self manage his therapeutic regimen, and his ability to recall the advice or instructions conveyed to him. The SN decided to meet with Mr. Jones to develop mutual goals that would prepare him to manage his care at home.

The SN was aware that without assistance, Mr. Jones was not equipped to self manage his illnesses based on *deficient knowledge* and difficulties reading instructions. For example, he did not understand the interrelationship between the amount of salt he ingested in his diet and his high blood pressure, nor did he link saturated fats found in the butter to his cholesterol levels. Mr. Jones thought that because he was taking the medication, he did not have to adhere to the diet. Based on the risk factors of lack of comprehension and low literacy, the diagnosis was *risk for ineffective self health management*.

Functional health literacy is the degree to which individuals have the capacity to obtain, process, and understand basic health information and services needed to make appropriate health decisions (Schillinger, 2001). Limited health literacy negatively impacts individuals' abilities to read prescriptions, food labels, and health education materials, and the time to take medications (White et al., 2008). Limited health literacy is particularly prevalent among the elderly, minority, low income, and recent immigrants groups (DeWalt, Berkman, Sheridan, Lohr, and Pignone, 2004; White et al., 2008). These groups are also the populations that are most likely to bear a disproportionate incidence of chronic diseases, have difficulty accessing formal health care systems, and, without appropriate assessment, do not disclose their limited literacy status (Mayer, 2007). A low level of literacy is a potential barrier to active participation in self management of chronic illness. Studies show that addressing health literacy is associated with better outcomes, such as reduced hospitalization, ED use, and overall management costs (Coleman and Newton, 2005).

NOC Outcomes

The NOC outcomes that were selected to help Mr. Jones self manage his illnesses were *knowledge: treatment regimen, diabetes self management,* and *cardiac disease self management.* The baseline score on *knowledge* was 2 (limited knowledge) and the target score was 4 (substantial knowledge). The baseline scores on the *diabetes* and *cardiac self management* outcomes were 2 (rarely demonstrated) and the target scores were 5 (consistently demonstrated).

NIC Interventions

The NIC interventions that were selected to address the outcomes were *health literacy enhancement, culture brokerage, active listening, emotional support, teaching: prescribed diet, teaching: prescribed medications,* and *teaching: prescribed activity/exercise.* Self management of chronic illness is the ability to deal with all aspects of chronic illness, symptoms, treatment, physical and social consequences, and life style changes (Redman, 2005). The ethical approach to care of Mr. Jones required that he receive adequate instruction that he understood. Interventions that improve health literacy are a prerequisite to reducing the costs of illness, closing the health disparity gap, and improving the quality of health care for all (Parker, 2006).

In the case of Mr. Jones, addressing the problem of literacy was further compounded because there were no family members to work with the SN to develop and implement the self-management teaching program. Because Mr. Jones was receiving the services of an HHC aid who regularly helped him, the SN involved the HHC aid in the teaching process, conducting assessment of the HHC aid's literacy during the process.

In supporting Mr. Jones, the SN elicited information about the meaning of chronic illness to him, his perceptions and beliefs about the origins of these illnesses, and the remedies that were prescribed (Degazon, 2008). The nurse relied on oral communication modes and identified problems from Mr. Jones's perspective by asking provocative questions and listening to his responses. Simple words were used to convey important teaching points, content was broken up into short sessions, and the teaching was spread over several visits. When it seemed necessary, the nurse used story scripts to teach self-management of chronic illnesses. The nurse shared personal experiences of people from similar backgrounds to provide a rich context for Mr. Jones to identify barriers, such as problems created by a multi-medications regimen. The "show me" approach used by the SN was a good way to elicit information about what Mr. Jones may or may not understand about the illness management process.

The SN developed a self management plan that would negate the shame associated with limited literacy. In the next visit with Mr. Jones, the SN began by discussing the possible goal of helping him to achieve his own health goals. The SN respectfully asked Mr. Jones to tell her what problems he had understanding the terms associated with his illness and communicating with health care professionals. Mr. Jones was able to convey his fears that he would suffer from complications of his illness as a result of the lack of understanding about how to prevent complications, and his uneasiness in sharing these fears with health care providers who might not respect him. The SN assured Mr. Jones that his fears were understandable and suggested that they establish a plan to help him become self sufficient. The SN solicited the HHC aid to be a partner in Mr. Jones's self health management plan. Mr. Jones agreed to be screened for functional health literacy. The SN reviewed a number of literacy assessment instruments and selected the Rapid Estimate of Adult Literacy in Medicine (REALM-66). The REALM-66 is the most frequently used instrument, it takes two to three minutes to administer, is non-threatening, and requires minimal training to use (White et al., 2008).

The HHC aid was included in the planning because if the knowledge was to be effective, it needed to be reinforced and used for every meal. Although HHC aids do not administer medications, they relay information about the purpose, frequency, importance, and untoward effects of medications. They also assist in diet management by preparing foods within the prescribed diet regimen.

The SN worked on ways to translate self-management support into daily practice for Mr. Jones and his aid. This involved reviewing meal preparation with the aid and encouraging him with self health management tasks. The SN demonstrated for the aid how to encourage Mr. Jones to continue toward his goal to effectively manage his therapeutic regimens.

Evaluation

The target scores for the outcomes were met. In time, Mr. Jones shared his experience of exposing his poor reading level to the SN. He expressed that the SN's matter of fact approach to the topic and her positive regard for him as a person had enabled him to talk about it and to use her help to learn self management of his chronic illness.

References

Coleman, M., and Newton, K. (2005). Supporting self-management in patients with chronic illness. *American Family Physicians, 72,* 1503–1510.

Degazon, C.E. (2008). Cultural diversity and community health nursing. In M. Stanhope and J. Lancaster (eds.), *Community health nursing* (7th ed.)(pp. 141–164). St. Louis: Mosby.

DeWalt, D.A., Berkman, N.D., Sheridan, S., Lohr, K.N., and Pignone, M.P. (2004). Literacy and health outcomes: A systematic review of the literature. *Journal of General Internal Medicine, 19,* 1228–39.

Mayer, V. (2007). Low health literacy: The impact on chronic management. *Case Management, 4,* 213–218.

Parker, R.M. (2006). What an informed patient means for the future of health care. *Pharmacoeconomics, 24* (Suppl. 2), 29–33.

Redman, B.K. (2005). The ethics of self-management preparation for chronic illness. *Nursing Ethics, 12,* 360–369.

Schillinger, D. (2001). Improving the quality of chronic disease management for a population with low literacy: A call to action. *Disease Management, 4,* 103–109.

U.S. Department of Health and Human Services. (2000). *Healthy People 2010.* Retrieved September 2, 2008, from http://www.healthypeople.gov.

White, S., Chen, J., and Atchison, R. (2008). Relationship of preventive health practices and health literacy: A national study. *American Journal of Health Behavior, 32,* 227–242.

6.6. Self Management of Chronic Illness and Financial Status

Tomoko Hasegawa Katz, RN, PhD and Edmont Katz, MA

Mrs. SK is a 72-year-old Japanese woman with type 2 diabetes mellitus (DM) and hypertension who was admitted to the hospital two weeks ago for a R femoral neck fracture. She suffered the fracture in a fall outside when cleaning a community refuse bin. She underwent surgery and recovered without complications. She was ready to be discharged to home.

Her fasting blood glucose at discharge was from 90 to 120 with 1,400 Kcal dietary therapy. She began rehabilitation two days after surgery for the hip fracture. She was able to ambulate with a walker and was training with a cane. She independently fed, toileted, and dressed herself, but required help with bathing.

Mrs. SK's family and lifestyle history included losing her husband to cancer five years ago. She now lived with a daughter and a grandchild. She had four other children who lived nearby. Before the accident, she did all of her own housekeeping. She often mentioned that she had to go home and take care of her family. She said, "My husband and I never made a lot of money, but we have good children and lovely grandchildren. I am proud of myself for being independent until now."

Mrs. SK's children are also concerned about her. Her daughter wanted Mrs. SK to come home, but worried about her health condition after discharge.

During hospitalization the nurses learned that 10 years ago Mrs. SK was diagnosed with hypertension and was advised by her physician to take antihypertensive medication. She had refused to take medication, however, because she was concerned about financial difficulties and tried to minimize health care costs as much as possible. Mrs. SK received Social Security every month, but it was only marginally sufficient to cover her living expenses. While hospitalized, her systolic blood pressure ranged from 150 to 160 mm/hg.

STOP. THINK. Which diagnoses, outcomes, and interventions would you select?

Submitter's Analysis and Use of NANDA-I, NOC, and NIC

In planning for discharge, the nurse was concerned that, in spite of care providers' urgings, Mrs. SK continued to refuse to take antihypertensive medications because of financial concerns. Without appropriate medications, future control of her hypertension was unlikely and she was at risk of stroke, heart attack, cognitive decline, renal complications, and other complications (Swartz, 2008).

Mrs. SK's advancing age would likely reduce the effectiveness of her current pattern of self management, placing her at increased risk of complications. For this reason, *risk for ineffective self health management* related to deficient knowledge and financial inability to regularly purchase drugs was selected as the nursing diagnosis. Mrs. SK was undergoing rehabilitation for independent living, so blood pressure control was important for her health.

NOC Outcomes

The NOC outcome that was selected was *discharge readiness: independent living*. The baseline score was identified as 3 (sometimes demonstrated) and the target goal was set as 4 (often demonstrated).

NIC Interventions

The NIC interventions chosen for Mrs. SK by the nurses were *health education* and *health system guidance*. Information can guide patients to the sources of health and social care, and enable them to manage their long term health and social care (Dodson, Bisnauth, and James, 2008). The nurses initially assessed Mrs. SK's current knowledge and found that she did not adequately understand the prognosis of hypertension and the actions of anti-hypertensive medications. The nurses subsequently taught Mrs. SK about the pathophysiology, prognosis, treatment, diet, medications, and secondary complications of hypertension.

Mrs. SK had not made use of the Japanese social welfare system. There is financial support available from local governments for the elderly, single parents, and people of low income. The nurse explained how the health system worked in her town and what health care services she was qualified to receive. The nurse introduced Mrs. SK to a medical social worker (SW) for education about appropriate community resources. The SW explained to Mrs. SK about the cost of medications for her hypertension and how much financial support she could receive from her local government. The SW also taught her how to apply for social support.

Mrs. SK became interested in learning from the nurses and the SW. She agreed to take oral medication for her hypertension. Through knowledge provided by the SW, Mrs. SK was empowered to register for social support from the local government.

Evaluation

Mrs. SK became comfortable in accepting social services to maintain her health. With help from the nurses and SW, she recognized that receiving services was a reward for her life efforts. On discharge, she could explain the pathophysiology, medications, side effects, and diet for hypertension. She could also describe how to safely perform activities of daily living at home. She promised to follow the treatment plan after returning home. Supported by nurses and the SW, she achieved the target score of 4 on *discharge readiness: independent living* and she reduced her *risk for ineffective self health management.*

References

Dodson, L., Bisnauth, R., and James, N. (2008). Information is power. *Nursing Management, 15*(4), 14–19.

Swartz, M.J. (2008). Managing hypertension in women. *Critical Care Nursing Clinics of North America, 20,* 305–310.

6.7. Case Management for Homeless Man with Severe Pancreatitis

Ellen R. Mitchell, RN, MA

VH is a 53-year-old Hispanic male who presented to the ED complaining of severe epigastric and abdominal pain that does not radiate. He had experienced nausea and vomiting "a lot" for four days prior to admission. He denied hematemesis or melena. He had had nothing to eat or drink for 24 hours and stated that he had been on a "rum binge" for five days. His health history included repeated admissions for acute pancreatitis, usually precipitated by excessive alcohol intake.

The physical examination was impressive for abdominal tenderness at the periepigastric area, without rebounding or guarding. His serum amylase was 149 Somogyi units, and lipase was 553 units per liter. His other lab values were within normal limits. VH was admitted to the hospital for management of acute pancreatitis. He was started on intravenous fluids and was kept NPO (nothing by mouth). An abdominal ultrasound was ordered which was negative for obstruction or stones.

On arrival to the inpatient unit, the advanced practice nurse (APN) case manager interviewed VH to determine his health care needs and to supplement the staff nurse's plan of care as indicated. Using a standardized interview tool, the APN case manager ascertained that VH had been homeless since he was "thrown out" by his family several months earlier for repeated and excessive drunkenness. He said that he slept in a "mission," where he has been able to get a hot meal, take a shower, and sleep. He reported having had "bad" experiences in the city shelter system and claimed to have been "robbed" on more than one occasion.

VH said he was jobless. When he needed cash, he panhandled or collected recycling cans for refunds. Last year, he received Medicaid and public assistance, but he was decertified from these programs for failure to provide updated financial and other documentation needed to renew these benefits.

VH said that he did not see the point of "not drinking." He felt that there was no value to his life, and that there was nothing he could do to change it. He said that he had "failed" his family, and "failed out" of rehabilitation programs, so "why not drink?". He did not want his next of kin notified of the hospitalization.

When asked about the present illness and pain, VH expressed lack of understanding of the connection between his symptoms and binge drinking. He did not know that acute pancreatitis is life-threatening and progresses to chronic pancreatitis accompanied by chronic pain and other symptoms.

STOP. THINK. Which diagnoses, outcomes, and interventions would you select?

Submitter's Analysis and Use of NANDA-I, NOC, and NIC

From the interview with VH, the APN case manager identified and validated three nursing diagnoses for the case management plan of care: risk of disease complications (this diagnosis needs to be developed for submission to NANDA-I) related to knowledge deficits and chemical dependency, *hopelessness*, and *social isolation*. These were in addition to two diagnoses identified by the staff nurse: *deficient fluid volume* and *acute pain*.

The APN case manager's perspective went beyond VH's immediate clinical needs to include the continuum of care after hospitalization. Case management is a multifunctional role that emphasizes assessment and interpretation of information, coordination of care, planning for care transitions, teaching for the continuum of care, and collaboration with other caregivers to facilitate and optimize communication throughout and beyond the hospital stay (Carr, 2007). The case manager focused on optimizing the quality of care while maintaining cost effective care over time. High quality and cost effective care can be achieved by envisioning the continuum of care and preventing recidivism, and not just by dealing with immediate problems. With VH, it was important that the case manager help him to avoid binge drinking, maintain hope for a meaningful life, and connect with other people, including his family, for social support and other needs (D'Amico, and Nelson, 2008). Mr. H's responses of *hopelessness* and *social isolation* confounded the difficulties of dealing with chemical dependency and the need to adopt a new lifestyle. *Hopelessness* is often associated with powerlessness (Miller, 2000), which was also demonstrated by VH.

NOC Outcomes

Two NOC outcomes selected for risk of disease complications were *knowledge: disease process* and *risk control: alcohol use*. On the *knowledge* outcome, VH was rated as 3 (moderate knowledge) and the target was to bring him to 4 (substantial knowledge). On *risk control: alcohol use*, his baseline score was 2 (rarely demonstrated) with a goal of at least 3 (sometimes demonstrated).

For the diagnosis of *hopelessness*, the NOC outcome of *hope* was selected. VH's baseline score for this outcome was 2 (limited hope), so the case manager's goal was to help him attain at least a level of 3 (moderate hope) before discharge.

For the diagnosis of *social isolation*, the NOC outcome of *social involvement* was selected. VH's baseline score was 2 (limited social involvement) and the goal score was 3 (moderate) before discharge.

NIC Interventions

The NIC intervention of *case management* was used to enhance VH's safety, productivity, satisfaction, and quality of life (Case Management Society of America, 2002). The APN case manager coordinated, integrated, and directed the delivery of services to VH. Emphasis was placed on early intervention, comprehensive care planning, and inclusive service referrals. The APN case manager identified existing and potential health problems by evaluating the health status of VH and intervening for holistic health outcomes. In collaboration with other members of the multidisciplinary team, The APN developed plans of care to meet VH's unique needs. Offering the best possible discharge plan was of utmost importance to reduce readmission and provide alternative care at less cost.

Using the interventions of *risk identification* and *teaching: disease process*, the APN case manager helped VH to understand the risks related to chronic pancreatitis and the implications of these risks to his lifestyle. The nurse explained the pathophysiology and etiology of pancreatitis and assisted him in understanding the connection between binge drinking and the onset of symptoms. His understanding of the relation of binge drinking to his present illness and future prognosis would probably be associated with increased stress because of the need to make lifestyle changes; therefore, the case manager also incorporated the NIC interventions of *presence* and *emotional support* to facilitate stress management and ability to deal with this new information.

The case manager used the NIC interventions of *active listening, presence, hope, inspiration, socialization enhancement, self esteem enhancement, counseling,* and *discharge planning* to achieve improved outcomes on *hope* and *social involvement*. Case managers often function in each of their varied, essential roles simultaneously, so it is not unrealistic for the case manager to pursue many interventional strategies in the course of a short hospital stay (Tahan, 1997). One of the best tools of an APN case manager in the planning of care for people who are chemically dependent and homeless is the ability to listen and be fully present with them. Listening to people with these problems is the foundation for meeting their needs. Advocacy, communication, education, and coordination of care become critically important as the APN case manager provides guidance to the patient (Carr, 2007). Hope inspiration and self esteem enhancement helped to provide VH with sufficient energy to make life changes. Counseling activities provided him with an empathic relationship and factual information to increase his trust in others and his ability to cope with lifestyle changes.

Starting the discharge plan on day one of hospitalization supported the ability of the APN case manager to complete the necessary activities, with a goal of hospital discharge in about three days.

Once VH's trust had been earned, the nurse case manager made a *referral* to the clinical social worker for assistance with reapplication for Medicaid and public assistance benefits. The social worker also was asked to investigate other options for better housing for VH.

During the course of the intake assessment interview, VH stated he had been estranged from his family as a direct result of his drinking. He felt powerless over the loss of family ties, felt no control over his alcoholism, thought that he had "failed" in not continuing in his treatment program, and thus, had chosen a life of homelessness. Using the interventions of *counseling* and *presence* reassured VH that he could start to turn his life around if he were willing to participate in an alcohol treatment program and follow up with *referrals* offered by the social worker to reinstate his much needed benefits. VH stated, "I really want to try again."

With his consent, the case manager made a *referral* to the hospital-based day treatment program for alcohol and substance abuse. VH agreed to participate, indicating a desire to pursue risk control of his alcohol use.

Evaluation

On day three of his hospitalization, VH tolerated a regular diet, and his amylase and lipase levels had returned to normal. The target goals for the NOC outcomes were met. When he was ready for discharge, the case manager completed the discharge plan as mutually agreed upon with VH and he was provided with an appointment for the day treatment program. VH was given a letter, written by the social worker, to the mission caseworker that focused on strategies to reinstate his benefits and encourage participation in the alcohol treatment program. Through the case manager's interactions with him, and the actions of the social worker, it was hoped that VH would be aware that holistic, multidisciplinary services were available to help him succeed in efforts to promote and protect his fragile health.

One month later, the case manager contacted VH at the mission and ascertained that he was keeping his appointments and had reapplied for benefits. He planned to try to reunite with his family with assistance of the program staff.

The care provided to VH was typical of the experiences of nurse case managers in large urban settings (D'Amico, and Nelson, 2008). Thankfully, it seemed that VH's story would have a positive ending, which may not always happen. It is important for case managers to try to effect these types of positive changes despite the unique challenges presented by chemical dependency and homelessness.

References

Carr, D.D. (2007). Case managers optimize patient safety by facilitating effective care transitions. *Professional Case Management*, 12(2), 70–80.

Case Management Society of America (2002). *Standards of practice for case managers*. Little Rock, AR: Author.

D' Amico, J.B., and Nelson, J. (2008). Nursing care management at a shelter-based clinic. *Professional Case Management*, 13(1), 26–36.

Miller, J.F. (2000). *Coping with chronic illness: overcoming powerlessness* (3rd ed.). Philadelphia: F.A. Davis.

Tahan, H. (1997). The role of the nurse case manager. In Cohen E.L. and Cesta, T.G. (eds.), *Nursing case management from concept to evaluation* (2nd ed.) (pp. 197–209). St. Louis: Mosby.

6.8. Psychiatric Care of an Adult Male with Poor Impulse Control

Mary Ellen McMorrow, RN, EdD, APN

Daniel, age 37, is a white male, the only son of Italian immigrants. From childhood intelligence tests, it was determined that Daniel's Intelligence Quotient (IQ) score was below normal at 60. Because Daniel was having many difficulties in school, when he reached the legal age permitted, his parents took him out of school and kept him home. He has never worked and has no hobbies other than watching television.

The police brought Daniel to the ED after a neighbor called 911 to report that Daniel was physically abusing his mother. From the ED, he was admitted to an acute psychiatric unit.

During the initial assessment of Daniel, he was shocked at the idea that he would hurt his mother. He was disheveled and smelled slightly of urine. His physical examination and laboratory and diagnostic tests were all within normal limits, except for a broken nose. Daniel said "the cops hurt me." The ED admission form indicated that Daniel struggled with the police when they were called to his home, which led to the broken nose. He was alert, aware, and oriented to time, place, and person.

Further assessment indicated that Daniel is bilingual and believes in Jesus. He denied any use of alcohol or substance use, other than "some wine" with holiday meals. Daniel's sole focus during the initial interview was on calling his mother to come and get him. He indicated little insight into his situation, refusing to discuss what precipitated his admission. Daniel said his mother is his only friend and did not mention his father during discussions with health care providers.

On the unit, Daniel was pleasant to the staff, but avoided the other patients. If other patients came too close to him, he pushed or shoved them away.

He often was heard shouting at his mother on the phone. Other patients said that he "hogs" the unit telephone. His roommates also complained that he "wets the bed" and "stinks up the room." When directed by the staff, Daniel showered and shaved, but usually he needed to be told.

Daniel's mother said that she did not want him discharged to home. The interdisciplinary team planned placement in an adult home.

STOP. THINK. Which diagnoses, outcomes, and interventions would you select?

Submitter's Analysis and Use of NANDA-I, NOC, and NIC

Daniel exemplified a common difficulty when caring for patients with mental illness and limited cognitive development, i.e., working with them to design a plan of care. The nurses did not assume that Daniel was not able to be involved in the decision making process, but, with assessment, they found that Daniel was unable to participate in identifying and prioritizing his responses. Continuous assessment of his responses was necessary to maximize his involvement. Recently, Daniel's behavior had been violent, so the nurse and the psychiatrist did everything according to the nursing diagnosis and Diagnostic and Statistical Manual of Mental Disorders (DSM) axis selected (Psychiatry Online, 2008): *risk for other-directed violence*, with a significant risk factor of history of violence.

Daniel's physical abuse of his mother was witnessed by a neighbor and verified by his mother. Additionally, he did not control his anger well enough to avoid fighting with the police. These were strong indications that he may potentially harm others, e.g., other patients or a staff member. This diagnosis was supported by the nurse's observation of Daniel's shoving and pushing other patients who Daniel perceived as threatening.

Daniel did not make verbal threats or self-directed signs of violence, but he had poor impulse control. His body language, e.g., rigidity and clenched fists, and his history of violence indicated aggressive behavior that was poorly controlled.

NOC Outcome

The NOC outcome that was selected for Daniel was *aggression self-control*. The baseline score on this outcome was 2 (rarely demonstrated) and the goal score was 5 (consistently demonstrated). To meet this outcome, multiple interventions were identified to prevent the reoccurrence of violence and help Daniel learn how to control his anger and frustration.

NIC Interventions

The NIC interventions that the nurses used were *impulse control training, self responsibility facilitation, anger control assistance, coping enhancement*, and *socialization enhancement*. The nurses began their interventions by monitoring Daniel's responses to various situations in the environment to see what triggered his anger and frustration. Increases in demands on Daniel were identified as potential triggers for violent behavior. Increased activity on the unit, physical closeness of other patients, and denial of privileges are likely to increase violence (Vittengl, 2002).

The staff noted that Daniel responded with other-directed physical force whenever another patient entered, or threatened to enter, his personal space or refused to comply with Daniel's express demands, e.g., change the television station to a show he wanted to watch. He also threw his arms about and approached others in a threatening manner when other patients teased or intimidated him. He acted angry as well when his roommates complained about his bedwetting.

The staff acknowledged to Daniel that anger was a normal response and that he would experience anger or frustration when threatened. For Daniel to successively live with other people, isolation was not used unless there was an immediate physical threat. The staff viewed it as important that he learn to recognize and control his anger in a socially acceptable manner. The nurses began by helping Daniel to identify his experience of anger as the basis of learning how to express the anger in a healthful way.

Because of Daniel's cognitive limitations, he was only able to identify a limited number of signs of anger. Daniel was able to recognize a sensation of "hot," clenching of fists, and tightness in his jaw as responses before he pushed someone. He also identified that he only pushed people who "didn't listen to me." He blamed others for his violence, including his mother. For patients with limited coping skills, externalizing blame is common. The nurse intervened by gently challenging this perception to help Daniel recognize the need for a more appropriate expression of his anger (Carson and Alvarz, 2006).

The nurses recognized the importance of *social enhancement* for Daniel to learn how to deal with the normal frustrations of life, especially since he would be placed in a group home. His protective and isolating home environment had prevented Daniel from developing the social skills necessary to interact with others. The staff encouraged Daniel to attend all group activities on the unit. The staff made it clear to Daniel that he was responsible for his behavior, but the staff was there to support him and direct other patients to respect Daniel's personal space.

Because bedwetting triggered several confrontations with Daniel's roommates, the staff worked with Daniel on this issue. Even though Daniel denied he wet the bed, he agreed to limit his fluid intake after dinner and to void before going to bed. Each night at "lights out," the staff reminded Daniel to use the bathroom. This limited the number of "accidents" and incidences with roommates.

The nurses encouraged Daniel to talk about his feelings, but he could only say he felt "bad" and was unable to differentiate between frustration and anger. With help, Daniel was able to recognize some of the triggers to his aggressive behavior. The nurses were empathetic. They listened to Daniel and expressed their concerns for his feelings. They focused on helping Daniel solve problems. Emphasis was on what Daniel could do, not on his limitations.

Daniel agreed to try alternative behaviors when he felt "hot" or his jaw got "hard." One technique that was encouraged was for Daniel to leave the room or situation. He was observed doing this a few times, after situations in which the staff reminded him of his agreement to leave the room.

Deep breathing was another technique that was attempted. Daniel, however, had difficulty with this relaxation method and would hyperventilate.

In community meetings and activity groups, Daniel was encouraged to speak up when he was unable to have things his way. While his vocabulary for verbalizing his feelings was limited, he did tell others what he wanted, and also began saying why he wanted certain things. The other patients began to respond more respectfully toward Daniel.

A significant issue for Daniel was discharge to a group home because Daniel wanted to go home. The psychiatric team focused on helping Daniel using *cognitive restructuring*. With redirection mostly through questioning (Coffin-Romig, 2008), Daniel was guided to re-evaluate this discharge plan as a positive opportunity. Two day visits and one weekend leave to the group home were arranged. The staff gave Daniel positive reinforcement for his stories of what happened during his visits.

Evaluation

Placement at a group home became available after Daniel was on the unit for three weeks. The group home was for adults with mental illness who were developmentally disabled. On discharge, Daniel's *aggression self-control* outcome score was 3 (sometimes demonstrated). This quantifiable improvement in behavior meant that it was possible for Daniel to live with others. The staff members were hopeful that, with continued reinforcement of behavioral control strategies, Daniel might reach a future goal of consistent demonstration of *aggression self-control*.

References

Carson, V.B. and Alvarz, C. (2006). *Anger and aggression*. In Varcaroles, E.M., Carson, V.B., and Shoemaker, N.C. *Foundations of Psychiatric Mental Health Nursing* (5th ed.). Philadelphia: Saunders.

Coffin-Romig, N. (2008). *Therapies in clinical practice*. In Fortinash, K.M. and Worret, P.A. *Psychiatric Mental Health Nursing* (4th ed.). St Louis: Mosby.

Psychiatry Online. (2008). DSM-IV-TR™ Diagnostic and Statistical Manual of Mental Disorders. Retrieved on September 13, 2008, from http://www.psychiatryonline.com/referral.aspx?gclid=CJqkoemX2ZUCFQK2Ggod80yjXw.

Vittengl, J.R. (2002). Temporal regulation in physical control at state psychiatric hospital. *Archives of Psychiatric Nursing, 16*, 80.

6.9. Response to a Diagnosis of Chronic Illness When Confounded by Other Life Events

Anne T. Lunney, RN, MS, MD

Dave, a 48-year-old Vietnam veteran, was recently discharged from prison for randomly shooting up his apartment and an incident of domestic violence. He has a known history of post traumatic stress disorder (PTSD), violence, and substance abuse. Prior to incarceration, his substance abuse was out of control and his interpersonal communication style was confrontational. His interactions with others, including health professionals, were strained.

Dave presented to the nurse practitioner at a VA clinic with a chief complaint of "I don't have any energy," and weight loss over the past two months. On exploration, it was determined that he had polyuria, polydypsia, intermittent blurred vision, and inability to attain an erection. A diagnosis of new onset diabetes was considered and the appropriate diagnostic tests were initiated. Patient teaching about diabetes consumed most of the initial visit since these were profound manifestations and it was expected that the diagnostic tests would confirm the clinical findings.

He returned the next day for follow up of laboratory results and initiation of a hypoglycemic agent. During this visit, it was necessary to provide Dave with detailed information about the balance of diet, exercise, and medication. When the nurse tried to teach Dave how to manage the diabetes, he did not seem to be listening, his affect was flat, and he avoided eye contact. These behaviors and knowledge of what Dave had experienced in the last year led the nurse to think that he might be overwhelmed. When she asked him whether he felt overwhelmed, he said "yes." With further discussion, he admitted that the thought of having another problem was more than he could handle.

With the disclosure of "feeling overwhelmed," the nurse and Dave discussed the changes that had occurred in his life over the last year. These included: incarceration; losing his wife, children, home, and car through domestic violence and substance abuse; going through a divorce; living with his mother; struggling to stay sober; and inability to attain an erection. In the discussion, he said "I cannot deal with any other problems." He said that he had difficulty sleeping, spent his time "hanging out" at his mother's, and did not go out with his friends.

STOP. THINK. Which diagnoses, outcomes, and interventions would you select?

Submitter's Analysis and Use of NANDA-I, NOC, and NIC

When Dave's symptoms of lethargy and weight loss were coupled with the classic symptoms of new onset diabetes, it seemed that the loss of energy was related to the diabetes and would resolve with treatment. It was important, however, that the extreme nature of Dave's lethargy be noted by the nurse and that other possible problems be considered. Other cues that indicated a need to explore alternative explanations were: the significant numbers and types of problems that Dave encountered in the last year, the verbal statement that he "could not deal with another problem," difficulty with sleeping, fatigue, depressed mood, decreased interest in social activities, weight loss, and feeling overwhelmed. The nurse practitioner considered the diagnosis of *major depressive episode* (American Psychiatric Association [APA], 2000) with an associated *risk for suicide* and then asked him if he was contemplating suicide. Dave responded "yes." Dave also verified that he had access to a firearm. The plan of care for Dave was also adapted to incorporate interventions for *powerlessness* and *hopelessness*.

This case heightened the awareness of the people involved regarding the challenges of the diagnostic process. Diagnostic biases that occur in relation to the patient's history and the overlap of cues to diagnoses might have prevented the nurse from thinking about and validating the nursing diagnoses of *risk for suicide, hopelessness*, and *powerlessness*. When there is a history of confrontational interactions, episodes of violence, and incarceration, it contributes to lack of trust and incidences of powerlessness among staff members (Lundström, Saveman, Eisemann, and Aström, 2007), which then can lead to doing nothing to diagnose and treat the person's real problems. The unspoken diagnosis that may guide the interactions of health professionals with people like Dave is *risk for violence to others*. This may lead health professionals to avoid unnecessary contacts and interact in ways to protect themselves from harm. Nurses might expect people like Dave to be aggressive, and, subsequently, avoid asking questions that provoke intense feelings. If this had happened, Dave's feelings of being overwhelmed and the subsequent risk of suicide would not have been identified. If the nurse's communication style, voice tone, or body language had communicated to Dave that she or he was not interested in knowing his feelings, he would not have talked about them. He would not have trusted the nurse with this information about himself and enabled the nurse to "know" him.

Another type of diagnostic bias was created by the overlap of symptoms among diagnoses. Although Dave exhibited six of the nine symptoms for a diagnosis of *major depressive episode* (APA, 2000), three of the six (weight loss, lethargy, and fatigue) are also symptoms of diabetes (Porth, 2005). In addition, other accurate nursing diagnoses could have prevented the nurse from perceiving *risk for suicide* as the highest priority. Dave had *deficient knowledge* regarding self management of diabetes and he had *sleep pattern disturbance*. If the nurse had continued teaching about how to manage the diabetes or improve sleep instead of seeing these problems as symptoms of a more significant problem, the *risk for suicide* would have been missed.

Ineffective coping and *ineffective self health management* are nursing diagnoses that are suggested by these data but should not be made because they are not highly accurate. Even though Dave was having problems with coping, the ineffectiveness of his coping is not the issue here. It is not the reason why he needs help. The diagnosis of *ineffective self health management* should not be made because he only just learned that he had diabetes. Because he should not be held accountable for effective management of therapeutic regimen, it is not appropriate to label these symptoms as ineffective management.

NOC Outcome

The most important outcome at this point in time was *suicide self-restraint*. Dave's overall baseline score was 3 (sometimes demonstrated) and the goal score was 5 (consistently demonstrated).

NIC Interventions

The NIC interventions that were initiated immediately were *emotional support, crisis intervention,* and *suicide prevention*. Besides providing emotional support and helping Dave to recognize the situation as a crisis, the nurse referred Dave immediately to a psychiatrist. The psychiatrist started Dave on a medication for depression and referred him to counseling two times a week. As part of suicide prevention, the nurse initiated a contract with Dave. In interviews with 40 people with various chronic illnesses who experienced powerlessness, investigators concluded that the process of helping people with powerlessness should be negotiated with the individual (Aujoulet, d'Hoore, and Deccache, 2007). In the contract, Dave agreed to: (a) call the nurse or psychiatrist if he was contemplating suicide, (b) remove the firearm from his place of residence, and (c) call the local suicide hotline if the nurse or psychiatrist were not available.

In scheduled meetings with Dave, the nurse used the interventions of *coping enhancement*, *hope instillation*, and *presence* to assist Dave in resolving feelings of powerlessness and hopelessness. During that time, the nurse also talked about his diabetes, slowly providing knowledge about methods to control the disease process through diet, exercise, and medication. Awareness of these modifiable factors helped to promote a sense of power (Miller, 2000). The preconceived ideas about diabetes that contributed to Dave's sense of being overwhelmed were explored and clarified. Dave was encouraged to discuss his problems with his PTSD group so he could obtain social support, an important source of power to manage chronic illness (Miller, 2000).

Evaluation

Dave responded to the nursing and medical interventions. Within one month, his overall score on *suicide self-restraint* was 5. He was self managing his diabetes with ongoing support from the nurse practitioner and clinic staff.

References

American Psychiatric Association. (2000). *Diagnostic and statistical manual of mental disorders* (4th ed.). Washington, DC: Author.

Aujoulat, I., d'Hoore, W., and Deccache, A. (2007). The perspectives of patients on their experience of powerlessness. *Qualitative Health Research, 17,* 772–785.

Lundström, M., Saveman, B.I., Eisemann, M., and Aström, S. (2007). Prevalence of violence and its relation to caregiver's demographics and emotional reactions: An explorative study of caregivers working in group homes for persons with learning disabilities. *Scandinavian Journal of Caring Science, 21* (1), 84–90.

Miller, J.F. (2000). *Coping with chronic illness: Overcoming powerlessness* (3rd ed.). Philadelphia: F.A. Davis.

Porth, C.M. (2005). *Pathophysiology: Concepts of altered health states.* Philadelphia: Lippincott, Williams and Wilkins.

7

Case Studies with a Primary Focus on Health Promotion Diagnoses and Associated Outcomes and Interventions

7.1. Support of a Mexican-American Woman in Postpartum Care

MaryAnne Levine, PhD, RN, SCM

Maria is a 16-year-old married Mexican female who 12 hours prior had a spontaneous vaginal birth, delivering a viable 3,500-gm male. Maria and her husband Carlos are recent immigrants to the United States and only speak Spanish. They live in an isolated rural region of the western U.S. in a town of 200 inhabitants where Carlos is employed as a manual laborer.

The night shift nurses reported the following information: Maria slept intermittently during the night. A female friend remained with her, although she, too, could not speak English. Maria does not have the requisite skills to care for a neonate. It was difficult for the nurses to work with her because there was a basic lack of communication. The nurses said that Maria was isolated and lacked family support, so they believed she would have a difficult time when discharged. They also expressed concern that Maria may soon have sore nipples because she kept the baby at her breast for too long at feedings. In addition, they reported that she had a painful perineum, which may hinder her overall activities, and that her husband did not participate as desired, which may lead to problems for Maria.

Next Day Observations and Assessment

Maria was resting comfortably; her uterus was well contracted and located 2 cm below and 3 cm lateral to her umbilicus. Lochia rubra was moderate. Maria walked to the bathroom without difficulty and voided sufficient quantities. Her episiotomy was well approximated with no erythema, ecchymosis, or discharge. Edema of the right labia minora and majora were noted. Breasts were soft; nipples and aureola were intact. Maria and her friend were busy talking to one another. Maria kept looking to her friend, watched her facial expressions, and attentively listened to her comments.

Day Nurses' Interactions with Maria and Her Friend

The day nurses who worked with Maria were able to communicate in simple Spanish and make full use of nonverbal communications. The nurses' interactions involved both Maria and her friend. Maria was able to initiate, maintain, and remove her son from the breast with no problems. She was confident in changing the baby's diapers, and with assistance was able to provide care to the umbilical cord stump. She declined analgesia for her perineum but wanted information about use of ice packs, and, after 24 hours, a sitz bath. Both Maria and her friend expressed desire to learn additional techniques about baby care, breastfeeding, and hygiene. They also asked about the well baby clinic at the health department. During visiting hours, family and many friends came to visit the mother and baby.

STOP. THINK. Which diagnoses, outcomes, and interventions would you select?

Submitter's Analysis and Use of NANDA-I, NOC, and NIC

The nursing diagnoses that the night nurses asked the day nurses to consider were *impaired verbal communication, interrupted family processes, social isolation, ineffective coping, compromised family coping, acute pain,* and *ineffective breastfeeding.* These diagnoses were ruled out because the day nurses obtained data that refuted the diagnoses through communication with Maria and her friend.

The shift report indicated the nurses' impression of *impaired verbal communication* because Maria did not speak English. Although this impression is supported by the defining characteristic—inability to speak or comprehend the dominant language—the day nurses disagreed with this interpretation for Maria and for others like her. This interpretation put the onus on Maria to communicate in English instead of on the hospital to have interpreters available as needed. It is common for nurses who speak only English to feel uncomfortable when they are unable to communicate with people who do not (Levine, Anderson, and McCullough, 2004). Great care needs to be taken that biased judgments, such as blaming the patient for not speaking English, are avoided when there are language and culture differences.

The impressions of *interrupted family processes* and *social isolation* were not supported by subsequent data collection. Maria and her husband were functioning well within their culture norms as a young married couple starting a family. Her husband was fulfilling his role by providing financially for them. Maria's husband was at work but her sister-in-law, a *doula*, was with her, and friends and relatives were visiting. *Doula is* a term derived from the Greek that means helper. Throughout history, female relatives have taken on this role, which is still prevalent in traditional cultures. Maria's *doula* had been married for several years and had two young children; she was an experienced mother who was well-suited to the role. Also, because they shared the same culture, they shared many similar childrearing practices. Maria and her doula were considered a dyad; thus all interaction, teaching, and planning was done predicated on this concept.

Maria and her husband were making the necessary discharge and transportation arrangements, thus the couple were appropriately adapting to a maturational crisis. Maria's social support systems were in place as evidenced by her *doula* and the support of her extended family and friends.

The diagnoses of *acute pain* and *ineffective breastfeeding* were refuted because Maria felt that her perineal discomfort did not affect her activities of daily living, mobilization, or breastfeeding. She prioritized focusing on her baby and her new role. Maria chose to use non-analgesic relief measures and stated that she was comfortable with using intermittent ice to her perineum. She walked about the maternity unit to promote comfort and perceived control, and took short, periodic rest periods in a side lying position. The nurses made a diagnosis of *readiness for enhanced comfort* and were alert to changes in Maria's comfort level.

The next day, the nursing diagnoses that guided the majority of nursing interventions for Maria were *health seeking behaviors: role change* and *effective breastfeeding*. The *health seeking behaviors* diagnosis was supported by many of the cues, especially expressed and observed desire to seek information for optimum care of newborn and self. Throughout the period of care, it was observed that Maria looked to her sister-in-law for approval and direction. She also asked for verbal feedback concerning her interactions with the baby.

The nurses used the nursing theory of modeling/role modeling as a basis of care for Maria (Erickson, 2006; Erickson, Tomlin, and Swain, 1983). Modeling consists of fully understanding another person's or group's view of their world from their perspective. The modeling/role modeling nursing theory says that nurses should meet their professional goal(s) by establishing the culture of each person because, if ignored, health care goals will not be attained. With this theory, therapeutic communication is one of the top priorities of the nurse. Role modeling then adds to the professional component of planning care that matches, yet expands, possibilities for the person. In doing so, alignment between care provider and care recipient occurs and the relationship is validated. In this case, Maria's world view and yearning for knowledge led to the nursing diagnosis of *health seeking behaviors* as the primary diagnosis.

NOC Outcomes

The NOC outcome of *health seeking behavior* was selected with Maria and her sister-in-law and the score on this outcome was 5 (consistently demonstrated). The mutual health directed goal (nurses and Maria) was that this outcome remained at 5.

For the diagnosis of *effective breastfeeding*, the outcome of *breastfeeding maintenance* was selected with a baseline score of 5 (totally adequate). The goal was to maintain a score of 5.

For the diagnosis of *readiness for enhanced comfort*, the outcome of *comfort status* was selected. The baseline score was 4 (mildly compromised); the goal score was to remain at 4.

NIC Interventions

The NIC intervention selected for *health seeking behavior* was *health education*. The priority activities for implementing this intervention were to determine personal context and social-cultural history of the individual's health behavior; determine current health knowledge and lifestyle behaviors; prioritize Maria's needs based on personal preferences, the nurses' skills and resources, and likelihood of successful goal attainment; and to consider the accessibility, Maria's preference, and cost of program planning. The expectation was that by establishing a therapeutic relationship (Erickson, 2006; Erickson, Tomlin, and Swain, 1983; Leenerts, 2003; Levine, 2006; Levine, in press; Paterson and Zderad, 1976; Peplau, 1952; Ramsden, 2000), *health seeking behavior* would be consistently demonstrated.

With the modeling/role modeling theory, establishing a true therapeutic relationship is the basis of nursing and by modeling the patient's world, trust occurs that contributes to the person's ability to adopt the health behaviors explained by the nurse. In this instance, the nurse sought to establish trust with both Maria and her sister-in-law or *doula*.

The interventions for breastfeeding maintenance were *teaching: infant nutrition 0 to 3 months, teaching: infant stimulation 0 to 4 months, teaching: infant safety 0 to 3 months*, and *anticipatory guidance*. These interventions also enhanced Maria and her doula's *health seeking behavior* with positive reinforcement. For the remainder of Maria's stay she continued to ask questions about infant care and take on more responsibility such as giving the baby a bath.

For the outcome of *comfort status*, the concern was Maria's edematous perineum. The NIC interventions of *heat/cold application* and *teaching: prescribed activity/exercise* were implemented. Maria was assisted in using intermittent ice and using positioning and walking to facilitate comfort.

Evaluation

At the time of discharge, all of the target goals were met. Maria was using the sitz bath every 4 to 5 hours and stated that this was very soothing to her perineal area. She continued to frequently ambulate and was able to comfortably sit in a bedside chair. She looked forward to being able to continue the sitz baths in her home. Maria's nipples and aerola remained intact without any soreness and she attained an excellent latch each time she breastfed. She thought that this was because it was such a natural thing for a mother to do because she had grown up watching numerous female relatives breastfeeding their infants, and her sister-in-law was with her if she needed direction.

Her family and friends had arranged to have dinners brought to her home for the next 10 days and her sister-in-law and her two children would be staying with Maria and her husband for the next two weeks to further help Maria and her family's transition to their new roles.

References

Erickson, H., Tomlin, E., and Swain, M. (1983). *Modeling and role-modeling*. Englewood Cliffs, NJ: Prentice Hall.

Erickson, H. (Ed.). (2006). *Modeling and role-modeling: A view from the client's world*. Cedar Park, TX: Unicorns Unlimited.

Leenerts, M. (2003). Teaching personal knowledge as a way of knowing self in therapeutic relationship. *Nursing Outlook, 51*, 158–164.

Levine, M.A., Anderson, L., and McCullough, N. (2004). Hmong birthing: Bridging the cultural gap in a rural community in northern California. *Lifelines, 8*, 147–149.

Levine, M.A. (2006). *Transforming experiences: A reflective topical autobiography of facilitating student nurse development through international immersion programmes*. Unpublished doctoral dissertation, Victoria University of Wellington, Wellington, New Zealand.

Levine, M.A. (In press). Transforming experiences: Nursing education and international immersion programs. *Journal of Professional Nursing*.

Paterson, J., and Zderad, L. (1976). *Humanistic nursing*. New York: Wiley and Sons.

Peplau, H. (1952). *Interpersonal relations in nursing*. New York: Putnam's Sons.

Ramsden, I. (2000). Cultural safety, Kawa whakaruruhau ten years on: A personal overview. *Nursing Praxis in New Zealand, 15*(1), 4–12.

7.2. Parenting of a Child with Spina Bifida

Maryanne Krenz, MA, RN

VA is a nine-year-old boy who was born with spina bifida and myelo-meningocele, resulting in paralysis at the first lumbar disk. After many different surgical interventions from birth, he was able to walk with braces and crutches but was still incontinent of bladder and bowel. When he was about seven and a half years old, VA had an episode of osteomyelitis, which occurred from a small laceration on his leg that did not heal. The osteomyelitis prevented him from walking with the braces and a walker for 18 months. The consequence of this was shortening of his leg tendons and eversion of both feet.

One day, VA's parents called the home care nurse who visited the family during the last period of recuperation. The family was faced with a difficult decision and was seeking guidance. VA's physicians had informed them that he would benefit by two types of surgery: (1) correction of orthopedic complications of immobility so he could resume walking with braces and a walker, and (2) urinary and bowel diversions to achieve continence. The dilemma of VA needing two additional surgeries, after having 14 surgeries since birth, led to feelings of confusion, worry, and frustration.

The purpose of many of the previous surgical interventions had been to achieve increased mobility. The family commitment to this goal was strong and the loss of VA's ability to walk was felt deeply by VA, his parents, and two teenage sisters. In addition, the necessity of wearing protective underwear and the embarrassment and shame associated with incontinence were also a concern. His mother said: "Now that he is getting older, the problem with elimination will have more of an effect on him."

The impact of each surgical procedure on his developmental status and well-being was also identified as a problem. He was unable to associate with friends as before the osteomyelitis and complained of boredom. Frustration was exhibited when his friends stopped by to see him because he wanted them to say longer. After a short visit, they ran out to play. His sisters tried to occupy him but school and work put limits on time.

VA became anxious during the 18 months of his illness. When invited to go for ice cream with neighbors, he expressed concern that they would not be able to manage him and the wheelchair. He became critical of others, worried about how others perceived him, and had made comments indicating low self worth. Schoolwork was also more of a struggle.

The family's adaptive resources for coping with repeated hospitalizations and recuperations were being challenged but they were still strong. His father stated, "We could go to doctors continuously if we permitted all the treatments they are willing to perform. These surgeries take a toll on all of us, including him. He needs to have time to just be a kid." VA was eligible for Little League baseball in the spring, which was a reason not to have both surgeries. Developmentally, being part of a team was important.

VA was aware of the issues and choices that were being considered. His parents felt that he was mature enough to participate in this decision making. He reminisced about times in the past when he was able to put on his braces and use a walker or crutches to go to school. He also expressed to his parents and sisters the need to be continent in the future. It was difficult for him to talk about these issues with health care professionals because of embarrassment. With the complexity of the developmental, physical, and emotional concerns facing this family, isolating an accurate focus of concern was a challenge. Anticipatory guidance was being sought because of the significance of the choice between having his mobility restored through surgery, extensive physical therapy, and braces, or the loss of ambulation and remaining wheelchair bound as well as having surgery for bowel and bladder diversions.

STOP. THINK. Which diagnoses, outcomes, and interventions would you select?

Submitter's Analysis and Use of NANDA-I, NOC, and NIC

The diagnoses of *anxiety, divisional activity deficit*, and *self esteem: situational low* were evident but were identified by the family as being managed effectively by the current coping strategies. They were able to calm VA and encouraged his participation in problem solving. Reinforcing his strengths was an ongoing approach and they were aware that expectations needed to be achievable. *Impaired physical mobility* and *bowel and urinary incontinence* were chronic conditions that all family members had adapted to handling and there were no nursing interventions that would improve the situation. Conversation about mobility being an essential component of his developmental status as a toddler and preschooler were reinforced using Erikson's Developmental Theory. The family agreed that VA had achieved the degree of autonomy and initiative needed to enable him to be a successful school-aged child.

As a school-aged child, industry versus inferiority was the developmental task at risk now. The heaviness of the braces and the strength needed to manage them with crutches or a walker were variables to be considered now that his height and weight were increasing each year. The degree of mobility would be limited because of this. The bowel and bladder incontinence were contributing to VA becoming self-conscious and feeling ashamed. Allowing both surgeries would impede his growth and development and diminish the coping resources of VA and his family.

The most accurate diagnosis was *readiness for enhanced decision making* because the family was seeking an improved state of well being in the face of severe disabilities (Pender, Murdaugh, and Parsons, 2006). Their point of view was health promotion even in the face of surgery and chronic dysfunction. In a literature review of decision making, O'Connor et al. (2003) identified that many people with chronic illnesses need help with decision making, even when it is not a problem.

NOC Outcomes

The two NOC outcomes selected with the family were *decision making* and *personal autonomy*. The baseline score for *decision making* was identified as 4 (mildly compromised) and the target score was 5 (not compromised). The baseline score on *personal autonomy* was 5 (consistently demonstrated for his developmental level) and the target score was 5.

NIC Interventions

The NIC interventions for *decisional conflict* were *decision making support* and *mutual goal setting*. There was a difference of opinion between the parents and the care providers because both surgeries were being recommended. Conflicts of family opinions with provider opinions can be common with complex management of chronic illness (Paterson, Russell, and Thorne, 2001). From the parents' point of view, agreeing to both interventions would hamper their child's emotional and developmental well being. The advantages and disadvantages of each alternative were identified during discussion and the goals for VA were articulated (Roelands, Van Oost, Stevens, Depoorter, and Buysse, 2004).

VA was eager to please his parents and tried to decipher what they wanted for him. *Mutual goal setting* was used to establish realistic expectations and not place the burden for the decision on a child, yet allow input to discover his needs and preferences. Often VA's father would take the lead in the conversation, yet he sought nonverbal input from his wife and VA or his two older sisters.

Evaluation

After three visits to discuss these issues with the family, the target scores on both *decision making* and *personal autonomy* were met. The family made the decision to have the surgery for the bowel and bladder incontinence during VA's school break in the summer. When the parents were absent, VA and his sisters had talked and his sisters facilitated the choice by helping VA prioritize what was most important to him. He had been unable to ambulate during the 18 months of healing from the osteomyelitis, so he realized that he cold live happily without being able to ambulate. The surgical procedures to establish bowel and bladder continence were extensive and he determined them to be the highest priority. VA expected to be wheelchair bound, which involved the loss of an achievement that in the past was considered essential. He would be able to participate in Little League baseball for the disabled in the wheelchair in the spring, but there was anticipatory grieving about this choice. In a follow-up telephone call, the family told the nurse that they were doing well.

References

O'Connor, A.M., Drake, E.R., Wells, G.A., Tugwell, P., Laupacis, A., and Elmslie, T. (2003). A survey of the decision-making need of Canadians faced with complex health decisions. *Health Expectations, 6,* 97–109.

Paterson, B.L., Russell, C., and Thorne, S. (2001). Critical analysis of everyday self-care decision making in chronic illness. *Journal of Advanced Nursing, 35,* 335–341.

Pender, N.J., Murdaugh, C.L., and Parsons, M.A. (2006). *Health promotion in nursing practice* (5th ed.). Upper Saddle River, NJ: Pearson Prentice Hall.

Roelands, M., Van Oost, P., Stevens, V., Depoorter, A., and Buysse, A. (2004). Clinical practice guidelines to improve shared decision-making about assistive device use in home care: A pilot interventions study. *Patient Education and Counseling, 55,* 252–264.

7.3. Woman Who Experienced Early Childhood Trauma

Jeanne Cummings, RN, MS, PMHNP-BC, PMHCNS-BC

AB is a 40-year-old unmarried, unemployed, heterosexual female who regularly visited the psychiatric outpatient clinic of a large city hospital to obtain medications and participate in therapy sessions with a nurse specialist. She was born in the United States and is the only child of parents from the Dominican Republic. AB reported a history of child-hood physical abuse by both parents who were alcoholics and past and current verbal abuse by her mother, so she minimized contact with her. Her father left the family when she was about five; later she learned that he had started another family. She saw her father infrequently, has had no contact with him in more than ten years, and had no desire to see him. Throughout childhood, AB was a witness to physical violence between her mother and a boyfriend. She also had a history of sexual and emotional abuse from ages six to eight by the mother's boyfriend. AB revealed this to her mother at the time of the abuse but was not believed. The abuse continued until the boyfriend left her mother. Other than these memories, AB has few other memories of childhood.

AB initially became distanced from her mother at age 16 when she dropped out of high school and moved in with a boyfriend who was alcoholic and abusive. After that, she fled the boyfriend and became homeless. She spent a few years living in shelters, working as a strip-per, and prostituting herself. Between the ages of 10 and 25, she exces-sively used alcohol, often blacking out. She used marijuana from ages 13 to 27. At that time, her substance abuse resulted in high-risk sexual behaviors and dangerous situations. She had been assaulted many times and had been arrested and incarcerated for prostitution.

AB eventually had a child and married. She separated from her husband; he was overly-controlling and abusive. Her daughter is 16 years old and lives with her. Six years ago, her daughter told AB that the long time live-in boyfriend of AB was sexually abusing her. The boyfriend denied this report but AB pressed charges. The boyfriend was convicted and incarcerated. After his conviction, the boyfriend and his family ostracized her. This was difficult for AB because she had developed a close relationship with the boyfriend's mother.

AB did not have any current intimate relationships and said that she had "sworn off" men. She had no friends and little social support; she felt that she could not trust anyone. She viewed her daughter as a friend. Yet, she said that looking at her daughter was "almost unbearable" because it reminded her of both her own and her daughter's childhood sexual abuse. She said that sometimes the two experiences got confused in her head.

AB had no evidence of thought disorder, psychosis, or mania. She denied any history of, or current, suicidal or homicidal ideation, plan, or intent. AB was adequately groomed, dressed plainly, and often wore a baseball hat, dark glasses, and no makeup. Her facial expressions were constricted, and her voice was hypo-phonic. She usually avoided eye contact by looking down at her lap while speaking. She frequently sat on the edge of the seat, often wringing her hands, and occasionally spoke through tears. AB usually arrived late for therapy sessions, often in a flurry, providing reasons why she was late.

AB had multiple vague somatic complaints. She frequently stopped all her medications and dropped out of treatment, after which she went to the ED in a crisis. The psychiatric treatment plan was for AB to attend and actively participate in weekly individual and group therapy sessions and monthly psychopharmacology visits. She also attended the hospital's medical clinic for her many vague somatic complaints. She had chronic back pain and irritable bowel syndrome but frequently missed her clinic appointments. Part of her psychiatric treatment plan was for her to attend clinic appointments as planned.

AB thought of herself as a perpetual victim. She felt permanently damaged, abandoned, helpless, and externally directed by her past and current situation. She felt transparent in that she thought her sexual abuse and abandonment wounds were visible to others. This belief contributed to feelings of worthlessness, chronic low self esteem, and feelings of being an outsider. She sometimes believed she would never get better and she could not remember being happy. In the past she avoided emotions through substance use and periodically self-created crises that served as avoidance behavior and provided her with temporary soothing by others.

AB initially had no insight into the part she played in perpetuating crisis-driven coping. She had a pattern of creating conflict with providers and frequently switched providers or treatment settings. This behavior led to a pattern of repeatedly starting psychiatric care services and not moving through treatment. Each time she returned for treatment she created a sense of urgency and crisis in relation to the need for care.

Based on her previous history, the psychiatric team continued outreach and encouraged her to move through these crises without a rupture in care. They continued aggressive outreach until AB agreed to participate in group and individual therapy.

The focus of treatment consisted of exploring what it would be like for AB to "be better." AB began to see a possibility that she could tolerate uncomfortable feelings. She began to trust that her providers would not abandon her as her mother and others had. AB became an active participant in health promotion and health protection strategies, not just in crisis care. She verbalized a desire to avoid running away from feelings as she had in the past and to start learning new ways of self care and not rely on others to rescue her. She decided to take her treatment one day at a time. She felt just getting herself to the clinic and attending sessions was the best way for her to experience what it would be like to create self care instead of crisis. AB believed this was the first step that would lead her to a healthy life.

STOP. THINK. Which diagnoses, outcomes, and interventions would you select?

Submitter's Analysis and Use of NANDA-I, NOC, and NIC

At this point in AB's care, the problem nursing diagnoses that were considered but ruled out were *ineffective coping, fear, powerlessness,* and *noncompliance. Ineffective coping* was ruled out because AB's coping techniques helped her to feel safe by avoiding consistent care and episodically seeking crisis-driven care. These coping strategies were effective for her at the time. For example, a defining characteristic of *ineffective coping* is inability to ask for help. AB did ask for help except when in a crisis mode.

Fear was ruled out because she was unable to define her feelings; she fled from them. This diagnosis requires a report of alarm, apprehension, and so forth. AB was disconnected from her feelings and generally expressed them somatically with no awareness of the connection between her feelings and the possible physical manifestations of them.

Noncompliance was ruled out because AB was actively engaged in care, even though it was in a crisis driven manner. She was seeking care in a way that felt safe to her. The *noncompliance* diagnosis should also be decided with AB and AB did not see herself as noncompliant.

Powerlessness was ruled out because AB participated in her care. She had previously sought to gain power by using crisis as a tool. AB agreed to look at the possibility of using her power in a more effective manner to enhance her sense of well being.

She expressed readiness to enhance power, which included readiness to enhance awareness of possible changes and a readiness to enhance participation in choices. She verbalized awareness that she had a choice about her care. She chose to engage in care that was different from the crisis-driven care of the past. She was aware that she had the freedom to participate in her care in a way that led to health. She became more aware and involved in her care, as shown by the health promoting choices she made.

Using Barrett's power theory, the nursing diagnosis of *readiness for enhanced power* was confirmed with AB (Barrett, 2000). Barrett's power theory proposes that the observable measurable pattern manifestations of power are awareness, choices, freedom to act intentionally, and involvement in creating change. Power as knowing participation is being aware of what one is choosing to do, feeling free to do it, and doing it intentionally.

Although AB was not yet ready to feel hopeful about whether the treatment would work, she was willing to engage more actively in self-directed care without it being crisis-driven. She verbalized a commitment to avoid episodes that require temporary rescuing by others. She felt she was ready to take responsibility for herself and attend all of her appointments. She was able to separate her pain from her daughter's pain. She verbalized a desire to work toward exploring issues of self care because she realized she had been stuck in a repetitive pattern that may have sabotaged her recovery. AB expressed a desire to enhance responsibility for her choices. By enhancing her self responsibility and becoming aware, she chose health-promoting behaviors instead of health defeating ones.

NOC Outcome

The NOC outcome that was agreed on by the nurse and AB was *health promoting behavior*. Her current score was 4 (sometimes demonstrated) and the goal score was 5 (consistently demonstrated). The plan for AB to achieve a goal of 5 was that she would continue visits to the clinic, avoid crisis-related episodes that resulted in ED visits, and agree to share feelings with providers in words instead of using crises to communicate. The goal of 5 was projected and agreed upon with AB because the goal was for her to at least come to her visits. Without trying to achieve a 5, very little progress would be made. AB felt strongly that she wanted a 5 as her goal. This active participation in her care was part of the power-enhancing goal, so the 5 was kept. AB said, "I know I can at least try to come to all my appointments and stay out of the emergency room."

NIC Interventions

The NIC interventions that were used to help AB were *health education, self-modification assistance, self-awareness enhancement, self responsibility facilitation,* and *coping enhancement.* The major approach to implementing these interventions was the use of Barrett's health patterning modalities. Barrett's power theory emerged from Rogers's (1970) premise that humans can knowingly participate in change.

Health education focused on the risks versus benefits of crisis-driven care as compared with regular planned participation in psychiatric care with her team. AB made the decision to knowingly participate in change by intentionally choosing to return for psychiatric care rather than returning to the ED in crises. In a study of menopausal women and exercise, for example, the motivation to exercise for health promotion came from overcoming the initial discomfort in order to experience the benefits to body and mind (Jeng et al., 2004).

In the past, AB had been unable to tolerate her uncomfortable feelings. She sought to end her discomfort by going to the ED in crisis. She began to make decisions that postponed the immediate gratification of the ED visit. Instead, she was able to tolerate some of the uncomfortable feelings and realized that feelings are not permanent, that they come and go. She chose to tolerate the temporary uncomfortable feelings in the present with the hope that they would eventually give way to more positive feelings in the future. She began to explore the possibility that by enduring some pain in the present, it may actually lead to long term health benefits, improved self esteem, and an increased sense of her own power.

AB began to believe that she had the capability to positively affect her own health for the long term. She began to realize her power by setting her own goals. She took responsibility for her appointment dates by writing them on a small calendar. She began to see that keeping her appointments enhanced her sense of well being. When she developed an awareness that she held the power to enhance her well being she began to believe more strongly in herself and she showed an increase in self-esteem.

Her use of coping skills such as using deep breathing and focusing on the present moment increased in frequency. According to Barrett (2000), changing beliefs through awareness and subsequent actions is a crucial method for power enhancement. AB was still not ready to say that she would be better one day but she was able to commit to attending all her appointments and take her medication as prescribed. This was important to her at this time, and her beliefs and values must be considered in order to continue to enhance her sense of power. Health, which includes manifestations of illness, is value–related and ultimately defined by the individual as that individual perceives it to be (Barrett, 2000).

Evaluation

AB and the nurse decided that her goal score was met. She regularly attended the clinic and took her medications as prescribed; she had no ED visits. She began to view her treatment as being optional, under her control, and meaningful. She made active decisions (*self-responsibility facilitation*), which led to enhanced self care. AB began to explore the possibility that she may feel better some day. She felt that this possibility may be related to her new-found self care behaviors and decisions. She began to trust that her providers would not abandon her when she shared her pain. She continued to demonstrate readiness for power by attending and actively participating in all of her psychiatric sessions. She began to trust herself and others. AB avoided her previous pattern of crisis-driven care and explored the possibility of hope as it related to her recovery.

References

Barrett, E.A.M. (2000). The theoretical matrix for a Rogerian nursing practice. *Theoria: Journal of Nursing Theory, 9*(4), 3–7.

Jeng, C., Yang, S., Chang, P., and Tsao, L. (2004). Menopausal women: Perceiving continuous power through the experience of regular exercise. *Journal of Clinical Nursing, 13,* 447–454.

Rogers, M.E. (1970). *An introduction to the theoretical basis of nursing.* Philadelphia: F.A. Davis.

7.4. Living with Multiple Health Problems

Debra Guss, RN, BS, ACRN

GG is a 52-year-old man of Puerto-Rican decent with multiple health problems. He was diagnosed with diabetes 20 years ago. Five years ago he suffered from a massive myocardial infarction (MI) requiring a quadruple bypass, and subsequently a cardiovascular accident (CVA) that left him with L-sided hemiparesis. He was currently receiving daily home health care (HHC) for the treatment of a large diabetic foot ulcer that affected his mobility. He is also legally blind in both eyes and is on dialysis for the treatment of kidney failure.

Previous to the beginning of his physical disability five years ago, GG worked as a social work supervisor in Manhattan and had a considerable amount of responsibility and financial success. He considered himself "an important person in the world who was respected and well regarded." After his first MI and then his subsequent CVA, GG could no longer work and almost lost his home and car. His illness progressed, so when admitted to HHC he was homebound and weak, unable to independently perform any of his activities of daily living (ADLs) or instrumental activities of daily living (IADLs). He was completely dependent on his wife, who also had health problems, and his 22-year-old son who lived with him and left school to take care of him.

GG liked to think of himself as one who took his illness in stride with a good sense of humor. GG suffered, however, when he considered the limitations that have occurred with his many chronic and debilitating illnesses. He lamented his loss of physical ability and resulting dependence on those around him. "Every day I discover something else that I cannot do. I hate depending on everybody to do things. I can't even open a bottle of water or press the numbers on the phone." He remembered the past when he was a runner and could run marathons and felt deep sadness as he looked at his atrophied legs. He reported "a sadness that never goes away."

His greatest sadness was the effect that his physical limitations had on his family. His inability to work, his loss of earning power and community status, as well as status within his family left him feeling "like I am not a man anymore." He stated that as a Hispanic man, he should be the patriarch of the family, and the loss of that role disturbed him. "If I was healthy my son would not act as he does. The kids don't obey me anymore." He also lamented that he has become a burden on his family. He was upset that his wife's health was deteriorating as she took care of him, and that his son is no longer in school or working in order to take care of him. He fears for the future of his family.

Despite his severe limitations, on most days GG remained upbeat, humorous, and interested in the world. He often tried to engage in some of his previous interests—playing the harmonica one day, the trumpet the next, and maintaining his antique guns. He sometimes tried to do small things for himself, e.g., shave, brush his teeth, and comb his hair. He spoke often of wishing he could do more, and he would take any suggestion given to him to improve his health. He dreamed of a time when he could walk again, and asked for a referral to start seeing a physical therapist so that he would be strong enough to walk once his foot healed.

STOP. THINK. Which diagnoses, outcomes, and interventions would you select?

Submitter's Analysis and Use of NANDA-I, NOC, and NIC

In considering the nursing diagnoses most appropriate for GG, diagnoses such as *self-care deficit, impaired tissue integrity,* and *impaired mobility* were immediately disregarded. Though physical limitation and limited self care were concerns, it was the response to these limits that was the core issue. Also considered was the diagnosis *ineffective role performance* with its defining characteristics of altered role perception and role strain. GG's current trajectory, however, is more focused on increasing control of illness than his ineffective role within it. Thus, the HHC nurse chose the health promoting diagnosis of *readiness for enhanced coping* to reflect GG's process of transforming himself to a person with personal power through his pursuit of information about his illness and participation in his care (Pender, Murdaugh, and Parsons, 2006).

NOC Outcomes

The NOC outcomes desired for GG were related to improving his coping, since the underlying chronic illness was not amenable to an immediate change that would influence his feeling of equilibrium. The variables that created a feeling of disequilibrium, his physical limitations and resulting dependence, could not be changed at this time. His response to these variables could be influenced, however, to help him have a greater feeling of well being. The goals for GG were to feel a greater sense of control and adapt more adeptly to life changes (Helgeson, 1992; Livneh, Lott, and Antonak, 2004). In her 1992 study of 96 cardiac patients, Helgeson found that realistic perceptions of positive control were correlated with positive adjustment to chronic illness. Livneh, Lott, and Antonak also found in a study of 121 patients with varying disabilities that psychosocial adaptation was associated with reaction to illness and perception of control over one's illness. This sense of positive control became the focus of GG's treatment plan.

The NOC outcome established with GG was *coping*. His overall baseline score was rated as 3 with a goal score of 4.

NIC Interventions

The nursing interventions that were selected to help GG to reach his goal of *coping* were *coping enhancement* and *learning facilitation*. These interventions were supported by the family and HHC nurse with a goal of assisting GG to achieve an increased sense of satisfaction and control. This model of *coping* was described in a review of literature by Livneh and Parker (2005) that examined patients with varied chronic illnesses. This review of literature correlated the use of coping strategies such as seeking information, treatment planning, and seeking social support with positive adaptation, lower psychological distress, and a higher perceived quality of life.

Initially, GG was encouraged to identify his strengths and abilities and increase participation in activities that he could do. GG was encouraged to focus on the aspects of his illness that were controllable such as participation in physical therapy, maintenance of his home exercise program, and self management of diet and medications.

The visiting nurse began to pre-pour GG's medication and set alarms on his watch so he could feel more in control of this activity. The family was instrumental in supporting this initiative, and GG began to participate in bathing, grooming, feeding, and dressing with the set up of these activities by family members. This improved GG's feeling of independence and feelings of self sufficiency.

GG started to feel like a participant in his care, and started to want more information regarding his illness, his treatments, and his options. The nurse was able to provide information that gave GG a greater feeling of understanding of his numerous illnesses and treatments, which enabled him to feel a better sense of the prognosis and expectations of the disease processes. GG learned the names and functions of all his medications and started carrying a list in his bag so he would not need to depend on family members to provide this information to health care providers. The visiting nurse also introduced GG to a woman with diabetes who had a kidney transplant three years earlier and who was working again and functioning well. They spoke together at length, and GG began to feel optimistic about his future. Whereas before he had outright dismissed the idea of a kidney transplant, he now felt that this was a viable possibility for improving his quality of life. He has since put his name on the transplant list and selected a hospital for transplantation.

Evaluation

GG did well in achieving his outcomes with the help and support of his family. His overall goal score of 4 was achieved. GG reached his goal in seeking information regarding disability and demonstrating a sense of control and surpassed his goal in increasing psychological comfort.

GG clearly demonstrated *readiness for enhanced coping* and was able to increase his sense of well being and control through the use of this specific outcome and nursing interventions. The conscious decision to enable GG's self sufficiency was supportive of a lifelong desire to increase his sense of well being and quality of life. If the nurse only focused on treatment of the medical diagnosis of diabetic foot ulcer, GG's life would not have sufficiently improved in quality. By working in partnership with GG to establish a diagnosis and decide on possible outcomes and interventions, the nurse was able to help GG to improve his quality of life.

References

Helgeson, V.S. (1992). Moderators of the relation between perceived control and adjustment to chronic illness. *Journal of Personality and Social Psychology, 63*, 656–666.

Livneh, H., Lott, S.M., and Antonak, R.F. (2004). Patterns of psychological adaptation to chronic illness and disability: A cluster analytic approach. *Psychology, Health and Medicine, 9*, 411–430.

Livneh, H., and Parker, R. (2005). Psychological adaptation to disability: Perspectives from chaos and complexity theory. *Rehabilitation Counseling Bulletin, 49*, 17–28.

Pender, N.J., Murdaugh, C.L., and Parsons, M.A. (2006). *Health promotion in nursing practice* (5th ed.). Upper Saddle River, NJ: Pearson Prentice Hall.

7.5. Response to Limitations Associated with Cardiac Disease

Bernadette Amicucci, RN, MS, CNE

Mrs. RP is a 61-year-old Italian-American woman who was just diagnosed with stage II CHF secondary to a septal myocardial infarction that occurred three years ago. For the past six years, since menopause, she has been treated for hypertension. She is overweight with a BMI of 31. Two years ago, she was diagnosed with type 2 diabetes. Mrs. RP was admitted to the telemetry unit for cardiac monitoring after presenting with symptoms of increased fatigue, dyspnea on exertion, cough, and palpitations. Her BP was 150/92, HR was 124, and RR was 28.

Mrs. RP has been married for 32 years and has two grown children. Her youngest, a 28-year-old son, lives at home. Her 31-year-old daughter is married and has a two-year-old girl who Mrs. RP "adores." Mrs. RP's husband works full time in a nearby city. Mrs. RP was retired from nursing after working as a registered nurse for 35 years in labor and delivery.

For Mrs. RP's diabetic regimen, she takes glucophage and attends yoga classes but said she was "inconsistent." She reported trying to maintain a lower carbohydrate diet, but complained that "it is really hard." She monitored blood glucose three times a day, with levels of 120 to 140 mg/dl.

Mrs. RP verbalized frustration with this new diagnosis of CHF, stating, "I have been trying to do everything I am supposed to and still I had a heart attack and now heart failure!" She added "What good did any of it do?"

She admitted to feeling a little upset but did not want her family to know. Mrs. RP felt overwhelmed at the thought of "having to worry about my heart failing." With her nursing experience, she was hesitant to ask questions. She said, "The physician thinks I know all about this because I'm a nurse but I never took care of anyone with heart failure."

Since her retirement, Mrs. RP had been taking cooking classes and has been trying to cook new dishes. She stated, "My husband never cooks. I prepare dinner unless we're going out."

Mrs. RP had always regarded herself as being healthy. She complained that the last six years have resulted in "menopause, high blood pressure, diabetes, a heart attack, and now this!" She became tearful when she talked about looking forward to retirement, but now she may not be able to enjoy life.

The increased fatigue was a concern. She stated "I have a two-year-old granddaughter I need to be able to play with!" She was concerned about limitations she may have when she was discharged and stated, "I know I should have been exercising more and losing weight; I hope I have the opportunity to make this a little better."

STOP. THINK. Which diagnoses, outcomes, and interventions would you select?

Submitter's Analysis and Use of NANDA, NOC, and NIC

Mrs. RP's concerns centered on her decreased activity tolerance and her need for optimum self management of her cardiac disease. Together Mrs. RP and the nurse identified nursing diagnoses that addressed these two primary concerns: *readiness for enhanced self health management of cardiac disease* and *activity intolerance* related to imbalance between oxygen supply and demand secondary to cardiac disease.

Mrs. RP had expressed some anxiety and depression but both are related to frustrations with her cardiac disease management and diabetes. The nurse determined that addressing these health management issues would in fact be the first step in eliminating these contributing factors to anxiety and depression.

NOC Outcomes

The NOC outcomes that were selected by Mrs. RP and the nurse were *knowledge: cardiac disease management* and *activity tolerance*. The outcome of *knowledge: cardiac disease management* was rated as 3 (moderate knowledge) with a goal of 4 (substantial knowledge) before hospital discharge. It was expected that, after returning home, it was possible for her knowledge level to increase to 5 (extensive knowledge).

The outcome of *activity tolerance* related to her ability to play with her grandchild; her personal goal was increased endurance during play activities. After rating the indicators for the outcome of *activity tolerance*, Mrs. RP and the nurse rated this outcome as 2 (substantially compromised) with a goal of 3 (moderately compromised) or 4 (mildly compromised).

NIC Interventions

The interventions for the outcome of *knowledge: cardiac disease management* were *teaching: disease process, teaching: prescribed medications*, and *emotional support*. Teaching included the pathophysiology and contributing factors to CHF, and how the disease could be managed. The need for cardiac rehabilitation to assist with exercise and weight management was reinforced. Mrs. RP was positive about activity, including walking, and verbalized the ability to incorporate this plan into her life. In a randomized control study of 552 women age 60 and older, heart disease self-management programs were shown to reduce long-term health care use and potentially decreased overall health care costs (Wheeler, 2003).

Teaching about the prescribed medications included the actions, scheduling, and possible side effects, and the need for self-monitoring of pulse and blood pressure. A low carbohydrate diet with no added sugar and limited to 2 mg of sodium was explained by the nurse and the dietician. The carbohydrate grams and the sodium content of her favorite foods were identified by the dietitian. Ideas about how to lower the carbohydrate and sodium content using cooking skills were provided by the dietitian.

Two interventions were selected for the diagnosis of *activity intolerance*: *energy management* and *referral*. For energy management, the nurse discussed the need for incremental change in Mrs. RP's exercise regimen to prevent increased cardiac workload. Each day, the nurse helped Mrs. RP to progressively increase her activity, e.g., changing positions in bed, moving to the chair, walking in the room, and walking in the hallway. The nurse also helped her to learn how to monitor her responses to activity and to alternate activity with rest.

The nurse used the NIC intervention of *referral* by contacting a local cardiac rehabilitation center and consulting with them on a plan for Mrs. RP. Once the consult was completed, the recommendation for a three-times-a-week exercise schedule was made. Mrs. RP was positive about the proposed schedule and verbalized her ability to incorporate this plan into her life. In a pre/post study of physical fitness with 119 people in a cardiac rehabilitation program, there were significant positive differences in psychological status and physical fitness after the program (McKee, 2008).

The nurse provided *emotional support* throughout the interventions with Mrs. RP to help her manage the anxiety of having this new illness that she perceived as a problem. The possibility of seeking a support group when she returned home was suggested and reinforced.

Evaluation

By the time Mrs. RP was discharged to home, her BP had decreased to 140/86 and her resting HR was 72 to 76. She no longer complained of dyspnea and her RR was 20 to 24.

Mrs. RP's target score of 3 was met for *activity tolerance* as indicated by her ability to ambulate the length of the hall without dyspnea, fatigue, or tachycardia. The goal of regular activity was set with the nurse and Mrs. RP collaborated to plan a workable activity and rest schedule. She made an appointment with the cardiac rehabilitation center prior to discharge.

Mrs. RP's *knowledge of cardiac disease management* increased from 3 to 4. She was able to explain the pathophysiology and contributing factors to heart failure. She verbalized an understanding of the need to take medication as prescribed and prior to her discharge she asked her physician to order prescriptions at the local pharmacy. She demonstrated self pulse checks and was beginning a journal to maintain heart rate, symptoms, and medication schedule. She planned to implement the ideas for food preparation and went home with menus planned for the week following discharge. She enlisted the help of her daughter to do the required shopping.

Mrs. RP was still hesitant about sharing the extent of her concern and anxiety with her family, but agreed that a support group might provide the forum she needed to share her concerns. At the time of discharge, RP considered attending the group as "a possibility." She had the meeting dates and times with her.

References

McKee, G. (2008). Predictors of fitness improvements in phase III cardiac rehabilitation exercise. *International Journal of Therapy and Rehabilitation, 15,* 138–142.

Wheeler, J.R.C. (2003). Can a self-management program reduce health care costs?: The case of older women with heart disease. *Medical Care, 41,* 706–715.

7.6. Living with Chronic Obstructive Pulmonary Disease

Dawn Fairlie, RN, MS, APRN-BC

FM is a 78-year-old Caucasian male with a history of chronic obstructive pulmonary disease (COPD). He has had three hospitalizations in the past six months for respiratory decompensation. The community health nurse made a home visit to evaluate his self health management.

FM lives in a modest private home with his 76-year-old wife. They have one married adult son who lives approximately 90 minutes away and "is very busy" with frequent travel for his job. Their daughter-in-law takes Mrs. M grocery shopping one time a month and drives them to their scheduled physician visits. Mrs. M prepares the meals and assists Mr. M as needed with his personal care and other activities of daily living.

Both FM and his wife received health care services at a private physician's office. They received annual flu shots and have had their pneumococcal vaccinations.

FM used a wheelchair for distance and used a walker and minimal assistance to transfer from a hospital bed to his recliner or commode. He had a urinal within reach, a tub transfer seat, and a handheld shower head.

FM was alert and oriented to time, place, and person. Vital signs were: T 98.7°F, BP 130/82 mm/hg, A/P 86/86 and regular, R 22 a minute, and dyspnea on exertion. FM used nasal oxygen (O_2) at 2 liters per minute, using an around-the-clock oxygen concentrator. Pulse oximetry on oxygen was 95%. Breath sounds were diminished with wheezing throughout and chronic coarse crackles at the bases, which sometimes clear with aggressive laborious coughing. Sputum was moderate in amount, thick and white.

FM managed his medications, self administered his metered dose inhalers (MDI), and appropriately scheduled his prescription and nonprescription medications. He explained to the nurse his scheduling, as well as the actions and side effects of his medications. He demonstrated the correct MDI technique. He stated that his brother used a peak flow meter "to measure his breathing," and reported that, although he felt better after his hospitalizations, it had been difficult for his family. He pragmatically stated that he wanted "to take better care" of himself. He asked the community health nurse if "measuring my breathing" might help to decrease the hospitalizations.

 STOP. THINK. Which diagnoses, outcomes, and interventions would you select?

Submitter's Analysis and Use of NANDA-I, NOC, and NIC

The home health care (HHC) nurse used Orem's theory of self care as a framework for nursing care. The HHC nurse, FM, and Mrs. M. agreed that this framework was consistent with their belief systems.

Several diagnoses were considered and ruled out by the nurse. *Activity intolerance* and *ineffective airway clearance* are often appropriate when an older person has COPD, but they were not priorities for intervention with FM. *Impaired gas exchange* did not apply because there was adequate compensation as indicated by the oxygen saturation level. *Deficient knowledge* was ruled out because the evidence indicated that FM had sufficient knowledge to manage his care. FM was doing his best to follow instructions, as indicated by his strict adherence to the medication regimen. Additionally, he sought information resources by discussing the use of a peak flow meter.

Of the health promotion diagnoses, *readiness for enhanced knowledge* was deemed inappropriate because FM was functioning at a more complex level than merely expressing an interest in learning. *Readiness for enhanced power* was considered because FM demonstrated the defining characteristics of the diagnosis, but was ruled out because interventions for this diagnosis would not be likely to produce the best outcomes.

FM's question regarding decreasing hospitalizations clearly indicated that the best nursing diagnosis to guide care at this time was *readiness for enhanced self health management*. The defining characteristics that were specific to FM included his explicit desire to manage the illness and prevent frequent hospitalizations. The HHC nurse, FM, and Mrs. M agreed to the diagnosis *readiness for enhanced self health management*. This diagnosis was consistent with a systematic review of previous research studies, showing that self management education for people with COPD was associated with a reduction in hospital admissions (Effing et al., 2007). People with COPD often experience a desire for self care performance related to their disease experience and its perceived severity, as well as with periods of disease exacerbation. In an experimental study in Sweden of 52 people with COPD, it was shown that a structured self care educational program was associated with a statistically significant increase in quality of life (Efraimsson, Hillervik, and Ehrenberg, 2008). These research findings were consistent with using Orem's model in nursing care with FM and Mrs. M.

NOC Outcomes

The NOC outcomes agreed upon by the HHC nurse, FM, and Mrs. M were *knowledge of treatment regimen* and *risk control*. FM, his wife, and the HHC nurse scored his current *knowledge of treatment regimen* as 4 (substantial knowledge) with a goal of 5 (extensive knowledge); and his *risk control* as 5 (consistently demonstrated) with a goal score of remaining at 5.

NIC Interventions

The family-focused NIC interventions of *teaching: procedure/treatment, respiratory monitoring*, and *risk identification* were identified by the HHC nurse, based on FM's unique self care strengths and needs and validated by FM and his wife. Mrs. M's role in assisting her husband was consistently integrated.

The HHC nurse instructed FM and his wife in the use of a peak flow meter so FM could use the data obtained from the peak flow meter readings to adjust his self management routine according to the written stepped-approach action plan. His wife agreed to remind him to test himself and would read the results for him to record in a journal. Together they agreed on a plan to monitor and record three times each day for one week. A personal best reading was established on a subsequent visit and an action plan formulated that included the use of green, yellow, and red zones with their corresponding readings and appropriate courses of action. A copy of the plan was taped to the refrigerator alongside the phone number of his pulmonary physician.

The nurse also implemented the intervention of *emotional support* and discussed the possibility with FM of him using *guided imagery*. Mr. M was initially skeptical about incorporating *guided imagery* into his care plan. In response, the HHC nurse explained to him a research study in which individuals who practiced guided imagery had an increase in oxygen saturation (Louie, 2004). FM agreed to "give it a try." The HHC nurse loaned him a guided imagery audiotape specifically written for individuals with COPD. He agreed to listen to it each morning and evening for one week. FM reported initially feeling awkward and then said that he looked forward to using the taped session.

FM and his wife were also instructed in monitoring fatigue levels and correct monitoring of the respiratory secretions. The wife agreed to purchase only white tissues and a florescent table lamp was brought up from the basement for improved visualization of the secretions. FM and his wife were advised that early morning secretions are usually darker than those expectorated during the daytime hours. They were advised to call the pulmonary specialist for changes in color, consistency, and amount, or if an odor or foul taste was noticed. Mrs. M was advised of early mental changes associated with respiratory decompensation and she agreed to contact the pulmonary specialist if she noticed any signs and symptoms.

Further management of risks that could exacerbate FM's COPD was explored. FM agreed to continue to have an annual influenza vaccination, and avoid extremes of temperature, dust, and individuals with respiratory infections. Mrs. M was instructed on procedures for cleaning the O_2 concentrator filter. Safe use of oxygen was discussed and an "Oxygen in Use" sign was placed on the foyer door. The electric company was notified that the FM household was oxygen-dependent in the event of a power outage. Storage and checking the emergency oxygen tanks was discussed.

Evaluation

FM and Mrs. M worked together to successfully achieve an outcome score of 5 for each NOC. Prior to discharge from the home care agency, the family demonstrated the ability to self monitor with a peak flow meter and could describe appropriate actions based on theoretical scenarios. They verbalized increased confidence with their ability to manage risks related to COPD and were assured by their ability to detect early warning signs of respiratory decompensation as well as feeling secure in appropriate actions established in the written plan.

References

Effing, T., Monninkhof, E.M., Van der Valk, P.D., Van der Palen, J., Van Herwaarden, C.L., Partidge, M.R., Walters, E.H., and Zielhuis, G.A. (2007). Self management education for patients with chronic obstructive pulmonary disease. *Cochrane Database Systematic Review, October 17*(4), CD002990.

Efraimsson, E.O., Hillervik, C., and Ehrenberg, A. (2008). Effects of COPD self-care management education at a nurse-led primary health care clinic. *Scandinavian Journal of Caring Sciences, 22*, 178–85.

Louie, S.W. (2004). The effects of guided imagery relaxation in people with COPD. *Occupational Therapy International, 11*, 145–59.

Case Studies with a Primary Focus on Strength Diagnoses and Associated Outcomes and Interventions

8

8.1. Mother Breastfeeding Her Newborn

Alda Valéria Neves Soares Gomes, RN, MNS, Gilcéria Tochika Shimoda, RN, MNS, and Ilva Marico Mizumoto Aragaki, RN, MNS

Mrs. IA was admitted by the nurse to the rooming-in unit after delivery of a male infant at the obstetric center. The nurses in the rooming-in facility used the construct of caring and Orem's theory as the foundation of nursing care. Mrs. IA is a normal, post-delivery, puerpera 26-year-old woman, married, and an elementary school teacher, and this is her second child. Her son's weight was adequate for a gestational age full-term newborn, which with the Capurro method was equal to 41 weeks and 1 day. His Apgar scores were 9 and 10; his weight was 3,410 gm.

During the physical examination and interview, the nurse identified the following data: contracted uterus with physiological vaginal bleeding and right mediolateral episiotomy with mild infiltration and swelling. Mrs. IA showed tiredness after her prolonged labor, although she was happy with the birth of her second child. Mrs. IA informed the nurse that the baby had already been breastfed in the labor room, latching on well, and she wanted to breastfeed him exclusively up to six months and continue at least until he reached one year old. She had breastfed her daughter for three years. She said she had mild uterine cramps.

During the physical examination of Mrs. IA's breasts, the nurse observed protruding nipples and the presence of colostrum in a small amount. Mrs. IA said that she wanted to breastfeed and that this practice was common in her family. Her cousins, aunts, mother, and grandmother on her mother's side all breastfed their children.

Initially, when the nurse helped her to breastfeed, it was observed that Mrs. IA placed herself inadequately because of discomfort in the perineal area, most likely from swelling of the episiotomy. She also told the nurse that she had uterine cramps but did not want any pain medication. She said that she expected them to subside in time and that they were no problem to her. Her position for breastfeeding was quickly corrected when she was more comfortable and the nurse reminded her of the posture to be adopted.

 STOP. THINK. Which diagnoses, outcomes, and interventions would you select?

Submitter's Analysis and Use of NANDA-I, NOC, and NIC

The nurse considered the diagnoses of *risk of infection* related to infiltration and swelling at the episiotomy site, *acute pain* related to recent delivery, and *effective breastfeeding* as evidenced by expressed satisfaction in the beginning of breastfeeding and good suction of the newborn to the mother's breast.

The nurse decided to rule out the diagnoses of *risk of infection* and *acute pain. Risk of infection* was ruled out because Mrs. IA's swelling at the episiotomy site was expected and was within normal limits. The swelling would automatically be treated with local cold application and analgesic medication as needed. The episiotomy site would be routinely observed for healing as long as Mrs. IA was hospitalized. *Acute pain* was ruled out because Mrs. IA said it was not a problem for her.

The diagnosis *effective breastfeeding* was selected and recorded so that other nurses would know that breastfeeding was determined to be effective. This would prevent other nurses from having to spend time and energy assessing Mrs. IA's breastfeeding and it would save Mrs. IA from having to answer the questions of every nurse about her breastfeeding. With the diagnosis of *effective breastfeeding*, nurses on this unit knew to continue supporting Mrs. IA's positive experiences of breastfeeding throughout her three-day stay on the unit. The benefits of breastfeeding for both the mother's and the child's health was well known to nurses on this unit (World Health Organization, 2003). Successful breastfeeding is mainly based upon the mother's decision and desire to breastfeed; the mother's actions are expected to focus on the establishment of this practice in an efficient way.

NOC Outcomes

The NOC outcomes that were selected for Ms. IA were *breastfeeding establishment: infant, breastfeeding establishment: mother*, and *breastfeeding maintenance*. The baseline scores were noted as 5 (totally adequate) and the target scores were to maintain scores of 5. Because this was only the beginning of the breastfeeding process, it was considered essential to frequently evaluate the indicators of these three outcomes to continue to maintain positive and effective breastfeeding.

NIC Interventions

Using Orem's nursing theory, the nurses' main focus was to select interventions that would promote Mrs. IA's self care and consequently, the care of the baby (Orem, 2001). During the three-day hospitalization, the nursing care was focused on the NIC interventions of *breastfeeding* and *counseling*. The nurses reinforced the mother's orientation to breastfeed her son. The nurses assisted Mrs. IA whenever indicated with the breastfeeding technique; Mrs. IA mentioned that her son was more eager in sucking the nipple compared to her daughter. At one point, Mrs. IA showed some concern related to the amount of milk produced. The nurse reassured her that her body would produce the amount of milk needed and provided instruction about the production of milk and the need for frequent fluid intake. This information alleviated IA's concerns.

In the first day after delivery, the nurse observed that Mrs. IA placed herself appropriately for breastfeeding, her pain had lessened, and the episiotomy swelling had subsided. Mrs. IA reported the many activities she recalled from the hospitalization when her daughter was born and she seemed to be satisfied with the breastfeeding process.

In Mrs. IA's daily evaluation, the nurse perceived the breasts presented an adequate amount of colostrum, as stimulated by the reflex of oxytocin; the newborn child sucked regularly on the breast, the latch-on position was correct, and the baby seemed satisfied with the amount of liquid he was getting.

Mrs. IA attended group guidance that focused on mothers and families, whose content addressed care of newborn children, mother self care, and breastfeeding techniques. She expressed that she had a good opportunity to recall and reinforce her knowledge, practice, and attitude regarding breastfeeding.

Evaluation

At hospital discharge, the nurse evaluated that Mrs. IA still presented with the diagnosis of *effective breastfeeding* and continued to score 5 on the selected outcomes. Mrs. IA showed confidence and satisfaction with the breastfeeding process and her breasts presented good milk drainage and intact nipples, and the baby's suction was correct.

In the 10th-day return appointment after discharge, the nurse verified that Mrs. IA continued to exclusively breastfeed her child, having good milk production and intact nipples. Her son gained 40 gm a day. Mrs. IA said she wanted to breastfeed as long as her son desired, and expressed no doubt about the process of breastfeeding.

References

Orem, D. (2001). *Nursing concepts of practice* (6th ed.). St. Louis, MO: Mosby.

World Health Organization (2003). Global strategy for infant and young child feeding.   http://www.who.int/nutrition/publications/gs_infant_feeding_text_eng.pdf.

8.2. Nursing Communication for Continuity of Care

Janice Pattison, RN, MS, ANP-C

Mrs. G, a 65-year-old woman, was admitted to the hospital after a car accident in which she sustained a compound fracture of her R leg. She was a passenger in the car and had been wearing her seatbelt. After evaluation in the ED, she was transferred to the operating room for repair of the fracture. After surgery, she was admitted to a post operative orthopedic unit where she received care for the fracture and was monitored for sequelae of the accident.

Within 24 hours of admission to the medical unit, the nurse conducted a comprehensive assessment using Gordon's functional health patterns (Gordon, 2008). In the category of management of health, Mrs. G explained that she takes medications for the following chronic illnesses and problems: arthritis, essential thrombocythemia, gastroesophageal reflux, overactive bladder, and hypertension. Both her mother and father died of heart disease; at age 52, her father died prematurely. Her mother had hypertension from age 47 to 88, when she died. Her sister was recently diagnosed with breast cancer. Mrs. G knows the names and dosages of her medications and has been taking them as prescribed. She visits a hematologist every three months for evaluation of the blood disorder and obtains new prescriptions as needed, generally walks two miles in 32 minutes four to seven times a week, adheres to a 2,000- to 2,500-calorie diet with low to moderate amounts of saturated fats, conducts a monthly self breast examination, and obtains a yearly mammogram. Assessment of the nutrition pattern showed a weight of 145 pounds with a height of 5 feet 7 inches. Her vital signs were stable with an average BP of 136/82 and a pulse of 72 to 74.

Mrs. G has a supportive family who will provide assistance with activities of daily living when she is discharged to home. Mrs. G considered herself in good health and looked forward to getting "back on her feet again."

A referral was made to a home health care (HHC) agency, which was part of the same health care system as the hospital. Both agencies were using the same electronic health record so the nursing plan of care was communicated electronically to the HHC agency. Mrs. G primarily needed home care services for a nurse to teach daily cleansing of the pin sites and to monitor for signs and symptoms of infection.

 STOP. THINK. Which diagnoses, outcomes, and interventions would you select?

Submitter's Analysis and Use of NANDA-I, NOC, and NIC

In the referral to the HHC agency, the nurses on the medical unit communicated their ongoing diagnoses, outcomes, and interventions so that HHC nurses would be able to continue the plan of care. In a comparison study of nurses' discharge notes with paper and electronic charting, the investigator found that the hospital nurses shared more detail and focus about their patients with HHC nurses with use of a language-specific template (Hellesø, 2006). The most important diagnosis of Mrs. G that they communicated was *effective self health management.* Another routine diagnosis for a person with pins and lacerations, such as Mrs. G, was *risk for infection*.

Because Mrs. G had so many health problems, each with specific therapeutic regimens, it was routine care for the HHC nurse to focus on the effectiveness of Mrs. G's *self health management*. With communication of this strength diagnosis, however, the admission visit was much easier. The HHC nurse did a sufficient assessment to validate the diagnosis and planned to be available if Mrs. G showed any evidence of needing additional support or help with her therapeutic regimens. In addition to easing the HHC nurses' workload, this helped Mrs. G because she did not have to review her self health management whenever new nurses from the HHC agency came to visit.

NOC Outcomes

The NOC outcomes communicated by the hospital nurses to the HHC agency were *treatment behavior: illness or injury* and *infection severity*. For the outcome of *illness behavior*, Mrs. G's baseline score was recorded as 5 (consistently demonstrated) and the target score was to remain at 5. For the outcome of *infection severity*, the baseline score was recorded as 5 (none) and the outcome score was to remain at 5.

NIC Interventions

Two NIC interventions were communicated to the HHC agency to support ongoing maintenance of *treatment behavior* at a level of 5 (consistently demonstrated); these were *risk identification* and *teaching: prescribed activity/exercise*. The HHC nurses were expected to observe for any risk factors that indicated a change in the outcome. The intervention of *risk identification* was also used to monitor for possible pain and the effects of immobility. Mrs. G and her family were instructed on the adverse effects of immobility and shown how to help Mrs. G increase mobility as able with a cast and pins, e.g., transfer to a wheelchair, change positions in bed, and so forth.

The NIC interventions that were selected to address Mrs. G's *risk for infection* were *wound care* and *infection protection*. *Wound care* involved pin site cleansing and observation. In a review of four studies that met specific inclusion criteria, 16% of pin sites became infected (Williams and Griffiths, 2004). It was unclear from this study which cleansing treatments were best to prevent infection. In this case, normal saline was used, followed by betadine. *Infection protection* would be implemented by daily aseptic care of the pins and modification of the environment to prevent the open skin area from being exposed to pathogens. The nurse performed the initial pin care and after that taught and supervised the *wound care* to be given by a family member. Thereafter, the nurse visited once or twice a week to observe the wound for changes and assess for possible infection.

Evaluation

The nurses in the HHC agency telephoned the nurses on the hospital medical unit to say that they followed the care plan as laid out by the hospital discharging nurse. Mrs. G was maintaining her outcomes at a level of 5. The nurses' communication of the care plan from the hospital to the HHC agency facilitated continuity of care and saved the HHC nurses time and energy, which was then used to serve other patients.

References

Hellesø, R. (2006). Information handling in the nursing discharge note. *Journal of Clinical Nursing, 15*, 11–21.

Williams, H., and Griffiths, P. (2004). The effectiveness of pin site care for patients with external fixators. *British Journal of Community Nursing, 9*, 206–209.

Appendix A

Webliography

www.nanda.org The official website for NANDA International. Join NANDA-I and use the Members Only section.

www.blackwellpublishing.com/journal.asp?ref=1541-5147 Site of the *International Journal of Nursing Terminologies and Classifications*, Official Journal of NANDA International.

www.nursing.uiowa.edu/excellence/nursing_knowledge/clinical_effectiveness/index Access the latest information about NOC and NIC through the Center for Nursing Classification and Clinical Effectiveness.

www.acendio.com Association for Common European Nursing Diagnoses, Outcomes and Interventions. Find the latest information about European nurses' use of standardized nursing languages.

www.aentde.com Association for Spanish Nursing Taxonomy and Diagnosis. This group works in Spain on nomenclature development and refinement.

www.icn.ch/icnp.htm Learn about the International Classification of Nursing Practice, an umbrella system for all standardized nursing languages. It can be used with NANDA-I, NOC, and NIC.

www.ihtsdo.org The International Health Terminology Standards Development organization, formerly SNOMED-CT. This is a comprehensive system of clinical terminology that includes NANDA-I, NOC, and NIC, with millions of other terms.

http://ncvhs.hhs.gov The National Committee on Vital and Health Statistics makes decisions for the U.S. on the organization of standardized languages for the electronic health record.

www.ahrq.gov U.S. government website that provides excellent information about the latest research findings on various health related topics.

www.cochrane.org The Cochrane Collaboration, originating from the U.K., provides systematic reviews of research on a variety of health-related topics.

www.ncqa.org/tabid/65/Default.aspx The National Committee for Quality Assurance is a private group that provides excellent insights on the measurement of quality care, including health outcomes.

www.nursingworld.org/MainMenuCategories/ThePracticeof ProfessionalNursing/PatientSafetyQuality/NDNQI/NDNQI_1. aspx Click on this web address to learn about ANA's National Database of Nursing Quality Indicators.

Appendix B

Assessment Tool: Functional Health Patterns

The purpose of this tool is to provide guidance in conducting and recording a health history of Functional Health Patterns (Gordon, 1994).[1]

Directions

1. The categories on the left provide guidance to the type of information that is included in the pattern description. The pattern of the client (data from the client) should be described on the right. The description as written should be understandable by others, for example,

   Correct: no hx. of related physical and psychological problems
   Incorrect: none

2. Use interviewing techniques as described in the literature, e.g., include silence and statements, not just questions.

3. Since all of the data represent subjective data, quotation marks should not be used. It will be assumed that every sentence represents the words of the client and family or the words of client and family are paraphrased.

4. Since the subject of every sentence is "I" or "we," the subject should not be repeated throughout. The client's responses can be written as incomplete sentences, e.g., attend church every day at 9 a.m. (the subject is assumed to be "I" or "We").

5. When clients have long stories to tell in relation to an assessment category, the data can be shortened by paraphrasing, but be careful

[1] Gordon, M.(1994). *Nursing diagnosis: process and application* (2nd ed.). New York: McGraw Hill.

339

to retain the essence of the client's response.

6. As much as possible, record your data in the form of cues, as opposed to inferences. Cues are units of sensory data. Inferences are the subjective meanings that persons apply to cues. Recognize the difference between cues and inferences.

7. Avoid interjecting diagnoses into the data base, e.g., anxious (a dx.) about her relationship with her family. This statement should only be in the data base if it is a statement made by the client.

8. Consider the assessment categories of this form as incomplete for any particular client. Follow through on cues that are raised in the assessment, e.g., if Mary states she smokes 1 pk. cigarettes per day, identify whether she knows the dangers of smoking, how she feels about smoking, what is her motivation to quit, does smoking affect other aspects of her life, are there other risk factors for heart and lung disease?

Assessment Tool: Functional Health Patterns**

Date_____Nurse_____

Consumer's Initials_____Age_____Gender_____Occupation_____

Physician(s)_____Pharmacist_____

Reason for Contact_____

Health perception/health management pattern	
Meaning of health	
Description of health status	
Health promotion: food and fluids, exercise, lifestyle and habits, stress management	
Health protection: screening programs, visits to primary health care professionals, diet, exercise, stress management, rest, economic factors	
Self examination of: breast and/or testicles, blood pressure, other	
Knowledge of self-examination	
Med history, hospitalizations and surgery, family med hx	

** Assess individual and family whenever possible. Assess congruence of individual and family perceptions. Incorporate bio-psycho-socio-cultural dimensions of each pattern.

Behaviors to manage health problems: diet, exercise, medications, treatments	
Names, dosage, and frequency of prescription and nonprescription drugs	
Risk factors rel. to health, e.g., family history, lifestyle and/or habits, poverty	
Relevant PE (physical exam) data: Complete.	
Nutrition/metabolic pattern	
Usual number of meals and snacks	
Types and amts.—foods and fluids	
24 hr. recall or 3 day diet hx	
Shopping and cooking habits	
Satisfaction with weight	
Influences on food choices, e.g., religious, ethnic, cultural, economic	
Perceptions of metabolic needs	
Related factors, e.g., activity, illness, stress	
Ingestion factors: appetite, discomfort, taste and smell, teeth, oral mucosa, nausea or vomiting, dietary restrictions, food allergies	
Hx. of related physical and/or psychological problems	
Relevant PE data: General survey—skin, hair, nails, abdomen	
Elimination Pattern	
Usual voiding pattern: frequency, amount, color, odor, discomfort, nocturia, control, any changes	
Usual defecation pattern: regularity, color, amount, consistency, discomfort, control, any changes	
Health/cultural beliefs	
Level of self care: toileting, hygiene	

Aids for excretion, e.g., medications, enemas	
Actions to prevent cystitis	
Hx. of related physical and/or psychological problems	
Relevant PE data: abdomen, genitals, prostate	
Activity/exercise pattern	
Typical ADL	
Exercise: type, frequency, duration, intensity	
Leisure activities	
Beliefs about exercise	
Ability for self care: dressing (upper and lower) bathing, feeding, toileting; independent, dependent, or assistance needed	
Use of equipment, e.g., cane	
Related factors, e.g., self concept	
Hx. of related physical and/or psychological problems	
Relevant PE data: Respiratory, cardio-vascular, musculo-skeletal, neurological	
Sleep/rest pattern	
Usual sleep habits—number of hours, time of sleep and awakening, bedtime rituals, sleep environment, rested after sleep	
Cultural beliefs	
Use of sleep aids, e.g., drugs, relaxation tapes	
Scheduled rest and relaxation	
Symptoms of sleep pattern disturbance, e.g., fatigue	
Related factors, e.g., pain	
Hx. of related physical and/or psychological problems	
Relevant PE data: General survey	

Cognitive/perceptual pattern	
Description of special senses: vision, hearing, taste, touch, smell	
Aids to senses, e.g., glasses	
Recent changes in senses	
Perception of comfort/pain	
Cultural beliefs re: pain	
Aids to relieve discomfort	
Educational level	
Decision-making ability	
Hx. of related physical, developmental, or psychological problems	
Relevant PE data: General survey—neurological	
Self perception/self concept pattern	
Social self: occupation, family situation, social groups	
Personal identity: description of self, strengths, and weaknesses	
Physical self: any concerns about body, likes/ dislikes	
Self esteem: feelings about self	
Threats to self concept, e.g., illness, changes in roles	
Hx. of related physical and/or psychological problems	
Relevant PE Data: General survey	
Role/relationship pattern	
Description of roles with family, friends, coworkers	
Role satisfaction/dissatisfaction	
Effect of health status	
Importance of family	

Family structure and support	
Family decision-making processes	
Family problems and/or concerns	
Child rearing patterns	
Relationships with others	
Significant relationships	
Hx. of related physical and/or psychological problems	
Relevant PE Data: General survey	
Sexuality/reproductive pattern	
Sexual concerns or problems	
Description of sexual behavior, e.g., safe sex practices	
Knowledge related to sexuality and reproduction	
Effect of health status	
Menstrual and reproductive hx.	
Hx. of related physical and/or psychological problems	
Relevant PE data: General survey—genitals, breasts, rectal	
Coping/stress tolerance pattern	
Nature of current stressors	
Perceived level of stress	
Description of overall and specific responses to stress	
Usual stress management strategies and their effectiveness	
Life changes and losses	
Coping strategies usually used	
Perceived control over events	
Knowledge and use of stress management techniques	

Relationship of stress management to family dynamics	
Hx. of related physical and/or psychological problems	
Relevant PE data: General survey	
Value/belief pattern	
Cultural/ethnic background	
Economic status, health behaviors that relate to cultural/ethnic group	
Goals in life	
What is important to client and family	
Importance of religion/spirituality	
Affect of health problems on spirituality	
Relevant PE data: General survey	

Appendix C

The Lunney Scoring Method for Rating Accuracy of Nurses' Diagnoses of Human Responses

1989 by Margaret Lunney, RN, PhD

This appendix describes a seven-point scale with criteria for each point on the scale that can be used by nurses to facilitate their own achievement of accuracy of diagnosing human responses or by judges of nurses' accuracy. The scoring method can be used to rate the accuracy of formally approved diagnostic labels, e.g., NANDA-I labels, or diagnoses that are not derived from formal classification systems. To score the accuracy of nurses' diagnoses of human responses, one or more raters decide the degree of accuracy using the predefined criteria of the scale (Appendix C Table 1). The scale is conceived as a continuum from high to low accuracy, with each level ordered according to how close a nurse's diagnosis is to approximating accuracy, e.g., the lowest level is viewed as the least accurate. Each of the seven levels on the scale is associated with a number from +5 to −1, one of which is assigned to a diagnosis. The criteria for assigning scores are defined by the degree of consistency between a diagnosis and the cues in a clinical case.

This scoring method can be used to rate the first part of a diagnosis and/or the second part of a diagnosis, i.e., the contributing factor (etiology) that is indicated by the cues. Both parts of a nursing diagnosis should be highly accurate in order to provide direction for nursing interventions. In clinical cases, all of the cues/data are considered as relevant to stating the most accurate nursing diagnosis. Some cues are highly relevant, i.e., they are specific to confirm a diagnosis or disconfirm an alternative diagnosis, while others are predictive or supportive.

For example, when Marian Hughes (see the box titled "Sample Nursing Case Study") states that she was not following her prescribed diet, this cue could *predict* the diagnosis *deficient knowledge regarding prescribed diet*. When Marian is able to describe what she should eat and

Appendix C Table 1. Scale for Degrees of Accuracy—Number Criteria

+5	Diagnosis is consistent with all of the cues, supported by highly relevant cues, and precise.
+4	Diagnosis is consistent with most or all of the cues and supported by relevant cues but fails to reflect one or a few highly relevant cues.
+3	Diagnosis is consistent with many of the cues but fails to reflect the specificity of available cues.
+2	Diagnosis is indicated by some of the cues but there are insufficient cues relevant to the diagnosis and/or the diagnosis is a lower priority than other diagnoses.
+1	Diagnosis is only suggested by one or a few cues.
0	Diagnosis is not indicated by any of the cues. No diagnosis is stated when there are sufficient cues to state a diagnosis. The diagnosis cannot be rated.
−1	Diagnosis is indicated by more than one cue but should be rejected based on the presence of at least two disconfirming cues.

how she can adjust her diet to her lifestyle and shows that the meals she eats at school are consistent with her diet, these cues are *highly relevant* to disconfirm, or rule out, the same diagnosis. When cues that are highly relevant to a specific diagnosis are ignored or misinterpreted, diagnostic statements are less accurate than when they are taken into account.

In diagnosing clinical cases, some nurses may decide on diagnoses by using predictive cues without considering cues that are highly relevant to confirm or disconfirm diagnoses or without considering other possibilities indicated by the cues. These nurses write statements that are less accurate than those who consider all of the cues to arrive at a diagnosis.

Levels of the Scale

+5 Level

A score of +5 is applied to responses that are consistent with all of the cues, supported by highly relevant cues, and precise. For example, in the sample case study, "communication gap between Marian and her mother" would be scored as +5. It is assumed that labels scored as +5 will be consistent with all of the cues because consistency or harmony is a characteristic of human beings. If a diagnostic label is high on a

Sample Nursing Case Study

(1) Marian Hughes is a 16-year-old female with a medical diagnosis of diabetes mellitus. (2) She was admitted three days ago for treatment of an acute episode of diabetic ketoacidosis. (3) When Marian discussed with you how she managed the therapeutic regimen before hospitalization, she stated that she was not adhering to her prescribed diet. (4) You decide that Marian needs assistance to improve her management of the therapeutic regimen, especially the types of foods she eats. (5) Marian's stay in the hospital unit is uneventful in that medical treatments are successfully resolving the crisis.

(6) Marian's daily habits include getting up for school about 7 am and rushing to get the bus by 7:30. (7) She says that she should get up about 6:30 but she likes to sleep. (8) She states that she does not want her mother to help her get up earlier. (9) The meal that she eats at school is consistent with her prescribed diet, while the two meals at home are not.

(10) In the morning she grabs whatever is quick and easy, usually toast and butter. (11) In the evening, her mother makes meals that comply with the diabetic diet but Marian states that she does not like them so she only eats part of her supper and then snacks on other foods later.

(12) Marian is able to explain to you what she should be eating and she can adjust her diet to her lifestyle. (13) The knowledge of the foods on her diet that she likes was not discussed with her mother because she doesn't want to sit down and talk with her. (14) In general, Marian and her mother argue over many of Marian's behaviors, such as school grades, smoking, and coming in late at night.

Nursing diagnosis: ineffective self health management related to_____. (Note: Fill in the blank by stating the most probable explanation for Marian Hughes's behavior.)

scale of accuracy, it will not be inconsistent with available data, even that which is not directly related.

The highly relevant cues for "communication gap between Marian and her mother" are sentence numbers 9, 11, 13, and 14. Responses that are scored as +5 are precise in that they reflect the specific nature of highly relevant cues in the clinical case and provide direction for nursing intervention. These are labels that would best portray to another nurse the focus of case management or treatment. This is the highest level of accuracy so only those responses that have the highest relevance, when considering all of the available data, should be scored as +5.

To be precise does not mean that the diagnosis is one particular word or phrase. For example, in the sample case study, the words "ineffective communication," "miscommunication," "noncommunication," "difficulty requesting support," and "lack of discussion" are similar in their meaning and would be scored as +5 as long as it is clear that the communication problem exists between Marian and her mother.

Responses should be rejected for the +5 level if there are cues in the clinical case that are inconsistent with the response. For example, in the sample case study, a response of *"powerlessness* of Marian's mother" would be inconsistent with the expected behaviors of teenagers and their mothers. Teenagers develop a separate identity from their parents and gain control over their own behaviors; therefore, to consider the power of Marian's mother as a priority would be inconsistent with the purpose of helping Marian.

Responses should also be rejected for the +5 level if they are less precise than are indicated by the cues. For example, in the sample case study, "poor relationship of Marian and her mother" would be consistent with all of the cues but would not be a precise match with the cues. This diagnosis does not reflect the specific dimension of the relationship that should be addressed, i.e., communication between Marian and her mother.

If responses are reflective of and consistent with the cues but are not as relevant as other responses, they should be rejected for the +5 level. For example, in the sample case study, "ineffective time management" is a precise interpretation of specific cues (cues 6, 7, 8, and 10), and is not inconsistent with other cues, but is a lower priority than the communication problem between Marian and her mother.

+4 Level

A score of +4 is applied to responses that are consistent with most or all of the cues and supported by relevant cues but fail to reflect one or a few highly relevant cues. For example, in the sample case study, "conflict in relation to mother" would be scored as +4. Responses to be scored at this level are those that do not reflect one or a few cues that have high relevance for understanding the situation, such as cues 9 and 13. These two cues indicate that Marian does not share important information with her mother. Marian and her mother have not agreed on ways that both of them can contribute to the objective: effective management of her therapeutic regimen. Statements at the +4 level, such as "conflict with mother" or "alteration in relationship with mother," are consistent with cues and adequately supported, but fail to reflect one or a few highly relevant cues.

Responses should be rejected for the +4 level if the criteria for one of the other levels is met more precisely. For example, in the sample case study, the diagnosis "alteration in family process" would be rejected for the +4 level because it meets the criteria for the +3 level.

+3 Level

A score of +3 is applied to responses that are consistent with many of the cues but fail to reflect the specificity of available cues. For example, in the sample case study, diagnoses such as *altered family dynamics, adolescent striving for independence,* and *inability to communicate with others* are consistent with many of the cues but do not reflect the specific dynamics of the family situation.

Responses should be rejected for the +3 level if the criteria for one of the other levels are met more precisely. For example, in the sample case study, the diagnosis *angry with mother* would be rejected for the +3 level because it meets the criteria for the +2 level.

+2 Level

A score of +2 is applied to responses that are indicated by some of the cues but there are insufficient cues relevant to the diagnosis and/or the diagnosis is a lower priority than other diagnoses. For example, in the sample case study, "knowledge deficit of mother regarding foods to cook," indicated by cues 9, 11, and 13, would be scored as +2 because there are insufficient highly relevant cues to support the diagnosis. A diagnosis of *ineffective time management*, indicated by cues 6, 7, 8, 9, and 10, would be scored as +2 because a diagnosis related to the communication of Marian and her mother is more relevant. Because the existence of one human behavior does not exclude the existence of other human behaviors, there can be diagnostic statements that are adequately supported but do not reflect highly relevant cues.

Responses should be rejected for the +2 level if the criteria for one of the other levels are met more precisely. For example, in the sample case study, "low self esteem" should be rejected for the +2 level because it meets the criteria for the +1 level, i.e., it is only suggested by the combination of Marian's age and the presence of a chronic illness.

+1 Level

A score of +1 is applied to responses that are only suggested by one or a few cues. For example, in the sample case study, "overeating snack foods" and "lack of motivation" would be scored as +1. Even though a diagnostician may consider these responses as possibilities, when there are not enough data to give them credibility, they should not be viewed as diagnoses. If hypotheses that are not supported by adequate data are accepted prematurely as diagnoses, it is likely that more accurate diagnoses will not be considered.

Responses should be rejected for the +1 level if the criteria for one of the other levels is met more precisely. For example, in the sample case study, "social isolation" should be rejected for the +1 level because it meets the criteria for 0.

0 Level

A score of 0 is applied to diagnoses that are not indicated by any of the cues. For example, in the sample case study, *hopelessness* and *hyperglycemia* would be scored as 0. Responses that are not indicated by cues may be written by nurses when they expect certain types of patients to exhibit these responses and do not consider whether or not cues are present to support the diagnosis. In practice situations, nurses may routinely associate certain nursing diagnoses with medical diagnoses, e.g., myocardial infarction may prompt nurses to write "decreased cardiac output" without considering whether there are cues to support the decision.

Responses are scored as 0 if no diagnosis is stated. For example, in the sample case study, if the space was left blank or the respondent repeated the cues in the case study, e.g., "arguments with her mother," the score would be 0. Responses are also scored as 0 if, for any reason, they cannot be rated.

Responses should be rejected for the 0 level if the criteria of one of the other levels is met more precisely, i.e., there are cues in the case study that suggest the diagnosis.

−1 Level

A score of −1 is applied to responses that are indicated by more than one cue but should be rejected based on the presence of two or more disconfirming cues. For example, in the sample case study, *knowledge deficit* regarding prescribed diet, for which there are three disconfirming cues (9, 12, and 13), would be scored as −1. Disconfirming cues are those that specifically relate to the diagnostic hypothesis and are highly relevant to directly rule out the hypothesis. Some research indicates that expert diagnosticians are able to rule out hypotheses when there are two disconfirming cues.

Responses should be rejected for the −1 level if the criteria for one of the other levels is met more precisely or if there are no disconfirming cues. It is an error to interpret cues as disconfirming for one diagnosis because they confirm another diagnosis. For example, in the sample case study, cues 9, 11, 13, and 14 support the diagnosis of "communication gap between Marian and her mother" but they do not disconfirm an alternative diagnosis such as "powerlessness."

Appendix C Table 2 shows how the scoring method was used to rate nurses' diagnoses of the sample case study.

Appendix C Table 2. Using the scoring method to rate nurses' diagnoses of the sample case study.

Diagnosis	Score
Ineffective communication between Marian and her mother	+5
Communication gap between Marian and her mother	+5
Intrafamilial communication problems	+5
Ineffective/inability to communicate with family	+5
Intrafamilial conflict	+4
Stressful mother-child/developmental tasks	+4
Unresolved conflicts with mother	+4
Intergenerational conflict with mother	+4
Conflict in relation to mother	+4
Alteration in relationship with mother	+4
Adolescent striving for independence	+3
Altered family processes	+3
Inability to communicate with others	+3
Poor familial coping—mother daughter dyad	+3
Striving for autonomy and independence	+3
Angry with mother	+2
Inability to cope—teenager	+2
Coping/developmental stage	+2
Ineffective coping mechanism	+2
Anger/rebellion/unresolved conflicts	+2
Conflict between priorities	+2
Knowledge deficit of mother regarding foods to cook for Marian	+2
Ineffective time management	+2
Developmental stage	+1
Low self esteem	+1
Rebellious behavior	+1
Self concept as different	+1
Adolescent image	+1
Overeating snack foods	+1
Lack of motivation	+1
Altered nutrition	0
Denial	0
Acceptance of diagnosis of DM	0
Altered fluid balance r/t DM	0
Knowledge deficit r/t meds	0
Noncompliance	0
Uncontrolled diabetes	0
Immaturity as evidenced by mother/daughter conflicts	0
Hyper/hypoglycemia	0
Hopelessness	0
Arguments with her mother	0
Deficient knowledge regarding prescribed diet	−1

Additional Guidelines for Raters of Nurses' Diagnoses

1. Keep in mind that the purpose is to rate the degree of accuracy of interpretations of clinical cases. Judge the degree of accuracy and not other characteristics of diagnoses.
2. Do the following as needed to choose the best score:
    *   Consider the "probable intention." If you are relatively sure of the intended meaning, rate the response accordingly.
    *   When you are not sure of the meaning of a diagnosis, use a reliable source such as the NANDA-I book.
    *   Consider the meaning of each word and the meaning of combinations of words, e.g., "ineffective communication" is not the same as "ineffective communication techniques."
    *   If there are two or more diagnoses, score each of them.
    *   If the requirements are to state one diagnosis but more than one diagnosis is given, use the highest score except if one of the diagnoses was a much lower score than the other. You may decide that the overall score should be an average of the two diagnoses.
3. Become aware of how you are applying the criteria. The goal is to be consistent, i.e., achieve test-retest reliability, so self awareness of ways that you make judgments is important.

Appendix D

Nursing Diagnosis Accuracy Scale (NDAS)

Fabiana Gonçalves de Oliveira Azevedo Matos, MS and
Diná de Almeida Lopes Monteiro da Cruz, PhD

The Nursing Diagnosis Accuracy Scale (NDAS; developed by Matos and Cruz and published in *Proceedings of the 6th European Conference of Acendio*, 2007. p. 144–145) was developed to retrospectively estimate the accuracy of nurses' diagnoses from data in patients' charts. Applying NDAS requires examining each diagnosis stated for a patient, taking into consideration the written assessment data. The study for the development of the NDAS is reported elsewhere (Matos, 2006).

Directions

The NDAS has five dichotomous items. Items 1 and 5 address whether the diagnosis should be scored or not. The scores on items 2 through 4 enable an interpretation of accuracy of the diagnosis.

- Read carefully the written assessment data in the chart from interviews, physical examinations, and other sources;
- Answer each NDAS item for each nursing diagnosis stated for the patient;
- Read each item and follow the specific directions;
- Whenever indicated, reread the written assessment data;
- Consult the NANDA-I classification to compare the match of assessment data with diagnoses;
- Use the NDAS Answer Table (Appendix D Table 1 to document your judgment).

Item 1

Is (are) there cue(s) for this nursing diagnosis?
☐ Yes   ☐ No

Directions

- Consider the definition of "cues" as patients' manifestations that represent signs, indicators, or characteristics of a nursing diagnosis.
- If there is at least one cue for the diagnosis, independent of its relevance, specificity, and coherence, answer YES.
- If your answer is NO, the remaining items are not applicable. Interrupt here the NDAS application for THIS DIAGNOSIS.

Item 2

The relevance of existing cue(s) is:
☐ High/Moderate   ☐ Low/Null

Directions

- Consider the definition of "cue relevance" as a cue property of being important as an indicator of a nursing diagnosis; rate the relevance level of the existing cue(s).
- If you judge that there is (are) cue(s) in both levels of relevance, point out only the highest one (High/Moderate).

Item 3

The specificity of existing cue(s) is:
☐ High/Moderate   ☐ Low/Null

Directions

- Consider the definition of "cue specificity" as a cue property of being proper and distinctive of a nursing diagnosis; rate the specificity level of the existing cue(s).
- If you judge that there is (are) cue(s) in both levels of specificity, point out only the highest one (High/Moderate).

Item 4

The coherence of existing cue(s) is:
☐ High/Moderate   ☐ Low/Null

Directions

- Consider the definition of "cue coherence" as a cue property of being consistent with the available data set; rate the coherence level of the existing cue(s).
- If you judge that there is (are) cue(s) in both levels of coherence, point out only the highest one (High/Moderate).

Item 5

Do you accept this diagnosis?
☐ Yes   ☐ No

Directions

- Consider that even having cues with some relevance, specificity, and coherence, the nursing diagnosis may not be a priority for the patient situation, may not guide adequate nursing intervention selection, or other diagnoses can better explain the patient response. In these cases mark "No."

Appendix D. Table 1. NDAS Answer Table.

Diagnoses[1]	Item 1		Item 2		Item 3		Item 4		Item 5	
	Are there cues?[2]		Relevance (cue × diagnosis)		Specificity (cue × diagnosis)		Coherence (cue × data set)		Do you keep the diagnosis?	
	Yes	No	High/ Mod. (1)	Low/ Null (0)	High/ Mod. (3,5)	Low/ Null (0)	High/ Mod. (8)	Low/ Null (0)	Yes	No
1.										
2.										
3.										

[1]List stated nursing diagnoses.
[2]When your answer is NO, fill the remaining cells for the diagnosis with n/a (= not applicable)

Appendix D. Table 2. NDAS Scoring Key

Item		Definition	Category	Score
1	Presence of cues	Presence of patients' manifestations that represent signs, indicators, or characteristics of a nursing diagnosis.	Yes No	None None
2	Relevance of cues	Cue property of being important as indicator of a nursing diagnosis.	High/Moderate Low/Null	1 0
3	Specificity of cues	Cue property of being proper and distinctive of a nursing diagnosis.	High/Moderate Low/Null	3, 5 0
4	Coherence of cues	Cue property of being consistent with the available data set.	High/Moderate Low/Null	8 0

Appendix D. Table 3. Apply scoring key to answers for each item, and sum all scores of each nursing diagnosis. Total score is interpreted as following:

Accuracy total score	Interpretation	Accuracy category
0	Assessment data presents no cues for the diagnosis OR cue(s) presented is(are) low in relevance, specificity, and coherence	Null
3,5 4,5	Cue(s) present in assessment data is (are) low/null in coherence, although there are either highly relevant cues or highly specific cues for the diagnosis.	Moderate
8,0 9,0 11,5 12,5	Cue(s) present in assessment data is (are) high in coherence, AND/OR high in relevance, AND/OR high in specificity for the diagnosis.	High

Reference

Matos, Fabiana Gonçalves de Oliveira Azevedo. (2006). Development of a tool to estimate diagnostic accuracy. Unpublished Master's Thesis. São Paulo—School of Nursing, University of São Paulo, São Paulo, Brazil.

Index